T0220803

Lecture Notes of the Institute for Computer Sciences, Social Informatics and Telecommunications Engineering 501

The LNICST series publishes ICST's conferences, symposia and workshops.

LNICST reports state-of-the-art results in areas related to the scope of the Institute. The type of material published includes

- Proceedings (published in time for the respective event)
- Other edited monographs (such as project reports or invited volumes)

LNICST topics span the following areas:

- General Computer Science
- E-Economy
- E-Medicine
- Knowledge Management
- Multimedia
- Operations, Management and Policy
- Social Informatics
- Systems

Shuihua Wang

Editor

IoT and Big Data Technologies for Health Care

Third EAI International Conference, IoTCare 2022
Virtual Event, December 12–13, 2022
Proceedings

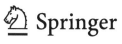 Springer

Editor
Shuihua Wang
University of Leicester
Leicester, UK

ISSN 1867-8211   ISSN 1867-822X (electronic)
Lecture Notes of the Institute for Computer Sciences, Social Informatics
and Telecommunications Engineering
ISBN 978-3-031-33544-0   ISBN 978-3-031-33545-7 (eBook)
https://doi.org/10.1007/978-3-031-33545-7

This Springer imprint is published by the registered company Springer Nature Switzerland AG
The registered company address is: Gewerbestrasse 11, 6330 Cham, Switzerland

Preface

We are delighted to introduce the proceedings of the third edition of the European Alliance for Innovation (EAI) International Conference on IoT and Big Data Technologies for HealthCare (IoTCare 2022). This conference brought together researchers, developers and practitioners around the world who are leveraging and developing technology for the Internet of Things and big data in Healthcare. The theme of IoTCare 2022 was the convergence of IoT and big data technologies for e-health, e-care, lifestyle, aging population, smart personal living applications, etc.

The technical program of IoTCare 2022 consisted of 23 full papers in the oral presentation sessions at the main conference tracks. The conference main track was on integrating healthcare with IoT. Aside from the high-quality technical paper presentations, the technical program also featured one keynote speech by M. Tanveer, who is Associate Professor and Ramanujan Fellow of the Department of Mathematics of Indian Institute of Technology Indore.

Coordination with the steering chairs, Imrich Chlamtac and Liangxiu Han, was essential for the success of the conference. We sincerely appreciate their constant support and guidance. It was also a great pleasure to work with such an excellent organizing committee team for their hard work in organizing and supporting the conference. In particular, the Technical Program Committee, chaired by Yu-Do Zhang, completed the peer-review process of technical papers and made a high-quality technical program. We are also grateful to Conference Manager Ivana Bujdakova for her support and to all the authors who submitted their papers to the IoTCare 2022 conference.

We strongly believe that the IoTCare conference provides a good forum for all researchers, developers and practitioners to discuss all science and technology aspects that are relevant to IoTCare. We also expect that the future IoTCare conference will be as successful and stimulating, as indicated by the contributions presented in this volume.

Shuihua Wang

Organization

Steering Committee

Imrich Chlamtac   University of Trento, Italy
Liangxiu Han   Manchester Metropolitan University, UK

Organizing Committee

General Chair

Shuihua Wang   University of Leicester, UK

TPC Chair

Yudong Zhang   University of Leicester, UK

Sponsorship and Exhibit Chair

Ziquan Zhu   University of Leicester, UK

Local Chair

Ziquan Zhu   University of Leicester, UK

Workshops Chair

Yuan Xu   University of Jinan, China

Publicity and Social Media Chair

Xujing Yao   University of Leicester, UK

Publications Chair

Dimas Lima   University of Santa Catarina, Brazil

Web Chair

Wei Wang   University of Leicester, UK

Technical Program Committee

Siyuan Lu	University of Leicester, UK
Xujing Yao	University of Leicester, UK
Xiang Yu	University of Leicester, UK
Vishnu Varthanan	Kalasalingam Academy of Research and Education, India
Muhammad Attique Khan	COMSATS University Islamabad, Pakistan
Yi Chen	Nanjing Normal University, China
Zhengchao Dong	Columbia University, USA
Jiangyi Zhang	Jiangnan University, China
Reham Mostafa	Mansoura University, Egypt
Muhammad Sharif	COMSATS University Islamabad, Pakistan
Muhammad Younus Javed	HITEC University Taxila, Pakistan
M. Hassaballah	South Valley University, Egypt
Shuihua Wang	University of Leicester, UK
Tallha Akram	COMSATS University Islamabad, Pakistan
Kashif Javed	National University of Sciences and Technology, Pakistan
Junaid Ali Khan	HITEC University Taxila, Pakistan
Mudassar Raza	COMSATS University Islamabad, Pakistan
Robertas Damasevicius	Vytautas Magnus University, Lithuania
Rameez Naqvi	COMSATS University Islamabad, Pakistan
V. Rajinikanth	St Joseph's College of Engineering, India
Jamal Hussain Shah	COMSATS University Islamabad, Pakistan
Dongye Liu	Inner Mongolia University, China
Weiling Bai	Inner Mongolia University, China
Na Ta	Inner Mongolia University, China
Huadong Wang	Inner Mongolia University, China
Gaocheng Liu	Inner Mongolia University, China
Chunli Guo	Inner Mongolia University, China
Shuihua Wang	Hunan Normal University, China
Tenghui He	Hunan Normal University, China
Xinyu Liu	Hunan Normal University, China
Chunguang	Henan Vocational College of Industry and Information Technology, China
Cui Jianfeng	Xiamen University of Technology, China

Ma Lei	Beijing Polytechnic University, China
Mingcheng Peng	Jiangmen Vocational and Polytechnic College, China
Yuling Jin	Chizhou Vocational and Technical College, China
Shuai Yang	Changchun University of Technology, China
Xinchun Zhou	Baoji University of Arts and Sciences, China
Dan Zhang	Xinyang Vocational and Technical College, China
Tian Hong	Baotou Iron & Steel Vocational Technical College, China
Li Heng	Henan Finance University, China
Wenda Xie	Jiangmen Polytechnic, China
Tong Xuanyue	Nanyang Institute of Technology, China
Sui Dan	California State Polytechnic University-Pomona, USA
Yanning Zhang	Beijing Polytechnic University, China
Xiaogang Zhu	Nanchang University, China
Xuechao Zhang	Hulun Buir Vocational Technical College, China
Feng Cheng	Xizang Minzu University, China
Keming Mao	Northeastern University, China
Jianwei Zhang	Zhengzhou University of Light Industry, China
Hao Xu	Xinyang Vocational and Technical College, China

Contents

Big Data Technologies for e-Health

A Review of Computer-Assisted Techniques Performances in Malaria
Diagnosis 3
    Ibrahim Mouazamou Laoualy Chaharou, Jules Degila, Lawani Ismaïl,
    and Habiboulaye Amadou Boubacar

Research on Cloud Health Privacy Information Protection Algorithm
Based on Data Mining 20
    Wennan Wang, Shiyang Song, Linkai Zhu, Junyu Su, Te Guo,
    and Jinhai Tang

Data Security Mining Method for Social Media Users' Mental Health
Status Test Based on Machine Learning Algorithm 35
    Junyu Su, Wenjian Liu, Hanxu Zhao, Wennan Wang, and Chiyu Shi

Early Warning Method of College Students Mental Subhealth Based
on Internet of Things 49
    Xiang Li

Automatic Assessment Method of College Students Psychological Stress
Based on Medical Big Data 61
    Xiang Li

Research on Medical Sensitive Data Protection Algorithm Based
on Differential Privacy 73
    Xiaofeng Li, Zhongwei Chen, and Zhichang Huang

Classification and Storage Method of Medical Health Monitoring Data
Based on Bayesian Algorithm 88
    Xiaofeng Li and Zhongwei Chen

Analysis on the Balance of Health Care Resource Allocation Based
on Improved Machine Learning 102
    Ying Wang and Helin Li

Data Acquisition Method of Human Injury in Sports Based on Internet
of Things 117
    Helin Li and Ying Wang

Big Data Technologies for e-Care

The Psychosocial Therapy Mode Intervened in the Emotion Management
of Property Management Staff 133
 Qianyi Wan and Changyan Liu

Personalized Recommendation Method of Maternal and Child Health
Education Resources Based on Association Rule Mining Algorithm 143
 Changyan Liu, Yu Wang, and QianYi Wan

Methods of Integrating Ideological and Political Education into Health
Management in Colleges and Universities Based on Internet of Things
Technology 159
 Wenjuan Xie and Jin Zhou

Data Mining of Psychological Tendency and Health of Ideological
and Political Students in Higher Vocational Tourism English Courses 178
 Jin Zhou and Wenjuan Xie

Intelligent Imaging Method of Nuclear Magnetic Resonance Medical
Devices Based on Compression Sensing 191
 Xuchu Deng, Zongying Lai, and Lizhi Chen

Evaluation of Post Fitness of Employees in Health Care Enterprises Based
on Big Data 206
 Lizhi Chen and Xuchu Deng

Design of Telemedicine and Health Care System Based on Embedded
Technology 221
 Shufeng Zhuo, Yi Hu, Xinyao Liu, and Zixiu Zou

Anomaly Detection Method of Healthcare Internet of Things Gateway
Supporting Edge Computing 239
 Zixiu Zou, Yi Hu, Xinyao Liu, and Shufeng Zhuo

Research on Fast Encryption of Electronic Health Record Data Based
on Privacy Protection 255
 Tianlin Fu, Juanfen Shi, and Haipeng Ke

Research on Secure Storage of Healthcare Data in the Environment
of Internet of Things 271
 Haipeng Ke, Juanfen Shi, and Tianlin Fu

Architecture of Wide Area Health Monitoring System 289
 Xiaohan Liu, Talatu Suri, Xiaoyun Zhao, Shilong Zhang, Ou Li,
 Yi Yang, Xiaochao Shi, Ping Liang, and Kuangyang Shu

Internet of Things Technologies in Healthcare for People with Hearing
Impairments 299
 Bader Alsharif and Mohammad Ilyas

Artificial Intelligence-Based Early Warning Method for Abnormal
Operation and Maintenance Data of Medical and Health Equipment 309
 Xuan Zhang, Yihan Ping, and Chao Li

Abnormal Signal Recognition Method of Wearable Sensor Based
on Machine Learning 322
 Chao Li and Xuan Zhang

Author Index 339

Big Data Technologies for e-Health

A Review of Computer-Assisted Techniques Performances in Malaria Diagnosis

Ibrahim Mouazamou Laoualy Chaharou[1]([✉]), Jules Degila[1], Lawani Ismaïl[1], and Habiboulaye Amadou Boubacar[2]

[1] University of Abomey Calavi, Abomey Calavi, Benin
`ibrahim.laoualy@imsp-uac.org`
[2] Air Liquide, Paris, France

Abstract. Malaria belongs to the class of the deadliest infectious diseases in the world. The generally available tools to diagnose this disease, the microscopy and rapid diagnostic test (RDT), have many limitations. Alternative diagnostic techniques with superior results are inaccessible to developing countries with more prevalent cases. Early detection of the infection is critical. Computer-assisted methods are needed. This study surveys the performance of the computer-assisted techniques used in malaria diagnosis and the preprocessing techniques to render the data usable. The survey illustrates, compares and discusses computer-assisted methods results, considering different performance metrics. It highlights how artificial intelligence can strengthen the fight against disease.

Keywords: Malaria · Diagnosis · Machine learning · Computer-assisted techniques · Performance metrics · Deep learning

1 Introduction

Malaria is an ancient disease whose first trace dates from the 5th century before Jesus Christ [1]. The parasite of this disease was discovered in 1880 by Alphonse Laverran, doctor and, French military [2]. Five Plasmodium species cause malaria in humans: Plasmodium falciparum, Plasmodium vivax, malariae Plasmodium, oval Plasmodium, and Plasmodium knowlesi. The most severe species is the Plasmodium falciparum, which causes the most significant number of deaths and is responsible for 97% of malaria cases globally. The World Health Organization (WHO) report of 2020 reported that malaria affected 229,000,000 people in 2019 while causing the death of 409,000 people [3]. To effectively treat this disease, it is imperative to go through an accurate diagnosis, given that its symptoms are found in many other febrile illnesses. Different diagnostic tools have been developed. The microscopic examination of the thick and thin blood smear is a reference used since 1904 to diagnose malaria [4]. However, the resulting performance depends on the quality of the smear (both light and thick), the availability of high quality and well-maintained optical microscope,

© ICST Institute for Computer Sciences, Social Informatics and Telecommunications Engineering 2023
Published by Springer Nature Switzerland AG 2023. All Rights Reserved
S. Wang (Ed.): IoTCare 2022, LNICST 501, pp. 3–19, 2023.
https://doi.org/10.1007/978-3-031-33545-7_1

and the practitioner's expertise. With these sensitive requirements, WHO recommends using RDTs, especially in limited resource areas [5]. However, more than 90 % of commercially available RDTs target the Plasmodium falciparum histidine-rich protein-2 (PHRP-2), a specific protein of Plasmodium falciparum. On the one hand, false negatives are common because of the parasites that can detect of the PHRP-2 gene. On the other hand, false positives can result from PHRP-2 presence in the blood 30 days after the elimination of the infection [6]. Polymerase chain reaction (PCR), and loop-mediated isothermal amplification (LAMP) molecular diagnostic tests have been developed and offer ultra-sensitivity in the field. However, PCR is limited to well-equipped laboratories distant from the remote endemic areas and is not ideal for quickly treating malaria cases [1,7]. As for the LAMP method, it requires moderately qualified personnel and presents a complex design of primers. In addition, there is no documentation for malaria LAMPs as a diagnostic tool in the population, and the price is high for commercial LAMP kits [1,6,8]. Overall, computer-assisted techniques are desirable to meet the requirements for early detection of the disease. In this study, we present the performance of the computer-assisted methods used for the early diagnosis of malaria via the images of a blood smear to encourage their uses in the fight against malaria. The rest of this document is organized as follows. Section 2 presents related works, and Sect. 3 describes the materials and methods used. Section 4 deals with the data acquisition process, while Sect. 5 discusses the images' pretreatment. In Sect. 6, the methods used to classify the malaria parasites are shown. Section 7 presents the discussions and the conclusion follows in Sect. 8.

2   Related Works

This part presents some survey studies on malaria diagnosis using computer-assisted techniques. Each survey was presented according to the authors' objectives. Thus, this study [9] presents an overview of the computer vision studies used to diagnose malaria while seeking to solve specific problems in the field. The authors of this survey [10] identified 112 articles addressing the diagnosis of malaria assisted by the computer published between 2000 and 2015. In addition, the study discussed various image-processing algorithms for blood smears, recognition forms, and malaria detection. [11] presents the analysis of different researchers' work in detecting malaria parasites using computer vision. This study examined the image processing methods, the classification of malaria parasites and their stages of life while discussing possible research prospects on existing challenges. Furthermore, [12] presents an investigation into the image acquisition process's different stages to classify the red blood cells infected with the malaria parasite. This study was carried out to supplement prior investigations in the diagnosis of malaria assisted by the computer and to provide the last update of state of the art in this area as it presents at the end of 2017. Each of these surveys has been presented to meet the objectives of the respective authors. But in general, there is a presentation of an overview of computer vision studies

used for the diagnosis of malaria while detailing image processing methods, clas
sification of infected and non-infected red blood cells with the malaria parasites
then the solutions found. In our case, the objective is to present the performance
of computer-assisted techniques used for the diagnosis of malaria and then to
propose a process to achieve this performance to motivate decision-makers to
invest in this area to get rid of malaria, which causes several deaths each year.

3   Materials and Methods

As part of this work, we collected more than 300 articles, including 229 articles
uploaded directly in to web of science database and other publications were
found by searching Google Scholar using the following research strings:

– methods of malaria diagnosis performed in laboratories;
– malaria diagnostic kits
– malaria diagnoses using machine learning
– image preprocessing techniques for malaria diagnosis.

   We sorted all the publications to keep 102 publications relevant to this work.
These publications were published in sources such as: The _American Journal
Of Tropical Medicine And Hygiene, Malaria Journal, Plos One, ScienceDirect,
IEEE Access, Springer Link,_International_Journal_of_Advanced_Research_in_
Computer_Science_&_Technology,_Journal_of_Microscopy, Journal of Physics:
Conference Series, IEEE Journal of Biomedical and Health Informatics, Open
Access Freely Available Online, Neural Computing & Applications, International
Conference of Advanced Computer Science and Information Systems, United
States National Library of Medicine.

4   Data Acquisition

Data acquisition is essential for implementing any efficient malaria prediction
system through blood smear images. Indeed, most prediction errors are due to
how the data were acquired. Many samples have information that contributes
to prediction errors. For example, before applying operations to the blood drops
on the slides, the variation of blood volumes on the slides used for training
and those used for testing causes prediction errors, as illustrated in the case
of a study in Peru [13]. It is also crucial to take suitable precautions in blood
preparation. As indicated here [12], inadequate blood preparations often lead to
artefacts commonly confused with malaria parasites, leading to false positives. In
addition, there is a possibility that errors come from the devices used to acquire
the images (as in [14], where it is specified that the lighting in a microscope
can considerably modify the information captured by the image sensor. Thus,
a microscope can substantially change the data captured by the image sensor)
and/or preprocessing not applied to the data. This section will give an overview
of the steps used in the literature to acquire the data.

4.1 Coloring Methods

To diagnose malaria based on the colors of blood components, it is essential to use a staining method. Thus, the staining method will stain the parasites to identify them on the microscopic images of the blood smears. Various staining methods have been used in the literature to identify malaria parasites. Therefore, our objective is not to present an exhaustive list of staining methods but instead to overview the most commonly used ones.

Giemsa Coloring Method

The Giemsa coloring method was developed in 1904 by Gustav Giemsa. This method has allowed blood smear microscopy to be the golden standard for diagnosing malaria [15]. The Giemsa solution is a mixture of eosin and methylene blue (azure). The eosin colors the chromatin of the parasite in red, while the methylene blue colors the parasitic cytoplasm in blue. This method has been recommended for coloring thin and thick blood smears [16]. Although widely used, this coloring method has disadvantages such as the need for much work with a delay that can exceed 45 min to have the result [17]. Nevertheless, referenced publications here [18–25] used the Giemsa coloring method to highlight the parasite of malaria.

Leishman Coloring Method

Although the Leishman staining method is less widely used than the Giemsa staining method, it offers better visualizations and sensitivity while taking less time than the Giemsa staining method to detect malaria parasites [26–28]. In addition, studies like [29–31] have used Leishman staining to identify malaria parasites in blood smears.

Fluorochrome Coloring Method

This coloring technique also performs better than Giemsa's coloring in detecting malaria parasites with thin and thick blood smears. However, the problem with this technique is that standard epi-lighted mercury vapor fluorescence microscopes are expensive, especially for tropical countries where malaria is endemic [32–34].

Acridine Orange Coloring Method

The orange coloring method with acridine also is better than the Giemsa coloring method. However, the disadvantage of this method is that the sensitivity depends on the parasitic density and the differentiation of space is often difficult [17]. Nevertheless, studies like [35–38] used the acridine orange coloring methods for blood smear coloring to diagnose malaria.

Wright Coloring Method

This technique (often combined with the Giemsa coloring technique) makes malaria parasites visible [39]. For malaria diagnosis, various studies, such as [40–43], used this technique to highlight the parasites.

Digitization of Blood Smear

After the blood smear coloring using an effective method, we move on to the scanning process of the blood smear using a digital camera. At this level, different tools were used to collect the images that would be processed before moving on to the learning phase. These references [11, 17, 44–47] indicate the example of some studies that described the various methods and tools used to acquire the images of blood smears.

5 Pretreatment of Images

The objective of the pretreatment process is to obtain images with low noise and a high contrast compared to the original images for the subsequent processing [48,49]. The pretreatment process contains operations such as the removal of unwanted noises, the increase in the picture contrast, the colors' conversion, the image's sharpness, the image filtering stretch [44,47,50], the correction of the bottom lighting of the microscopic images of a peripheral blood smear, that varies from one slide to another due to the variation of coloration [51]. [52] specified the need for pre-treatment to eliminate white blood cells confused with red blood cells by the implemented algorithm for the best classification of malaria parasites. Even with Convolutional Neural Networks (CNN) that are algorithms designed for image recognition tasks, which have been successfully applied in different areas as detailed in [53,54], the authors went from poor performance to excellent performance by using preprocessing on the data as shown in [55]. The process of image preprocessing is so crucial that it is found in almost all studies involving artificial intelligence with image data. For example, these references [52,56–59] present studies that have used some preprocessing methods to improve the quality of images. Concerning the state of the data, some of the techniques below will be used to have better performances.

5.1 Segmentation Methods

A microscopic image of a thin blood smear contains various blood components such as erythrocytes, leukocytes, platelets, and staining artefacts. Segmentation of a digital image allows the separation of the image into constituent regions. It aims to isolate individual erythrocytes from the rest of the blood constituents and then locate the probable plasmodium parasites from infected erythrocytes. It provides the ability to detect the object of interest in blood cell images while allowing separation of the foreground (object) from the background, i.e., red blood cells, blood cells, other components, and parasite from the image's background help separate overlapping malaria parasites. This is one of the most challenging tasks in image processing because it determines the success or failure of the subsequent classification process [50,57,60–62]. Some examples of specific segmentation methods usage are given in [11,47–49,63].

5.2   Feature Extraction Methods

Malaria parasite infection causes microstructural changes in erythrocytes. Thus, feature extraction selects appropriate parameters that correctly describe the image information. These parameters are grouped in vector form and are called feature vectors. Parasites and other colored components are flexible objects with significant shapes, sizes, and morphologies. Therefore, color information is valuable but insufficient to distinguish between other colored things, such as Plasmodium, and different species. Nevertheless, geometric features are still essential for recognizing complex shapes, and many researchers have used them to identify parasites [11,50,64]. In studies like [30,47,57,61,65], examples of the use of feature extraction methods have been presented.

5.3   Feature Selection Methods

As specified in the previous section, malaria infection causes shape changes in red blood cells. Thus, feature selection plays a crucial role in finding the most significant features among many extracted features in pattern recognition. In addition, this technique reduces redundant and irrelevant data to increase predictive performance, as the original feature set may contain unrelated data leading to an overlearning problem [30,57,64].

6   Classification Methods

After the ready-to-use data is acquired, an algorithm will be trained to create a model capable of classifying infected and uninfected red blood cells. Depending on the literature, machine learning and/or deep learning methods were used for classification. Therefore, we present the performance of different methods used in classifying red blood cells in the tables below. Each table line gives essential information to gauge the performance of automatic or deep learning methods used for detecting of malaria parasites on the blood smear images (Tables 1 and 2).

Table 1. The performance of machine learning technologies

References	Methodologies	Number of samples	Accuracy (%)	Sensitivity (%)	Specificity (%)	Precision (%)	Recall (%)	F1 Score (%)	MCC (%)	AUC (%)
[71]	ANN	70	99	–		88	91	90		
[56]	Bayesian approach	600	84.0							
[71]	Bag of Features and SVM	27 558	85.6	–	–	–	–	–		93.2
[67]	CNN-SVM	26 161	98.93	99.16		99.21	–	99.18		
[67]	CNN-KNN	26 161	99.12	99.23		99.11	–	99.28		
[73]	C4.5	500	–	99.2	–			99.0		100.0
[75]	GB, RF and SC	27 558	96	–		97	97	97		
[57]	hybrid classifier	200	98.50	95.68	98.81	–	–	93.82		
[73]	IB1	500	–	99.8	–	–	–	99.0		99.0
[57]	KNN	200	97.35	83.64	99.07	–	–	88.05		
[76]	KNN	9	93.3	72.4	97.6					
[57]	Naive Bayes	200	97.23	95.68	97.38	–	–	89.21		
[73]	Naive Bayes	500	–	84.5	–	–	–	87.0	–	95.0
[74]	RF	27 558	–	–		82	86	84		
[66]	SVM	47	–	99.0	99.8	–				
[56]	SVM	600	83.5							
[68]	SVM	2565	91.66	–						
[53]	SVM	765	–	92.95	93.82	–			44.35	
[69]	SVM	450	–	94	99.7	–	–			
[57]	SVM	200	98.38	94.59	98.81	–	–	93.12		
[70]	SVM	15	–	93.12	93.17					
[72]	SVM	70	98	–		83	91	87	–	
[77]	SVM	60	93.33	93.33	–					
[44]	VGG19-SVM	1530	93.13	93.44	92.92	89.95	–	91.66		
[44]	VGG16-SVM	1530	89.21	89.80	89.81	84.47	–	87.05		

Table 2. The performance of deep learning technologies

References	Methodologies	Number of samples	Accuracy (%)	Sensitivity (%)	Specificity (%)	Precision (%)	Recall (%)	F1 Score (%)	MCC (%)	AUC (%)
[68]	AlexNet	2 565	95.79	-	-	-	-	-	-	-
[71]	AlexNet	27 558	96.4	-	-	-	-	-	-	99.2
[67]	Autoencoder	26 161	99.5	98.80	99.17	99.29	-	99.51	-	-
[78]	CNN	27 578	97.37	96.99	97.75	97.73	-	97.36	94.75	-
[53]	CNN	765	-	97.06	98.50	-	-	70.33	-	-
[79]	CNN	27 558	98.85	98.79	98.90	98.90	-	-	-	-
[71]	CNN	27 558	96.0	-	-	-	-	-	-	99.1
[80]	Custom CNN	27 558	99.09	-	-	99.56	-	99.08	98.18	99.3
[55]	CNN	27 558	99.96	-	-	100.0	99.928	99.96	-	-
[85]	CNN	27 558	97.30	-	-	97	97	97	94.17	97.04
[86]	CNN	27 558	98.23	96.44	99.99	99.09	-	97.74	-	-
[75]	CNNs and mini-VGGNet	27 558	-	-	-	99	96	97	-	-
[71]	DenseNet	27 558	96.6	-	-	-	-	-	-	99.1
[82]	DenseNet121	10 000	95.6	94.8	96.5	-	-	-	-	99.0
[88]	DBN	4 100	-	97.60	95.92	-	-	89.66	-	-
[84]	Faster R-CNN (InceptionV2)	643	-	-	-	72.29	93.03	-	-	-
[89]	FLANN/SSAE	1 182	89.10	93.90	83.10	-	-	94.50	-	-
[68]	GoogLeNet	2 565	98.13	-	-	-	-	-	-	-
[80]	InceptionResNet	27 558	98.79	-	-	99.56	-	98.77	97.59	99.2
[82]	InceptionV3	10 000	92.8	92.5	93.0	-	-	-	-	97.6
[82]	InceptionResNetV2	10 000	93.5	93.2	93.8	-	-	-	-	98.0
[68]	LeNet-5	2 565	96.18	-	-	-	-	-	-	-
[82]	MobileNetV2	10 000	94.8	94.1	95.5	-	-	-	-	98.7
[71]	ResNet	27 558	96.0	-	-	-	-	-	-	99.2
[81]	ResNet-50	27 558	95.4	-	-	-	-	-	-	-
[82]	ResNet50V2	10 000	93.8	93.5	94.0	-	-	-	-	98.2
[84]	RetinaNet (SSD ResNetFPN)	643	-	-	-	86.97	60.86	-	-	-
[80]	SqueezeNet	27 558	98.66	-	-	99.44	-	98.64	97.32	98.85
[84]	SSD (InceptionV2)	643	-	-	-	91.50	37.53	-	-	-
[71]	VGG-16	27 558	96.5	-	-	-	-	-	-	99.3
[80]	VGG-19	27 558	99.32	-	-	99.71	-	99.31	98.62	99.31
[82]	VGG19	10 000	95.9	95.6	96.3	-	-	-	-	99.1
[82]	VGG16	10 000	96.0	95.6	96.4	-	-	-	-	99.2
[90]	WELM/AlexNet_FC7	23 248	96.18	-	-	-	-	-	-	-
[82]	Xception	10 000	94.6	94.3	94.8	-	-	-	-	97.9

6.1   Interpretation of Results

The main objective of this study is to present the performance of computer-assisted techniques used to diagnose malaria to motivate their use in the fight against malaria. Therefore, we have collected in tables the results of several articles illustrating the performance of computer-assisted techniques in identifying malaria from blood smear images. Each row of a table gathers the essential information to judge the ability of a machine learning or deep learning methodology to identify malaria parasites. Each table has eleven columns: the first one represents the reference of the different papers, the second one shows the methods used, the third one represents the number of image samples used in the study, and from the fourth to the last one, we have different results of performance metrics according to the publications. These performance metrics are defined as follows:

- Accuracy: accuracy is a standard metric that is the percentage of the number of correct predictions [90].
- Sensitivity or Recall: the rate of correctly identified true positive predictions to all positive outcomes [90].
- Specificity is the rate of correctly identified negative predictions to all negative outcomes [90].
- Precision: the precision is the fraction of the correctly classified instances from the total classified instances [91].
- F1-score: this score is a harmonic mean of precision and sensitivity; it can be used as an overall performance metric [90].
- MCC: Matthew's correlation coefficient (MCC) is a metric formulated to evaluate the quality of binary classification; it was designed to be used as a balanced measure that can be used on imbalanced datasets [90].
- AUC: the area under the receiver operating characteristic curve (AUROC) is the area under an angle of true positive rate versus false-positive rate that can be used as a metric for methods working on imbalanced datasets [90].

These performance metrics provide the information expected by the doctor to make good decisions in the fight against malaria while pushing to replace existing tools. These continue to show their failings while plunging the world into more serious consequences. Indeed, the report on malaria published on December 6, 2021, by the WHO showed that the number of cases and deaths from malaria increased by 14,000,000 and 69,000 respectively in 2020 compared to the number of cases respectively. and the number of deaths observed in 2019 [96]. Moreover, according to WHO data, a few years ago, there was a shortage of more than 7 million doctors worldwide, and in 2035 this shortage will reach 13 million. This will mean that almost half of the world's population will not be able to get medical help, and access to a specialist will take a few weeks or more, even in the world's richest countries [97].

Therefore, computer-assisted techniques are urgently needed in the eradication of this disease. When data of sufficient quality and quantity are available, computer-assisted techniques offer better results than even the most advanced human expertise. These techniques have the quality of allowing the prediction of the parasite density which is essential information to know the severity of the infection to better guide the doctor in the choice of the appropriate treatment. The convincing results of these techniques and their successful use in various fields have made it possible to estimate that the proportion of professional tasks performed by intelligent robots will reach 52% in the world by 2025 [98].

7   Discussions

Techniques to eradicate malaria require an accurate diagnosis of the disease. Most failures in the fight against malaria are caused by an incorrect diagnosis of this disease, presenting the same symptoms as other febrile diseases. Misdiagnosis is widespread with all the tools currently available. As reported in [75], studies have shown that 46 laboratory professionals diagnosed 6 malaria slides for Plasmodium falciparum and Vivax with an error rate of 43.5% and 37%, respectively. Another similar study reported an overall malaria diagnosis error rate of 40.4%. The microscope has been used for more than a century. However, such a tool gives results that depend on the microscopist's expertise. More than half of all malaria diagnoses worldwide are performed by microscopy [72], mainly because of its low cost. The creation of rapid RDT tools has circumvented the problem of test performance being dependent on human expertise. However, RDTs can present many false positives with the detection of the pHRP-2 protein which can be present in the blood for up to 30 days after clearance of the infection. In addition, RDTs cannot detect malaria infections with very low parasitemia. RDTs have gained popularity mainly because of their ease of use [92], despite these weaknesses. The ultra-sensitives diagnostic tests like the PCR and LAMP tests are not practical for the reasons indicated in the introduction. The World Health Organization has recommended a minimum standard of sensitivity and specificity of 95% so diagnostic tools are clinically helpful when assessing patients infected with Plasmodium falciparum densities of 0.0002% [93]. Computer-assisted techniques provide much more advanced performance than these indications when data is used in quality and in sufficient quantity on deep learning algorithms.

Obtaining the best performance for malaria diagnosis using these techniques depends entirely on the data quality. In addition, many challenges affect the data depending on their acquisition conditions. These challenges have inhibited the achievement of the best performance in various studies. The best way to overcome this problem is to apply preprocessing on the data before running it through the chosen algorithm for training. As an illustration, in this study [55], the impact of pretreatment has considerably changed the performance measures in detecting malaria parasites, as presented in Table 3 below.

Table 3. Example of the impact of images preprocessing

Model	Accuracy	Precision	Recall	F1-score
Stacked CNN-5 layers with preprocessing	99.879	99.976	99.783	99.879
Stacked CNN-5 layers without preprocessing	49.61	50.14	50.14	50.14

In other cases, the effect of pretreatment [94, 95] improved the accuracy and F1-score in detecting malaria parasites via blood smear images. In some cases, the performance of computer-assisted techniques presented in the performance of machine learning or deep learning technologies sections has shown undeniable capabilities in the early identification of malaria, facilitating its eradication. In this sense, the present manuscript tries to draw the attention of the primary decision-makers to control deadly diseases such as malaria to invest in research using machine learning techniques for early and accurate malaria diagnosis. The lack of diagnostic experts further supports the integration of these techniques into easy-to-use tools. This problem has been considered in some studies that have developed malaria diagnostic systems that can be used in smartphones. In addition, studies like [45,52,67,72,87,99–101] have shown the possibilities of integrating diagnostic systems with smartphones and achieving better performance.

8 Conclusion

Malaria is one of the deadliest diseases worldwide. The performance of neural networks for malaria diagnosis through blood smear images is unbeatable in this era of Big Data. In some publications, the maximum potential of neural networks has not been reached, mainly because of some gaps in the available data. However, studies that consider the preprocessing operations on the data obtained rates are trending towards 100% on specific performance metrics. With these results, if the diagnostic method is easy to use, this will provide a compelling way to rid the world of malaria. Our future work will implement all processes to develop an efficient and usable system for diagnosing malaria.

References

1. Pham, N.M., Karlen, W., Beck, H.P., Delamarche, E.: Malaria and the last parasite: how can technology help? Malaria J. **17**(1), 1–16 (2018)
2. Cox, F.E.: History of the discovery of the malaria parasites and their vectors. Parasites Vectors **3**(1), 1–9 (2010)
3. WHO. https://www.who.int/docs/default-source/malaria/world-malaria-reports /world-malaria-report-2020-briefing-kit-fre.pdf?sfvrsn=69c55393_7. Accessed 26 July 2021
4. Jain, P., Chakma, B., Patra, S., Goswami, P.: Potential biomarkers and their applications for rapid and reliable detection of malaria. BioMed Res. Int. (2014)
5. Leski, T.A., et al.: Use of real-time multiplex PCR, malaria rapid diagnostic test and microscopy to investigate the prevalence of Plasmodium species among febrile hospital patients in Sierra Leone. Malaria J. **19**(1), 1–8 (2020)
6. Mbanefo, A., Kumar, N.: Evaluation of malaria diagnostic methods as a key for successful control and elimination programs. Tropical Med. Infect. Dis. **5**(2), 102 (2020)
7. Picot, S., Cucherat, M., Bienvenu, A.L.: Systematic review and meta-analysis of diagnostic accuracy of loop-mediated isothermal amplification (LAMP) methods compared with microscopy, polymerase chain reaction and rapid diagnostic tests for malaria diagnosis. Int. J. Infect. Dis. **98**, 408–419 (2020)
8. Grossenbacher, B., et al.: Molecular methods for tracking residual Plasmodium falciparum transmission in a close-to-elimination setting in Zanzibar. Malaria J. **19**(1), 1–12 (2020)
9. Tek, F.B., Dempster, A.G., Kale, I.: Computer vision for microscopy diagnosis of malaria. Malaria J. **8**(1), 1–14 (2009)
10. Das, D., Mukherjee, R., Chakraborty, C.: Computational microscopic imaging for malaria parasite detection: a systematic review. J. Microsc. **260**, 1–19 (2015)

11. Jan, Z., Khan, A., Sajjad, M., Muhammad, K., Rho, S., Mehmood, I.: A review on automated diagnosis of malaria parasite in microscopic blood smears images. Multimedia Tools Appl. **77**(8), 9801–9826 (2018)
12. Poostchi, M., Silamut, K., Maude, R.J., Jaeger, S., Thoma, G.: Image analysis and machine learning for detecting malaria. Transl. Res. **194**, 36–55 (2018)
13. Torres, K., et al.: Automated microscopy for routine malaria diagnosis: a field comparison on Giemsa-stained blood films in Peru. Malaria Journal **17**(1), 1–11 (2018)
14. Chaware, A., Cooke, C. L., Kim, K., Horstmeyer, R.: Towards an intelligent microscope: adaptively learned illumination for optimal sample classification. In: ICASSP 2020–2020 IEEE International Conference on Acoustics, Speech and Signal Processing (ICASSP), pp. 9284–9288. IEEE (2020)
15. Joanny, F., Löhr, S.J., Engleitner, T., Lell, B., Mordmüller, B.: Limit of blank and limit of detection of Plasmodium falciparum thick blood smear microscopy in a routine setting in Central Africa. Malaria J. **13**(1), 1–7 (2014)
16. WHO. https://www.who.int/fr/publications-detail/HTM-GMP-MM-SOP-07a. Accessed 26 July 2021
17. Keiser, J., Utzinger, J., Premji, Z., Yamagata, Y., Singer, B.H.: Acridine Orange for malaria diagnosis: its diagnostic performance, its promotion and implementation in Tanzania, and the implications for malaria control. Ann. Tropical Med. Parasitol. **96**(7), 643–654 (2002)
18. Tek, F.B., Dempster, A.G., Kale, I.: Parasite detection and identification for automated thin blood film malaria diagnosis. Comput. Vision Image Underst. **114**(1), 21–32 (2010)
19. Le, M.T., Bretschneider, T.R., Kuss, C., Preiser, P.R.: A novel semi-automatic image processing approach to determine Plasmodium falciparum parasitemia in Giemsa-stained thin blood smears. BMC Cell Biol. **9**(1), 1–12 (2008)
20. Walliander, M., et al.: Automated segmentation of blood cells in Giemsa stained digitized thin blood films. In: Diagnostic Pathology, vol. 8, no. 1, pp. 1–5. BioMed Central (2013)
21. Abbas, N., et al.: Plasmodium life cycle stage classification based quantification of malaria parasitaemia in thin blood smears. Microsc. Res. Techn. **82**(3), 283–295 (2019)
22. Ouangre, A., Sangare, I., Bado Nebon, D., Bamba, S.: Prévalence de la dengue et du paludisme chez les patients fébriles au CHU Souro Sanou de Bobo-Dioulasso. Journal de la Société de Biologie Clinique du Bénin (2019)
23. Heraud, P., et al.: Infrared spectroscopy coupled to cloud-based data management as a tool to diagnose malaria: a pilot study in a malaria-endemic country. Malaria J. **18**(1), 1–11 (2019)
24. Mustare, N.B.: Rapid diagnosis of malaria using images of stained blood smear. CVR J. Sci. Technol. **18**(1), 88–93 (2020)
25. Abad, C.S., Tellkamp, M.P., Amaro, I.R., Spencer, L.M.: Incidence of avian malaria in hummingbirds in humid premontane forests of Pichincha Province, Ecuador: a pilot study. Veter. World **14**(4), 889 (2021)
26. Sathpathi, S.: Comparing Leishman and Giemsa staining for the assessment of peripheral blood smear preparations in a malaria-endemic region in India. Malaria J. **13**(1), 1–5 (2014)
27. Loddo, A., Di Ruberto, C., Kocher, M.: Recent advances of malaria parasites detection systems based on mathematical morphology. Sensors **18**(2), 513 (2018)
28. Kocher, M., Prod'Hom, G.: MP-IDB: the malaria Parasite image database for image processing and analysis (2019)

29. Shujatullah, F., Khan, H. M., Malik, A., Malik, A.: Evaluation of ParaSight F test in dignosis of plasmodium falciparum infection. J.K. Sci. **11**(1), 1–4 (2009)
30. Das, D.K., Maiti, A.K., Chakraborty, C.: Automated system for characterization and classification of malaria-infected stages using light microscopic images of thin blood smears. J. Microsc. **257**(3), 238–252 (2015)
31. Maity, M., Maity, A.K., Dutta, P.K., Chakraborty, C.: A web-accessible framework for automated storage with compression and textural classification of malaria parasite images. Int. J. Comput. Appl. **52**(15), 31–39 (2012)
32. Kawamoto, F.: Rapid diagnosis of malaria by fluorescence microscopy with light microscope and interference filter. The Lancet **337**(8735), 200–202 (1991)
33. Malinin, G.I., Malinin, T.I.: Rapid microscopic detection of malaria parasites permanently fluorochrome stained in blood smears with aluminum and morin. Am. J. Clin. Pathol. **95**(3), 424–427 (1991)
34. Sodeman, T.M., World Health Organization.: The use of fluorochromes for the detection of malaria parasites (1969)
35. Zhou, M., et al.: High prevalence of Plasmodium malariae and Plasmodium ovale in malaria patients along the Thai-Myanmar border, as revealed by acridine orange staining and PCR-based diagnoses. Tropical Med. Int. Health **3**(4), 304–312 (1998)
36. Gay, F., Traoré, B., Zanoni, J., Danis, M., Fribourg-Blanc, A.: Direct acridine orange fluorescence examination of blood slides compared to current techniques for malaria diagnosis. Trans. Roy. Soc. Tropical Med. Hyg. **90**(5), 516–518 (1996)
37. Rickman, L., et al.: Rapid diagnosis of malaria by acridine orange staining of centrifuged parasites. The Lancet **333**(8629), 68–71 (1989)
38. Kimura, M., et al.: Improvement of malaria diagnostic system based on acridine orange staining. Malaria J. **17**(1), 1–6 (2018)
39. Abanyie, F.A., Arguin, P.M., Gutman, J.: State of malaria diagnostic testing at clinical laboratories in the United States, 2010: a nationwide survey. Malaria J. **10**(1), 1–10 (2011)
40. Lawrence, C., Olson, J.A.: Birefringent hemozoin identifies malaria. Am. J. Clin. Pathol. **86**(3), 360–363 (1986)
41. Cutts, T.A., Cook, B.W., Poliquin, P.G., Strong, J.E., Theriault, S.S.: Inactivating Zaire Ebolavirus in whole-blood thin smears used for malaria diagnosis. J. Clin. Microbiol. **54**(4), 1157–1159 (2016)
42. Shin, H.I., et al.: Diagnosis and molecular analysis on imported plasmodium ovale curtisi and P. ovale wallikeri Malaria Cases from West and South Africa during 2013–2016. Kor. J. Parasitol. **58**(1), 61 (2020)
43. Arispe Angulo, K.R., Harrington, A.M.: Fever in a kidney transplant patient From Nigeria. The Hematologist **17**(1) (2020)
44. Vijayalakshmi, A.: Deep learning approach to detect malaria from microscopic images. Multimedia Tools Appl. **79**(21), 15297–15317 (2020)
45. Yu, H., et al.: Malaria Screener: a smartphone application for automated malaria screening. BMC Infect. Dis. **20**(1), 1–8 (2020)
46. Molina, A., Alférez, S., Boldú, L., Acevedo, A., Rodellar, J., Merino, A.: Sequential classification system for recognition of malaria infection using peripheral blood cell images. J. Clin. Pathol. **73**(10), 665–670 (2020)
47. Karthik, G., Muttan, S., Saravanan, M.P., Seetharaman, R., Vignesh, V.: Automated malaria diagnosis using microscopic images. In 2019 Third International Conference on Inventive Systems and Control (ICISC), pp. 514–517. IEEE (2019)
48. Razzak, M.I.: Automatic detection and classification of malarial parasite. Int. J. Biometr. Bioinf. (IJBB) **9**(1), 1–12 (2015)

49. Arco, J.E., Górriz, J.M., Ramírez, J., Álvarez, I., Puntonet, C.G.: Digital image analysis for automatic enumeration of malaria parasites using morphological operations. Expert Syst. Appl. **42**(6), 3041–3047 (2015)
50. Memeu, D.M., Kaduki, K.A., Mjomba, A.C.K., Muriuki, N.S., Gitonga, L.: Detection of plasmodium parasites from images of thin blood smears. Open J. Clin. Diagnost. **3**, 183–194 (2013)
51. Das, D., Chakraborty, C., Mitra, B., Maiti, A., Ray, A.: Quantitative microscopy approach for shape-based erythrocytes characterization in anaemia. J. Microsc. **249**, 136–149 (2013)
52. Moallem, G., Poostchi, M., Yu, H., Silamut, K., Palaniappan, N., Antani, S.: Detecting and segmenting white blood cells in microscopy images of thin blood smears. In: 2017 IEEE Applied Imagery Pattern Recognition Workshop. IEEE (2017)
53. Opakumar, G.P., Swetha, M., Siva, G.S., Saisubrahmanyam, G.R.K.: Convolutional neural network-based malaria diagnosis from focus stack of blood smear images acquired using custom-built slide scanner. J. Biophotonics **11**, e201700003 (2014)
54. Rajaraman, S., et al.: Pre-trained convolutional neural networks as feature extractors toward improved malaria parasite detection in thin blood smear images. PeerJ **6**, e4568 (2018)
55. Umer, M., Sadiq, S., Ahmad, M., Ullah, S., Choi, G.S., Mehmood, A.: A novel stacked CNN for malarial parasite detection in thin blood smear images. IEEE Access **8**, 93782–93792 (2020). https://doi.org/10.1109/access.2020.2994810
56. Das, D.K., Ghosh, M., Pal, M., Maiti, A.K., Chakraborty, C.: Machine learning approach for automated screening of malaria parasite using light microscopic images. Micron **45**, 97–106 (2013)
57. Devi, S.S., Roy, A., Singha, J., Sheikh, S.A., Laskar, R.H.: Malaria infected erythrocyte classification based on a hybrid classifier using microscopic images of thin blood smear. Multimedia Tools Appl. **77**(1), 631–660 (2018)
58. Fatima, T., Farid, M.S.: Automatic detection of Plasmodium parasites from microscopic blood images. J. Parasitic Dis. **44**(1), 69–78 (2020)
59. Maqsood, A., Farid, M.S., Khan, M.H., Grzegorzek, M.: Deep malaria parasite detection in thin blood smear microscopic images. Appl. Sci. **11**(5), 2284 (2021)
60. May, Z., Aziz, S.S.A.M.: Automated quantification and classification of malaria parasites in thin blood smears. In 2013 IEEE International Conference on Signal and Image Processing Applications, pp. 369–373. IEEE (2013)
61. Gatc, J., Maspiyanti, F., Sarwinda, D., Arymurthy, A.M.: Plasmodium parasite detection on red blood cell image for the diagnosis of malaria using double thresholding. In: 2013 International Conference on Advanced Computer Science and Information Systems (ICACSIS), pp. 381–385. IEEE (2013)
62. Aris, T.A., et al.: Colour component analysis approach for malaria parasites detection based on thick blood smear images. In: IOP Conference Series: Materials Science and Engineering, vol. 557, no. 1, p. 012007. IOP Publishing (2019)
63. Abbas, N., et al.: Plasmodium species aware based quantification of malaria parasitemia in light microscopy thin blood smear. Microsc. Res. Techn. **82**(7), 1198–1214 (2019)
64. Das, D.K., Mukherjee, R., Chakraborty, C.: Computational microscopic imaging for malaria parasite detection: a systematic review. J. Microsc. **260**(1), 1–19 (2015)

65. Abbas, N., Saba, T., Mohamad, D., Rehman, A., Almazyad, A.S., Al-Ghamdi, J.S.: Machine aided malaria parasitemia detection in Giemsa-stained thin blood smears. Neural Comput. Appl. **29**(3), 803–818 (2018)
66. Linder, N., et al.: A malaria diagnostic tool based on computer vision screening and visualization of Plasmodium falciparum candidate areas in digitized blood smears. PLoS One **9**(8), e104855 (2014)
67. Fuhad, K.M., et al.: Deep learning based automatic malaria parasite detection from blood smear and its smartphone based application. Diagnostics **10**(5), 329 (2020)
68. Dong, Y., et al.: Evaluations of deep convolutional neural networks for automatic identification of malaria infected cells. In: Proceedings of the 2017 IEEE EMBS International Conference on Biomedical & Health Informatics (BHI), Orlando, FL, USA, 16–19 February 2017, pp. 101–104 (2017)
69. Diaz, G., Gonzalez, F.A., Romero, E.: A semi-automatic method for quantification and classification of erythrocytes infected with malaria parasites in microscopic images. J. Biomed. Inf. **42**(2), 296–307 (2009)
70. Savkare, S.S., Narote, S.P.: Automatic detection of malaria parasites for estimating parasitemia. Int. J. Comput. Sci. Secur. (IJCSS) **5**(3), 310 (2011)
71. Narayanan, B.N., Ali, R., Hardie, R.C.: Performance analysis of machine learning and deep learning architectures for malaria detection on cell images. In: Zelinski, M.E., Taha, T.M., Howe, J., Awwal, A.A.S., Iftekharuddin, K.M. (eds.) Applications of Machine Learning (2019)
72. Poostchi, M., et al.: Malaria parasite detection and cell counting for human and mouse using thin blood smear microscopy. J. Med. Imaging **5**(4), 044506 (2018)
73. Maity, M., Dhane, D., Mungle, T., Maiti, A.K., Chakraborty, C.: Web-enabled distributed health-care framework for automated malaria parasite classification: an E-health approach. J. Med. Syst. **41**(12), 1–18 (2017). https://doi.org/10.1007/s10916-017-0834-0
74. Khan, A., Gupta, K.D., Venugopal, D., Kumar, N.: CIDMP: completely interpretable detection of malaria parasite in red blood cells using lower-dimensional feature space. In: 2020 International Joint Conference on Neural Networks. IEEE (2020)
75. Gezahegn, Y.G., Gebreslassie, A.K., Hagos, M.A., Ibenthal, A., Etsub, E.A.: Classical machine learning algorithms and shallower convolutional neural networks towards computationally efficient and accurate classification of malaria parasites. In: Mekuria, F., Nigussie, E., Tegegne, T. (eds.) ICT4DA 2019. CCIS, vol. 1026, pp. 46–56. Springer, Cham (2019). https://doi.org/10.1007/978-3-030-26630-1_5
76. Tek, F., Dempster, A., Kale, I.: Parasite detection and identification for automated thin blood film malaria diagnosis. Comput. Vision Image Underst. **114**, 21–32 (2010)
77. Suryawanshi, S., Dixit, V.V.: Comparative study of Malaria parasite detection using euclidean distance classifier & SVM. Int. J. Adv. Res. Comput. Eng. Technol. (IJARCET) **2**(11), 2994–2997 (2013)
78. Liang, Z., Powell, A., Ersoy, I., et al.: CNN-based image analysis for malaria diagnosis. In: International Conference on Bioinformatics and Biomedicine (BIBM), pp. 493–496. IEEE (2016)
79. Alqudah, A., Alqudah, A.M., Qazan, S.: Lightweight deep learning for malaria parasite detection using cell-image of blood smear images. Revue d'Intelligence Artificielle **34**(5), 571–576 (2020)

80. Rajaraman, S., Jaeger, S., Antani, S.K.: Performance evaluation of deep neural ensembles toward malaria parasite detection in thin-blood smear images. PeerJ **7**, e6977 (2019). https://doi.org/10.7717/peerj.6977
81. Reddy, A.S.B., Juliet, D.S.: Transfer learning with ResNet-50 for malaria cell-image classification. In: 2019 International Conference on Communication and Signal Processing (ICCSP), pp. 0945–0949. IEEE (2019)
82. Zhao, O.S., et al.: Convolutional neural networks to automate the screening of malaria in low-resource countries. Peerj **8** (2020). https://doi.org/10.7717/peerj.9674
83. Singla, N., Srivastava, V.: Deep learning enabled multi-wavelength spatial coherence microscope for the classification of malaria-infected stages with limited labelled data size. Opt. Laser Technol. **130**,(2020). https://doi.org/10.1016/j.optlastec.2020.1063
84. Nakasi, R., Mwebaze, E., Zawedde, A., Tusubira, J., Akera, B., Maiga, G.: A new approach for microscopic diagnosis of malaria parasites in thick blood smears using pre-trained deep learning models. SN Appl. Sci. **2**(7) (2020). https://doi.org/10.1007/s42452-02
85. Masud, M., et al.: leveraging deep learning techniques for malaria parasite detection using mobile application. Wirel. Commun. Mobile Comput. (2020)
86. Kumar, R., Singh, S.K., Khamparia, A.: Malaria detection using custom convolutional neural network model on blood smear slide images. In: Luhach, A.K., Jat, D.S., Hawari, K.B.G., Gao, X.-Z., Lingras, P. (eds.) ICAICR 2019. CCIS, vol. 1075, pp. 20–28. Springer, Singapore (2019). https://doi.org/10.1007/978-981-15-0108-1_3
87. Jaeger, S., et al.: Reducing the diagnostic burden of malaria using microscopy image analysis and machine learning in the field. Am. J. Tropical Med. Hygiene (2017)
88. Bibin, D., Nair, M.S., Punitha, P.: Malaria parasite detection from peripheral blood smear images using deep belief networks. IEEE Access **5**, 9099–9108 (2017)
89. Pattanaik, P.A., Mittal, M., Khan, M.Z.: Unsupervised deep learning CAD scheme for the detection of malaria in blood smear microscopic images. IEEE Access **8**, 94936–94946 (2020). https://doi.org/10.1109/access.2020.2996022
90. Kudisthalert, W., Pasupa, K., Tongsima, S.: Counting and classification of malarial parasite from giemsa-stained thin film images. IEEE Access **8**, 78663–78682 (2020). https://doi.org/10.1109/access.2020.2990497
91. Towards Data Science. https://towardsdatascience.com/performance-metrics-for-classification-machine-learning-problems-97e7e774a007. Accessed 07 Jan 2022
92. Eshel, Y., et al.: Evaluation of the parasight platform for malaria diagnosis. J. Clin. Microbiol. **55**(3), 768–775 (2017). https://doi.org/10.1128/jcm.02155-16
93. Park, H.S., Rinehart, M., Walzer, K.A., Chi, J.T.A., Wax, A.: Automated detection of P. falciparum using machine learning algorithms with quantitative phase images of unstained cells. PLoS ONE **11**(9) (2016). https://doi.org/10.1371/journal.pone.0163045
94. Swastika, W., Kristianti, G.M., Widodo, R.B.: Effective preprocessed thin blood smear images to improve malaria parasite detection using deep learning. In: Journal of Physics: Conference Series, vol. 1869, no. 1, p. 012092. IOP Publishing (2021)
95. Engelhardt, E., Jäger, S.: An evaluation of image preprocessing for classification of Malaria parasitization using convolutional neural networks (2019)
96. WHO. https://www.who.int/fr/publications/m/item/WHO-UCN-GMP-2021.08. Accessed 15 Nov 2022

97. AI at the bedside of medicine. https://www.europeanscientist.com/fr/opinion/lintelligence-artificielle-au-chevet-de-la-medecine/. Accessed 15 Nov 2022
98. BFM. https://www.bfmtv.com/tech/vie-numerique/en-2025-les-robots-realiseront-52-des-taches-professionnelles_AV-201809170102.html. Accessed 15 Nov 2022
99. Guo, X., et al.: Smartphone-based DNA diagnostics for malaria detection using deep learning for local decision support and blockchain technology for security. Nat. Electron. **4**(8), 615–624 (2021)
100. Yang, F., Yu, H., Silamut, K., Maude, R.J., Jaeger, S., Antani, S.: Smartphone-supported malaria diagnosis based on deep learning. In: Suk, H.-I., Liu, M., Yan, P., Lian, C. (eds.) MLMI 2019. LNCS, vol. 11861, pp. 73–80. Springer, Cham (2019). https://doi.org/10.1007/978-3-030-32692-0_9
101. Yang, F., et al.: Deep learning for smartphone-based malaria parasite detection in thick blood smears. IEEE J. Biomed. Health Inf. **24**(5), 1427–1438 (2019)

Research on Cloud Health Privacy Information Protection Algorithm Based on Data Mining

Wennan Wang[1]([✉]), Shiyang Song[2], Linkai Zhu[3], Junyu Su[4], Te Guo[2], and Jinhai Tang[2]

[1] Academy of Management, Guangdong University of Science and Technology, Dongguan 523083, China
wwwwennan@sina.com
[2] Alibaba Cloud Big Data Application College, Zhuhai College of Science and Technology, Zhuhai 519099, China
[3] Information Technology School, Hebei University of Economics and Business, Shijiazhuang 050061, China
[4] Institute of Data Science, City University of Macau, Macau 999078, China

Abstract. In the process of selecting privacy evaluation indicators, the original algorithm did not set the degree of protection risk, which resulted in a little error in the protection of privacy information, which affected the efficiency of data operation. A data mining-based cloud health privacy information protection algorithm was studied. Build a differential privacy information protection model, establish the connection relationship between users and information, and use trapezoidal distribution membership function to determine the sensitive attributes of privacy information. Set up health privacy information protection indicators on the cloud, evaluate the risks of privacy information protection, and classify them into three levels: high, medium and low. Based on data mining, the information privacy mode is extracted, and the minimum support threshold is used to judge the support of private information in the database. Set the privacy information protection algorithm in the way of data support estimation. Experimental results: in the given data set, the support error of the algorithm in this paper is within 1.5%, and the error of the traditional algorithm is more than 5%. With the increasing size of the data set, the execution time of the traditional algorithm is much higher than that of the algorithm in this paper, which shows that the design is effective.

Keywords: Data mining · Information protection · Health privacy · Protection algorithm · Data set · Support

1 Introduction

Health information is a record of a resident individual's various health conditions in the entire life process, including records of information resources such as diseases and medical visits, and is a long-term dynamic process record. Health information involves residents' diagnosis and treatment information in hospitals, such as various inspection

S. Wang (Ed.): IoTCare 2022, LNICST 501, pp. 20–34, 2023.
https://doi.org/10.1007/978-3-031-33545-7_2

reports, etc., as well as residents' core health records. Health information records contain a large amount of data and are widely used in various fields. Users are most concerned about data security and privacy protection, including data leakage, loss and tampering during data storage, transmission and processing. With the rapid rise of network technology, the continuous development of database technology and the wide application of large-scale database management systems, a large amount of data information has been generated. A wealth of knowledge is hidden in these massive data, and people are eager to obtain useful knowledge from these data [1]. As a powerful data analysis tool, data mining can automatically extract from a large amount of heterogeneous data hidden, unknown and valuable knowledge, and realize the transformation from "data grave" to knowledge wealth, this knowledge is expressed as rules or patterns. They can provide valuable intellectual information for business decision-making, scientific exploration, and medical research.

The knowledge discovered by data mining can not only be used to derive sensitive information from non sensitive information, but also some knowledge discovered by data mining may be sensitive information itself, involving national security, trade secrets and personal privacy. With the continuous progress of information technology, information has gradually evolved into a kind of commodity, which can be collected and stored in database equipment for others to use with or without compensation. This information is easily collected and processed, and finally sold to some intermediary companies and marketing companies [2]. But what follows is that a large amount of personal information becomes more transparent, which makes personal safety feel damaged, and thus brings great harm to personal personality. In the current information age, privacy protection is much more complex than traditional privacy protection. How to prevent the leakage of users' privacy information and reduce the damage and loss of information assets caused by objective or human factors while publishing and applying big data is a widely concerned issue in the field of big data research, which will directly affect the safe application of big data. Based on data mining technology, this paper studies the cloud health privacy information protection algorithm. The overall research technical route of the algorithm is as follows:

(1) First, through the differentiated privacy information protection model, the connection between users and information is analyzed. The membership function is used to calculate the membership of information, and the sensitive attributes of privacy information are obtained.
(2) According to the sensitive attributes of privacy information, build indicators of cloud health privacy information protection, and assess the risk of privacy information protection.
(3) Set the minimum support threshold of privacy information protection, and judge the support of privacy information in the data through data mining methods. Set privacy information protection algorithm in the way of data support estimation.
(4) In the test experiment, the performance of the text algorithm is tested with the support error and operation time as the test indicators.

2   Health Privacy Information Protection Algorithm on the Cloud

2.1   Build a Differential Privacy Information Protection Model

The problem of health information privacy protection includes the user set and the connection relationship between users. In order to protect privacy reasonably and effectively, the data content and social structure are combined to build a differentiated privacy information protection model, that is, based on the social network structure model CVB, the value of users in sensitive attributes is extracted as attribute nodes, and the connection between users and attribute nodes is used, represents the specific attribute value of the user on the sensitive attribute.

The social network in reality is modeled as a simple graph with no authority and no direction, and its mathematical expression is:

$$C = (V, O, B, M) \tag{1}$$

Among them: $V = \{V_1, V_2, \ldots, V_w\}$ represents the user node set. V_q represents the q node, which corresponds to a real user in the network on the cloud. $N \subseteq V \times V$ represents a set of user relationships, any $O_{qp} \in O$ represents a social link between users V_q and V_p, and all relationships are of the same type and are not considered sensitive information.

$B = \{B_1, B_2, \ldots, B_w\}$ represents the set of sensitive attribute value nodes, that is, any $B_q \in B$ represents a specific value of sensitive attribute. For example, in the attribute "disease information", hepatitis and cold are two different attribute values, so two attribute value nodes are formed in the social graph model. M represents the mapping relationship between the sensitive attribute value and the user node. The dotted line indicates that the user has this attribute value, that is, the sensitivity function of the attribute value B_q. The mapping relationship is:

$$M(B_q) : B_q \rightarrow M_q \tag{2}$$

Therefore, the attribute tag of health user information on the cloud consists of two parts: sensitive attribute value and attribute value sensitivity, namely:

$$e_{V_q} = (V_q, B_q, V_q, M_q) \tag{3}$$

In the formula: e is the attribute label [3]. e_{V_q} represents the sensitive attribute value of user node V_q and the sensitivity of the attribute value. From this, a privacy information protection model with simple attributes is constructed, as shown in Fig. 1.

Figure 1 shows a simple privacy information protection model, including three user nodes $V = \{V_1, V_2, V_3\}$, three attribute nodes $B = \{B_1, B_2, B_3\}$, and the three social relationships in the network are O_1, O_2, and O_3. The attribute label of user V_1 is $e_{V_1} = (B_1, M_1)$, and the corresponding sensitivities are $e_{V_2} = (B_2, M_2)$, $e_{V_3} = (B_3, M_3)$.

In order to reduce the information loss caused by anonymous algorithm and improve the data utility of publishing graph, considering the sensitivity of attribute values has differences, the attribute value sensitivity function is proposed. By measuring the sensitivity of sensitive attribute values, the sensitive attribute values are divided into three

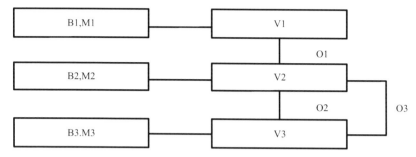

Fig. 1. Privacy information protection model for simple attributes

privacy levels, so that all values under the sensitive attribute category can be differentiated privacy protected.

Different attribute values have different degrees of privacy. When users enter their own health information, for example, the privacy degree of HIV is much greater than that of the common cold. Therefore, the privacy degree of sensitive attribute values is defined as the attribute value sensitivity, and accordingly The user's information privacy level is divided [4]. This time, a trapezoidal distribution membership function is used to determine the sensitivity of the sensitive attribute, and the thresholds r and t. The function value range is $[0, 1]$. Then exists:

$$\varsigma(u) = \begin{cases} u, u \leq r \\ \frac{u-r}{t-r}, r < u \leq t \\ 1, u > t \end{cases} \tag{4}$$

$$\varsigma \begin{cases} u \leq r, \varsigma = low \\ r < u \leq t, \varsigma = middle \\ u > t, \varsigma = high \end{cases} \tag{5}$$

In the formula: the sensitivity of sensitive attribute is $\varsigma(u)$. Privacy protection thresholds r and t are two constants, which reflect the extent to which the respondent can accept privacy disclosure. Their size is set by the data publisher according to different application backgrounds or the privacy protection requirements of the respondent. By default, $r = 0.5, t = 1$. In addition, data publishers can set privacy protection thresholds in real time according to the dynamic status of the network environment. The lower the threshold, the higher the demand for privacy protection.

The user's disease information "HIV" is not sensitive information in the AIDS friendly communication network, but is high-level sensitive information in ordinary social groups. Accordingly, users' information privacy levels are divided into three categories: high, middle, and low. There are certain differences in the protection forms of the three information privacy levels, which are processed through the principle of anonymity protection. The process is shown in Fig. 2 below.

In the above figure, the publisher initiates a publishing request in the network service to request the information of users in the database to be published. The protection model obtains the information of the publisher from the database, and combines the privacy

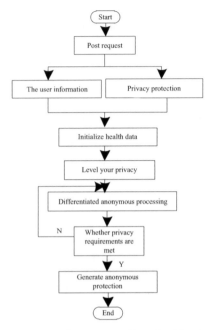

Fig. 2. Anonymous processing process of user health privacy information

protection requirements set by the publisher in the account to obtain the set of privacy information and the corresponding privacy protection requirements.

Generally, a simple form of anonymity is used to replace the user's unique identity with serialized symbols, build a social graph, obtain the sensitivity of each attribute value in the privacy information according to the sensitivity function, divide the privacy level, store the level in the user's attribute tag, and adopt the corresponding anonymity strategy. However, how to choose anonymous processing criteria requires selecting specific indicators in the protection model.

2.2 Setting up Health Privacy Information Protection Indicators on the Cloud

In order to ensure that the health information on the cloud is in a safe state, a risk assessment method is used to protect the privacy information, and a risk early warning protection index is proposed. Qualitative or quantitative evaluation of possible risk events, and privacy risk situation assessment based on the release of health information, can find out the main risk factors of privacy leakage, the state of each risk factor and the development trend, which is the design of health information release. Prerequisites for privacy-preserving algorithms.

With reference to ITSEC and in combination with the characteristics of health information release and its application mode, privacy assets, privacy threats and privacy vulnerabilities are combined to form the possible sources of privacy risk. The three are taken as the first level elements for evaluating privacy risk, and the second level evaluation elements and third level privacy risk evaluation factors are selected for them to design a privacy information protection system [5]. See Table 1 for details.

Table 1. Health privacy information protection system on the cloud

First-level indicator	Secondary indicators	Three-level indicator
Privacy assets	Degree of confidentiality	Data encryption
		Quarantine data
		Manage keys
		Data confidentiality
	Completeness	Backup data
		Destroy data
		Upgrade software
	Available value	Migrate data
		Identify risks
Privacy threat	Technical risk	Deliberate attack
		Network control
		Vulnerability Handling
	Human risk	Staff member
		Verify identidy
		Wrong operation
Privacy vulnerability	Organizational vulnerability	Approval system
		Network system
		Liability Regulations
	Technical vulnerability	Service Content
		Degree of access
	Other vulnerability	Regulations
		Privacy treatment
		Risk report

On the basis of the above indicators, through the research and analysis of a large number of privacy leaks and authoritative reports at home and abroad, and referring to the risk assessment indicators of the world's most authoritative IT research and consulting company Gartner, European network and information security agency ENISA, cloud computing security alliance CSA and other world authoritative organizations, sort out and summarize the privacy risk assessment indicators.

On the basis of fuzzy mathematics, Vague set theory, and intuitionistic fuzzy theory, a method for analyzing and processing uncertain information is developed. It uses the connection number to reflect the fuzzy, certain, uncertain and other phenomena between things and the changes between them. With the help of ternary or multivariate connection number, the various factors affecting privacy risk can be concentrated, effectively classified and reasonably described. Among them, factors that have a positive and obvious impact on system privacy risk can be expressed as support; Factors unrelated to privacy risk can be expressed as opposition; Other factors with uncertain impact on privacy risk can be expressed as a concentration is the uncertainty, or is further refined into the partial identical component, the neutral component or the partial inverse component of the uncertainty.

From the perspective of privacy risk assessment, "homeopathy" indicates that the result of privacy risk assessment tends to be in the same trend state with the ideal standard risk, that is, it is in "low risk"; "Balance of power" reflects that the privacy risk assessment results and the ideal standard risk are close to each other, that is, they are at "medium risk"; "Counter trend" indicates that the result of privacy risk assessment tends to be opposite to the ideal standard risk, that is, it is at "high risk". The results of privacy risk assessment can be simply "clustered" through potential value. The risk indicators of the above privacy protection are evaluated, and their levels are shown in Table 2.

Table 2. Health and privacy protection index levels on the cloud

Index	Influencing factors	Privacy assets	Privacy threat	Privacy vulnerability
Degree of confidentiality	Data encryption	High risk	Medium risk	High risk
	Quarantine data	Low risk	Low risk	High risk
	Manage keys	High risk	High risk	High risk
	Data confidentiality	Medium risk	High risk	High risk
Completeness	Backup data	High risk	High risk	Medium risk
	Destroy data	Low risk	Medium risk	High risk
	Upgrade software	High risk	High risk	Low risk
Available value	Migrate data	High risk	Low risk	High risk
	Identify risks	High risk	High risk	Low risk
Technical risk	Deliberate attack	High risk	High risk	High risk
	Network control	High risk	Low risk	High risk
	Vulnerability Handling	Low risk	High risk	Medium risk
Human risk	Staff member	Low risk	Low risk	High risk
	Verify identidy	Medium risk	Low risk	High risk

(*continued*)

Table 2. (*continued*)

Index	Influencing factors	Privacy assets	Privacy threat	Privacy vulnerability
	Wrong operation	High risk	Low risk	Medium risk
Organizational vulnerability	Approval system	High risk	High risk	Low risk
	Network system	Low risk	Low risk	Low risk
	Liability Regulations	Medium risk	High risk	High risk
Technical vulnerability	Service Content	High risk	High risk	High risk
	Degree of access	High risk	High risk	Low risk
Other vulnerability	Regulations	Low risk	Medium risk	Medium risk
	Privacy treatment	High risk	High risk	Low risk
	Risk report	High risk	High risk	Low risk

With the help of many experts, we will evaluate the level of risk factors in the current privacy in the process of health privacy data release, so as to complete the construction of privacy risk assessment index system. According to the principle of maximum membership, the results are divided into corresponding evaluation levels, corresponding to different risk levels, and information privacy patterns are extracted based on data mining.

2.3 Extracting Information Privacy Patterns Based on Data Mining

Mining itself is also an effective means of knowledge expression. The goal is to retain as many non sensitive patterns as possible in the result data set without disclosing sensitive patterns, especially some non sensitive patterns containing important information, so as to improve the availability of the result data set, that is, frequent pattern mining can be used to find non sensitive patterns containing important information. Figure 3 shows the process of processing the original data set to get the result data set.

The original dataset contains all frequent patterns, while the resulting dataset contains only non-sensitive patterns. First, on the original data set, frequent pattern mining is performed to obtain the corresponding set of frequent patterns. Through analysis, the data owner determines which of the frequent patterns obtained by mining contain sensitive information, which are called sensitive patterns or private patterns [6]. Then, according to the frequent patterns obtained by mining, some of which have been identified as sensitive patterns by the data owner, the original data set is processed by applying the privacy protection algorithm to obtain a new result data set.

Mining schemas typically target datasets stored in transactional databases, also known as transactional databases. Health privacy information on the cloud is a typical transaction database. A transactional database is usually described as follows: Let $S = \{S_1, S_2, ..., S_N\}$ be a set of N items [7]. A transaction record D, also called a transaction record, is a subset of the items in S. Table 3 is a simple transaction database.

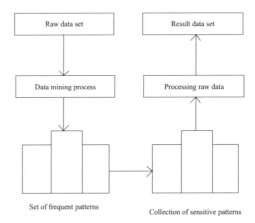

Fig. 3. Schematic diagram of the privacy protection process in frequent pattern mining

Table 3. Simple transaction database

Health information records	Item in info record
S1	z, x, c
S2	v, z, b, x
S3	v, z, b, x
S4	z, b, x, n
S5	v, z, b, m

In the table above, each transaction record has a unique identifier. A transaction database is a collection of transaction records. In this way, the database schema is defined, and the schema is called an item set, which is set as F, which is a subset composed of items in S, and F is included in transaction record D. If F contains G items, then the length of F is called G, denoted as:

$$|F| = G \tag{6}$$

Therefore, for convenience, we abbreviate the mode like $F = \{c, n, m\}$ as:

$$F = cnm \tag{7}$$

When there are two modes, rewrite them as F and H. If F is a subset of H, then F is said to be a sub-pattern of H. Correspondingly, H is said to be a supermode of F. Obviously, for a pattern of length 1, its subpatterns do not exist. And when there are two modes J and K, if J is a sub-mode of K, and there is no mode L, such that J is a sub-mode of L and L is a sub-mode of K, then J can be said to be a direct sub-mode of K, K is the direct supermode of J.

On this basis, to obtain the sensitivity support, a transaction record D supports mode F if and only if the transaction record D contains mode F [8]. If there are N multiple transaction records in transaction database S, and the number of transaction records including F is Z, then the absolute support degree of mode F on S is Z, which is denoted as $ZF_S(F)$. The relative support, referred to as support, is Z/N, and denoted as $Z \cup F_S(F)$.

When the private information database S is clear in the context, we also abbreviated the support degree $Z \cup F_S(F)$ and support number $ZF_S(F)$ of pattern F as $Z \cup F(F)$ and $ZF(F)$, respectively. Therefore, given the transaction database and the minimum support threshold, set it to λ, if the support $Z \cup F(F)$ of pattern F on S is greater than or equal to the minimum support threshold λ, then F is a frequent pattern on S.

Set the minimum support threshold λ to the value of 50%. According to the definition of frequent patterns, the support of all frequent patterns in the transaction database in Table 3 can be given, as shown in Table 4.

Table 4. Frequent mining patterns of single-transaction databases

Pattern length	Frequent pattern
1	(v,50%), (z,100%), (b,70%), (x,70%)
2	(vz,50%), (vb,50%), (vx,30%), (zb,70%) (zx,70%), (bx,50%)
3	(vzb,50%), (vzx,50%), (vbx,30%), (zbx,70%)
4	(vzbx,30%)

The task of frequent pattern mining is to find all frequent patterns whose support is not less than λ and their corresponding support when the minimum support threshold λ is given. Given a transaction database and a minimum support threshold λ, let $X(S, Z \cup F_S(F))$ denote the frequent pattern mining results on S, then:

$$X(S, Z \cup F_S(F)) = \{p, Z \cup F_S(F) | Z \cup F_S(F) \geq \lambda\} \tag{8}$$

In the formula: for convenience, when the transaction database S and the minimum support λ are clear in the context, $X(S, \lambda)$ is also simply marked as X [4]. Therefore, through the frequent patterns in data mining, the privacy pattern of health information on the cloud is given, and with the help of data support, the algorithm of privacy protection of data information is designed.

2.4 Data Support Setting Privacy Information Protection Algorithm

Suppose a database tuple is composed of Q and W, Q indicates that the attribute appears, and W indicates that the attribute does not appear. The probability of each data item remaining at the original value is E, and the probability of flipping is $Q - E$. All database tuples are distorted in the same way to form a new database. Data mining is performed on databases formed after distortion. For different properties, different values of E can be used to distort. For simplicity, all probabilities E are assumed to be equal in this paper.

Let the real data set matrix be represented as R, the matrix obtained by R after the distortion operation is T, and the distortion probability is E. The number of Q in column U of R is recorded as I_Q^R, the number of W is recorded as I_W^R, the number of Q in column U of T is recorded as I_Q^T, and the number of W is recorded as I_W^T. It can be seen from the data distortion process that:

$$\begin{cases} I_Q^R \times E + I_W^R \times (1 - E) = I_Q^T \\ I_W^R \times E + I_Q^R \times (1 - E) = I_W^T \end{cases} \tag{9}$$

This leads to:

$$I^R = P^{-1} I^T \tag{10}$$

Of which:

$$P = \begin{bmatrix} E & 1 - E \\ 1 - E & E \end{bmatrix} \tag{11}$$

$$I^T = \begin{bmatrix} I_Q^T \\ I_W^T \end{bmatrix} \tag{12}$$

$$I^R = \begin{bmatrix} I_Q^R \\ I_W^R \end{bmatrix} \tag{13}$$

In the formula: P is a matrix of order N. From Eq. (9), the true matrix one-item set support I_Q^R can be estimated from the distorted matrix T.

The calculation method of the support of N item set is similar to that of item set. at this time:

$$P = \begin{bmatrix} p_{0,0} & p_{0,1} & \cdots & p_{0,2^N-1} \\ p_{1,0} & p_{1,1} & \cdots & p_{1,2^N-1} \\ \cdots & \cdots & \cdots & \ddots \\ p_{2^N-1,0} & p_{2^N-1,1} & \cdots & p_{2^N-1,2^N-1} \end{bmatrix} \tag{14}$$

$$I^T = \begin{bmatrix} I_{2^N-1}^T \\ \vdots \\ I_Q^T \\ I_W^T \end{bmatrix} \tag{15}$$

$$I^R = \begin{bmatrix} I_{2^N-1}^R \\ \vdots \\ I_Q^R \\ I_W^R \end{bmatrix} \tag{16}$$

In the formula: I_A^T is defined as the number of N itemsets in the distorted database, the itemsets are in the form of N-bit binary numbers, and the decimal value A [9] corresponding to the N-bit binary numbers. $p_{i,j}$ is the probability that N itemset j (represented as N-bit binary) is distorted into N itemset i (represented as N-bit binary). The binomial set $p_{0,1}$ represents the probability that the itemset 11 is distorted to 00, which is $(1 - E)^2$. Then the support degree of the N itemset in the original data set is $I_{2^N-1}^R$. So far, the design of the cloud health privacy information protection algorithm based on data mining is completed.

3 Experimental Studies

3.1 Experiment Preparation

In the above, based on data mining technology, a new algorithm is designed for the privacy protection of health information on the cloud. In order to verify the effectiveness of this method, experimental testing method is used to demonstrate. Taking the noise protection algorithm as the control group, the effectiveness and efficiency of different algorithms are verified by comparing with the method in this paper. In the experimental test, first, given the minimum support threshold, in 50 groups of original data sets, obtain all the health information of users, randomly select 20 sensitive data sets, and take the remaining non sensitive data sets as the release data sets.

The first part uses the support error index to measure the effectiveness of the two algorithms. The larger the support error value, the greater the impact of the algorithm on the result data set, the worse the processing of sensitive data in health information, and it is difficult to complete the precision. Data protection.

Define the calculation method of the support error degree, and assume that there are $f = [f_1, f_2, ..., f_g]$ modes in the published data set, then:

$$k = \sum_{i=1}^{g} \frac{h(f)' - h(f)}{h(f)} \qquad (17)$$

In the formula: k is the support error degree. $h(f)$ represents the support of different modes in the result data set, while $h(f)'$ represents the support of different modes in the original data set.

In the second part of the test, the privacy protection threshold is taken as a constant, and the size of the original data set is gradually increased, so as to compare the efficiency of the two algorithms.

3.2 Results and Analysis

In the first part of the test, the number of transactions in the original data set is 200,000, the original data set remains unchanged throughout the process, the minimum support threshold is set to 4%, and the privacy protection threshold is gradually increased from 5% to 40%. In this case, the effectiveness of the two algorithms is compared, and the results are shown in Fig. 4.

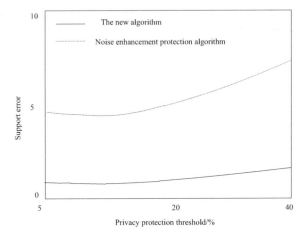

Fig. 4. Compares the support error under different privacy protection thresholds

It can be seen from the figure that a small privacy protection threshold means a higher degree of protection for sensitive modes. For the noise protection algorithm, as the privacy protection threshold increases, more sensitive transactions are processed, so the support error becomes higher. However, the variation range of this method becomes smaller, and the error degree is basically kept within 1.5, which has application effect.

In the second part of the test, keep the privacy protection threshold unchanged, set it to 30%, and the minimum support threshold is 2.0%, gradually increase the size of the original data set, and compare the efficiency of the two algorithms. The results are shown in Fig. 5.

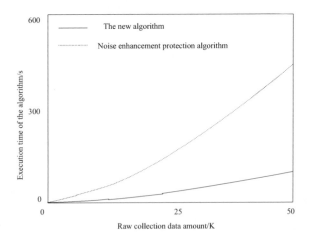

Fig. 5. Compares the execution time of the algorithm under different original data sets

In the figure, when the original data set is the same, the execution time of the algorithm in this paper is less than the execution time of increasing the noise privacy protection algorithm, and with the continuous increase of the original data set, increasing the execution time of the noise protection algorithm will increase the speed of its growth. It is much larger than the algorithm in this paper, indicating that the method designed this time is more effective.

4 Conclusion

With the development of network information technology and database technology, data mining technology shows an increasingly broad application prospect and plays an increasingly important role in more and more fields. However, as a large number of private data are widely collected and analyzed, the application of data containing sensitive information will pose a threat to personal privacy security. Therefore, this paper designs a new protection algorithm on the basis of data mining technology on how to deal with the privacy protection problem.

On the one hand, it deals with the privacy information contained in the health dataset itself, and on the other hand, it deals with the sensitive knowledge generated after the application of the dataset. The experimental results show that the error degree of this method is significantly reduced, and the error degree of this method is basically kept within 1.5; The execution time of the algorithm in this paper is significantly reduced, and the maximum is only about 150 s.

However, due to the limitation of time and energy, the research results that have been achieved still need to be further improved, and can be further expanded in the process of combining with relevant research directions and fields. Specifically, an algorithm will have more vitality only if it is applied in real life. It will be our important work in the future to apply our algorithm to realistic datasets and solve problems that arise in reality.

Acknowledgment. The authors are grateful to the support of the Guangdong Universities' Innovation Team Project (2021KCXTD015) and Guangdong Key Disciplines Project (2021ZDJS138).

References

1. Liu, Y., Yang, Y.: A Data mining algorithm for matrix and sort index association rules. Comput. Technol. Dev. **31**(2), 54–59 (2021)
2. Jia, X.: Time series data mining algorithm based on multiobjective decision. Electron. Design Eng. **29**(17), 45–49 (2021)
3. Yao, R., Fei, Y., Ding, Y., et al.: Research on engineering data information prediction model based on intelligent data mining algorithm. Electron. Design Eng. **30**(7), 63–67 (2022)
4. Lu, P., Ge, S., Wu, X., et al.: Design of personal health information management and privacy protection system based on ZigBee. Comput. Meas. Control **29**(4), 170–174 (2021)
5. Wei, W., Xin, Z., Wang, S., Zhang, Y.: Covid-19 diagnosis by WE-SAJ. Syst. Sci. Control Eng. **10**(1), 325–335 (2022)
6. Tang, C., Lin, X.: Protocol of privacy-preserving set intersection computation. Netinfo Secur. **1**, 9–15 (2020)
7. Huang, C., Wang, W., Zhang, X., Wang, S. -H., Zhang, Y.-D.: tuberculosis diagnosis using deep transferred EfficientNet. IEEE/ACM Trans. Comput. Biol. Bioinf. (2022)

8. Song, X., Gai, M., Zhao, S., et al.: Privacy-preserving statistics protocol for set-based computation. J. Comput. Res. Dev. **57**(10), 2221–2231 (2020)

9. Zhang, G., Tang, Z., Li, S., She, F.: Measurement and simulation of risk tolerance of medical privacy big data disclosure. Comput. Simul. **38**(12), 480–484 (2021)

10. Wang, J.: Back-propagation neural network learning algorithm based on privacy preserving. Comput. Sci. **49**(z1), 575–580 (2022)

Data Security Mining Method for Social Media Users' Mental Health Status Test Based on Machine Learning Algorithm

Junyu Su[1], Wenjian Liu[1], Hanxu Zhao[2], Wennan Wang[3], and Chiyu Shi[1(✉)]

[1] Faculty of Data Science, City University of Macau, Macau, China
sjy2166@163.com
[2] Alibaba Cloud Big Data Application College, Zhuhai College of Science and Technology, Zhuhai, China
[3] Academy of Management, Guangdong University of Science and Technology, Dongguan, China

Abstract. Users who frequently use social media can easily lead to changes in their mental health status. In order to accurately predict users' mental health status, a data mining method for testing social media users' mental health status is designed based on machine learning algorithms. Perform clustering processing on the test data, calculate the centroid of each cluster and the sum of squared errors of the data set, and obtain the clustering result of the test data; extract the characteristics of social media users' mental health status, and calculate the abnormal score of the object's mental health status, Use this to distinguish the user's psychological state; build a data mining model based on machine learning algorithms, build a one-dimensional convolutional neural network framework, record the activation functions of the convolutional layer and the pooling layer, and obtain the output value of the fully connected layer; design social media user psychology Health state test data analysis algorithm to obtain a safe mining method for social media users' mental health state test data. Obtain the best period of social media users' mental health status observation through experiments. It can be seen from the experimental data that the correlation of the mental health state mining results obtained by this method is higher than 0.91, and the prediction accuracy is higher than 92%, which improves the effectiveness of mental health state prediction. The best observation period is one month to two months before the expected time.

Keywords: Machine Learning Algorithm · Social Media Users · Mental Health Status Test · Data Security Mining Method

1 Introduction

At present, with the massive Internet big data information, our society has developed into an information society, and it has gradually developed into a trend in the whole world. In the current information society, the generation, dissemination, processing and use of

S. Wang (Ed.): IoTCare 2022, LNICST 501, pp. 35–48, 2023.
https://doi.org/10.1007/978-3-031-33545-7_3

information are inseparable from the effective construction of the whole society. At the same time, the progress of information technology further provides a strong guarantee for the normal operation of the whole society. The overall level of informatization in Chinese society has basically reached the level of moderately developed countries, and China is entering a period of accelerated transformation of the information society [1]. At present, China has entered the era of big data, and this rapid development is due to the lightning-fast progress of the Internet. Countless individuals or groups have studied the massive Internet data and information, and regard it as a huge treasure, hoping to dig out their own wealth. And social media is one of the most worthy of study among these sectors. Social media represents a class of websites and technologies on which users can write, comment on, share, and communicate with each other on the Internet. At the same time, Social Media is also a type of tool and platform, where users can share insights, opinions, experiences or suggestions with each other. At present, social media covers a wide range, including Weibo (Sina Weibo, Tencent Weibo), social networking sites (Facebook)., Twitter, Renren, Friends), blogs (Sina Blog), forums (Shui Mu Nianhua), WeChat, etc.

The rapid development of social networks has dramatically changed the way people communicate. With the rapid development of society, huge work and life pressures are coming, which not only brings a heavy burden to our body, but also a variety of psychological problems are gradually increasing [2]. Especially in the university campus, events such as jumping off the building, suicide, running away, depression, etc. often occur, and some vicious injuries occur from time to time. The mental health of large objects has become one of the focuses of social concern, and has received extensive attention from all walks of life. Mental health problems are showing a growing trend around the world. Therefore, it is particularly important to use Internet big data to discover people's mental health problems in time. To this end, this paper studies data security mining methods for testing the mental health status of social media users based on machine learning algorithms. The module designed for the study method is shown in Fig. 1:

As shown in Fig. 1, the research process designed in this paper is as follows: cluster the test data and calculate the clustering results of the test data; Extract the characteristics of users' mental health, and mine abnormal scores of mental health; The data mining model based on machine learning algorithm is Innovatively constructed, the optimal classification value is calculated, and the optimal classifier is used to realize the safe mining of users' mental health test data. The test results show that the contribution of this method lies in improving the accuracy of the mental health state prediction of social media users, which can better reduce people's psychological stress and reduce the incidence of psychological problems such as depression.

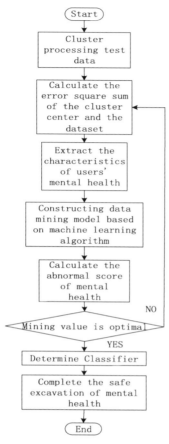

Fig. 1. Study module flow

2 Test Data Clustering

After years of development, data mining technology has achieved good results in the wide application of various fields, which is unmatched by other technical methods. Data mining technology is to dig out the hidden rules and value content in data to solve specific problems. People can also use computer applications to complete the same functions when they do not master the technology. Therefore, this paper proposes to introduce data mining technology into mental health data to mine and analyze the causes of the object's mental health problems, which provides a scientific basis for early prevention and early intervention to control the emergence of campus psychological crises.

The purpose of clustering is to group objects with similar properties together. In most cases, the data that people collect is unlabeled, and clustering can divide the data into multiple distinct groups. The data in each group has greater similarity, and the data between groups has greater exclusivity, that is, "similarity within a group and exclusivity between groups" [3, 4]. Clustering algorithms are mainly divided into partition-based clustering, hierarchical-based clustering, grid-based clustering, density-based clustering, and model-based clustering. As one of the commonly used methods in traditional machine learning algorithms, cluster analysis is widely favored due to its practicality, simplicity and efficiency. It has been successfully applied in many fields, such as: document clustering, market analysis, image segmentation, feature learning Wait. In this study, we choose the KMeans clustering algorithm, which is a partition-based clustering algorithm, to divide the meal times and entropy of the objects. First, randomly select k sample points from the sample set and use them as the center of the cluster. Then, according to the distance of each sample to the k centroids, it is divided into the nearest clusters, and the centroid of each cluster is recalculated. This article uses the Euclidean distance, and the calculation formula is:

$$D(s_t, M_g) = \sqrt{\frac{\sum_{i=1}^{n} X_{ij}^2}{M_g}} \tag{1}$$

In formula, $D(s_t, M_g)$ represents the Euclidean distance of each sample from the initial point to the cluster; s_t is the number of sample points; M_g is the centroid position; and X_{ij} represents the cluster entropy of the data.

In the sum of error squares for all datasets, the formula is:

$$G_{SSE} = \frac{\sum_{i=1}^{k} |D(s_t, M_g)|^2}{\sum_{i=1}^{k} M_g^2} \tag{2}$$

In formula (2), G_{SSE} represents the sum of squared of the dataset.

By initialization, you can randomly select k sample points from the original N samples and treat them as the hearts of the cluster. The eucoid distance of the remaining sample to the cluster center was calculated according to formula. Based on the results of the sum of squares calculation, each sample was divided into the nearest cluster cluster cluster to obtain the clustering results of the test data.

3 Feature Extraction of Mental Health Status of Social Media Users

Some studies have found that people with mental health problems develop eating disorders, especially those with depression. Based on this fact, the consumption records of the subjects in the canteen can be extracted by the store name to analyze their eating patterns. Pay particular attention to the subject's breakfast, lunch/dinner routine. In this study, the breakfast time period is set from 6:00 to 9:00, the lunch time period is set from 11:00 to 13:00, and the dinner time period is set from 17:00 to 19:30 [5, 6]. Since there are often multiple records for each meal, the first card swiping time in a meal is taken as the meal time of the meal. For example, there are 3 records in a breakfast, and their occurrence times are 7:20, 7:21 and 7:22, then use 7:20 as the breakfast time. The regularity of a behavior can be thought of as repeatable and will be measured by the entropy of the probability of the behavior occurring within a specific time interval.

Assuming n time interval $T_n = \{t_1, t_2, \cdots, t_n\}$, for any given object, the probability of behavior $F_m = \{f_{bre}, f_{lun}, f_{din}\}$ occurring within the time interval t_i is:

$$P_d(T_n = t_i) = \frac{D_f(t_i)}{\sum\limits_{i=1}^{n} D_f(t_i)} \tag{3}$$

In the formula, $P_d(T_n = t_i)$ indicates the probability of breakfast, lunch and dinner at any time interval; $D_f(t_i)$ indicates the frequency of any meal of the three meals in the time interval t_i [7]. According to the calculation of consumption characteristics of $P_d(T_n = t_i)$, the calculation formula is:

$$E_s = -\frac{\sum\limits_{i=1}^{n} P_d(T_n = t_i)}{\lg P_d(T_n = t_i)} \tag{4}$$

In formula, E_s indicates the entropy of meal consumption. The smaller E_s, the more concentrated the time interval of the probability distribution. Therefore, in the clustering process of entropy value and number, the clustering results of the measured meals can be obtained.

The goal of the above methods is to discover subjects with an abnormal diet. Suppose that the smaller an object is in the cluster, and the farther away it is from the center of the cluster, the higher the anomaly score is. Calculate the exception score of the object according to the formula:

$$Y_c = dis(h_k, p_c) \times \left(1 - \frac{\sum\limits_{i=1}^{n} d_i}{\sum\limits_{i=1}^{n} f_i}\right) \tag{5}$$

In formula, Y_c represents the score of the object diet abnormality; $dis(h_k, p_c)$ represents the Euclidean distance between the object and the centroid, where h_k represents the number of objects, p_c represents the centroid point of the cluster; d_i represents the consumption entropy of the i object and the diet, and f_i indicates the regularity coefficient of the object eating.

The abnormal score is mainly aimed at the difference of dining behavior between the object, as well as the dining difference of the object in different time periods, and finally the overall diet data of the object is obtained.

4 Building a Data Mining Model Based on Machine Learning Algorithms

According to the browsing history of the object, the characteristics of the Internet are mined. According to the order of access time, a time series of Internet access is established for each object. It is hoped to dig out the online pattern of the object from the online time series. In this study, the overall framework of the designed one-dimensional convolutional neural network is shown in Fig. 2.

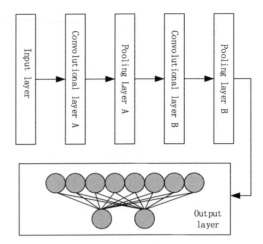

Fig. 2. One-dimensional Convolutional Neural Network framework

As shown in Fig. 1, there are five neural network layers except for the input layer. The first and third neural network layers use the convolutional layer, the second and fourth layers use the pooling layer, and the last output layer is the fully connected layer. Record the activation functions of the convolution and pooling layers separately, as shown in formula (6):

$$\begin{cases} Y_k^p = \dfrac{\sum\limits_{i=1}^{n} y_i^{p-1} * h_i^p}{\sum\limits_{i=1}^{n} b_p^i} \\[4ex] \hat{Y}_k^p = \dfrac{\sum\limits_{i=1}^{n} y_i^{p-1} \times down\left(f_k^p + k_i\right)}{\sum\limits_{i=1}^{n} b_p^i} \end{cases} \tag{6}$$

In the formula, Y_k^p and $\hat{Y}_k^p$ represent the activation functions of the convolutional layer and the pooling layer respectively, which are also the results obtained by training each tested data in different stages of the model; y_i^{p-1} represents the feature parameter corresponding to the convolution kernel; $*$ represents the multiplication operation; h_i^p represents the bias position of the convolution kernel; b_p^i represents the vector dimension of the convolution kernel in the online sequence; $down\left(f_k^p\right)$ represents the bias matrix downsampling function in the pooling layer; k_i represents the input value.

Within the full connection layer, you can get the activation function:

$$f(m) = \frac{f\left(Y_{(4)} * Y_{(3)}^2 + Y_{(1)}\right)}{f\left(Y_{(2)}^2\right)} \tag{7}$$

In formula, $f(m)$ represents the output value of the fully connected layer in a 1 D convolutional neural network; $Y_{(1)}$, $Y_{(2)}$, $Y_{(3)}$, $Y_{(4)}$ represent the output values of the first, second, third, and fourth layer, respectively. Through the above functions, a standard model of the mental health status test data of social media users can be established.

5 Design the Data Analysis Algorithm for Social Media Users' Mental Health State Test

Due to the implicit characteristics of mental health, it is impossible to directly observe the mental health status of individuals, so we can only use some explicit "behavioral samples" to measure indirectly. At present, traditional psychological testing of mental health or clinical application of patients prefers indirect methods using these phenotypes. Each assessment method consists of thousands of items, each of which can be regarded as an abstract description of a series of individual behavioral characteristics. Correspondingly, these behavioral characteristics have a certain relationship with psychological characteristics. When using these methods to assess the mental health status, firstly, the individual needs to select the corresponding options according to the fit degree of his specific situation and the content of the options; secondly, the assessor calculates the score according to the individual scoring method provided by the specific basis; finally, the evaluators put forward conclusions based on the overall evaluation results, and explain the meaning in detail, and then notify the relevant personnel in the form of text or reports.

Which of so many Internet behaviors could reflect significant effects on mental health issues is clearly critical to our research. Even different mental health issues target different internet behaviors. However, on the other hand, this particularity of cyberspace has led to a complicated trend in the relationship between Internet behavior and users' psychological characteristics. We cannot simply apply the traditional psychology research conclusions on a certain dimension of mental health to correspond to the characteristics of Internet behavior, but should first establish the most complete network user behavior type guidelines, and gradually screen and reconfirm effective Internet users on the basis of these guidelines. Correspondence patterns of the relationship between behavior and psychological traits.

In data mining technology, the algorithms used mainly include decision tree algorithm, association rule algorithm, neural network algorithm, genetic algorithm, Bayesian network algorithm and statistical analysis method. In the data analysis research of social media users' mental health, this paper chooses to use decision tree algorithm and association rule Apriori algorithm. Decision tree algorithm is a relatively classic classification data mining algorithm. It generally uses a top-down recursive form to build generative decision trees from a large number of cases. The classification model of the decision tree algorithm is a directed acyclic tree consisting of a root node, parent nodes, child nodes and leaf nodes. Typical decision tree algorithms include ID3 algorithm C4.5 algorithm and CART algorithm. Using the ID3 algorithm and the C4.5 algorithm to generate decision trees for studying mental health problems is a common method. The decision tree algorithm is used to predict and analyze the mental health data of social media users. The general idea is to first analyze and calculate which attribute has the greatest correlation with the psychological problem, as the root node of the decision tree, and then use the iterative recursive method to analyze the rest in the same way. Attributes are classified, a decision tree is formed and a classification tree model for predictive analysis is constructed, as shown in Fig. 3.

As shown in Fig. 3, the overall identification algorithm of social media users' mental health problems based on mining algorithm is mainly divided into three parts, including

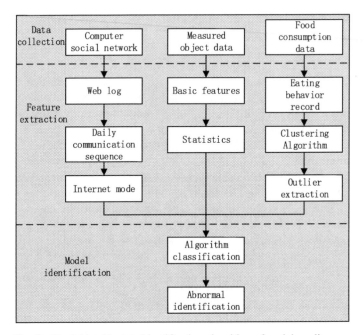

Fig. 3. Mental health state identification algorithm of social media users

data acquisition, feature extraction and model identification. In the data acquisition and preprocessing stage, we obtained three data sources, namely computer social network, basic information of the tested object, and dietary consumption data. In the feature extraction stage, relevant features such as students' online patterns and abnormal consumption scores are extracted from the above three data sources. In the model identification stage, the optimal classifier is screened out, and the abnormal points of social media users' mental health status are obtained. At this time, through the above method, a safe mining method for the test data of social media users' mental health state based on the machine learning algorithm can be obtained.

6   Experimental Test

In order to combine the social media behavior of Internet users with mental health assessment, and to integrate machine learning methods into the field of mental health assessment, this paper designs and studies a depression prediction model based on social media behavior of Internet users. This method better explores the effective way to combine the two modes. The core idea of the whole process is based on the most extensive psychological assessment methods at present, trying to replace the traditional method by using the user behavior of Internet users on social media to achieve basically the same purpose.

6.1 Acquisition and Preprocessing of Raw Data

In the acquisition and preprocessing part of raw data, on the one hand, the user's mental health assessment results are obtained through traditional scales, and on the other hand, the user's raw data on social media is obtained through Internet means, and then through step-by-step processing, the final result is formed. User network behavior characteristics are stored in the database. In the part of network behavior characteristics, it can be divided into three parts according to its process: social media API port call, data preprocessing, feature extraction and selection. In the acquisition of mental health status data, it is mainly divided into two parts: scale evaluation and data processing.

Application programming interfaces, or APIs for short, are functions that are pre-defined and encapsulated by website developers. Third-party personnel can directly call these functions without accessing the source code or understanding the details of the internal working mechanism of the website. At present, many social networking sites provide API interfaces. On the one hand, it is convenient for third-party personnel to develop more meaningful applications to enrich the website itself. On the other hand, it also provides a good opportunity for researchers to make it more convenient. to get the desired data.

Since the API ports provided by each website are different, the data formats of the obtained Internet users' network behavior are also different, so the data needs to be preprocessed before the next step to form the format required in the machine learning process. In the traditional machine learning process, data preprocessing is generally divided into three parts: data fusion, data cleaning and data transformation. Data fusion is to combine data from multiple data sources and store them uniformly, in other words, to realize the initialization of the data warehouse itself. The purpose of data cleaning is to remove errors or abnormal data in user data, remove redundant data, and standardize data formats. Data conversion is to convert user data into a custom normalized format, so as to facilitate the re-expansion and continuous transmission of user data.

According to the network behavior index system and the definition of specific psychological problems (such as depression, anxiety, etc.) in traditional mental health, the Internet behavior characteristics of individuals are extracted from the Internet behavior data of users. These Internet behavior characteristics can represent the overall behavior of individual users in the process of Internet communication, and are universal and specific. Then, according to the user's mental health status evaluation results, the characteristics that can represent the user's network behavior are selected.

The basic support for the establishment of the mental health model based on the social media behavior system of Internet users is the scale evaluation method in traditional psychology. Summarize. Therefore, as the establishment and evaluation standard of the model, the mental health status of some users must be obtained through the scale. There are many scales for comprehensive assessment of mental health commonly used in psychology at present, and different types of mental health have their own one or more assessment scales.

The data processing of the mental health measurement link is the same as the data preprocessing function of the network behavior part. After obtaining the mental health assessment scales of some users, the obtained scale scores need to be counted, summed and screened. Invalid or redundant assessment results will be removed.

A group of target users who are very active on social media and study in the same school are selected as the main subjects of this experiment, and the experiment time is from May 1, 2015 to May 15, 2015. Set the time period to 0.5 H_m, 1 H_m, 2 H_m, 3 H_m when the time point of May 1, 2015 is P_1, the time of 0.5 is from April 15, 2015 to May 1, 2015, and the time point of 1 is April 1, 2015 May 1, 2015; that is, the time period is the forward half month, one month, two months, and three months. Time point P_2 is half a month before P_1, that is, April 15, 2015, and the same time period is set under time point P_2. Time points P_3, P_4, and P_5 are April 1, 2015, March 15, 2015, and March 1, 2015, respectively. According to the above time points, the collected data and data can be divided into 20 data sets, as shown in Table 1.

Table 1. Time points and time periods

	0 Hm	0.5 Hm	1 Hm	2 Hm	3 Hm
P1	2015.05.01	2015.04.15	2015.04.01	2015.03.01	2015.02.01
P2	2015.04.15	2015.04.01	2015.03.01	2015.01.01	2014.11.01
P3	2015.04.01	2015.03.15	2015.02.01	2014.11.01	2014.08.01
P4	2015.03.15	2015.03.01	2015.01.01	2014.09.01	2014.05.01
P5	2015.03.01	2015.02.15	2014.12.01	2014.07.01	2014.02.01

These data are initially stored in text format and then transferred to the database. In the experiment, these time points are respectively used as test points for the user's mental health status.

6.2 Model Accuracy Test

Set the number of convolution kernels of the two convolutional layers to 16 and 32 respectively, use reLU as the activation function, and use adam as the optimization algorithm. Furthermore, to prevent overfitting, we use three dropout layers with parameters of 0.15, 0.15, and 0.5. In the model training phase, we selected 70 positive samples and 70 negative samples to train the model. In the feature extraction stage, all experimental samples are input into the trained model, and finally the result of the fully connected layer is used as the output value. According to the trend of model accuracy level, we can analyze from both vertical and horizontal aspects. First, at the longitudinal level, we observe different time periods at the same time node (P1, P2, P3, P4, P5), as shown in Fig. 4.

The performance test results of the time node model at the longitudinal level are shown in Fig. 4. We can see that with the increase of the observation period, the correlation coefficient script presents an "inverted U"-shaped change trend. This means that in a period of time, as the observation period becomes longer, each node of the model will continuously accumulate behavior data of the user network. Compared with a smaller amount of information, these accumulated data can better describe the The behavioral habits of bloggers and the psychological factors hidden behind them. Therefore, the

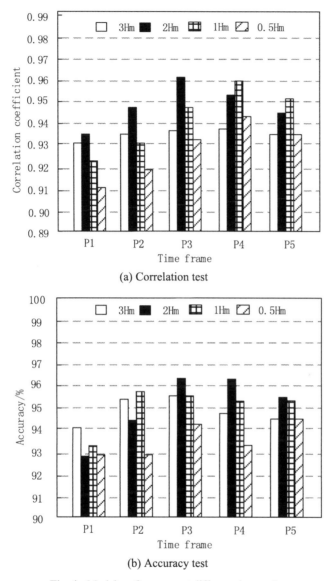

(a) Correlation test

(b) Accuracy test

Fig. 4. Model performance at different time nodes

correlation between the data of social media users' mental health status test and the three-meal data gradually increased. It can be seen from Fig. 4(a) that the optimal time period is usually between one month and two months, and the most relevant data in this image is 2 Hm at time node P34. However, since depression in mental health is an unstable psychological variable that changes with time, with the further growth of original data, the correlation between online user data and mental health status gradually weakens. Predictive power is gradually diminishing. Therefore, too long observation

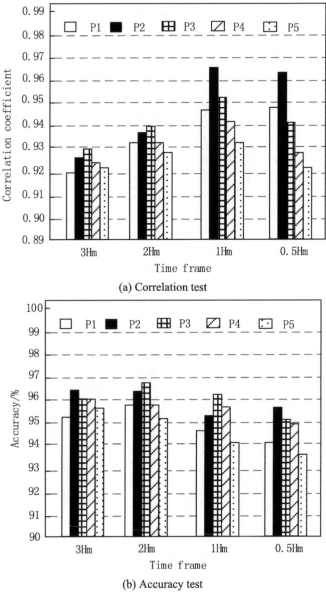

Fig. 5. Model performance for different time periods

period is not conducive to the prediction of depression state of Weibo users. In Fig. 4(b), the prediction results under all time periods are also in the "inverted U" shape, and the accuracy rate of P3 in the 2 Hm period is also the highest overall. Therefore, the accuracy trend of the classification model can be seen in this experimental test. However, under

this trend, the mining results of the present method can still maintain over 0.91 correlation and over 92% accuracy, indicating that the mining level of the present method is
relatively high.

At the lateral level, for the continuous value prediction of depression, we observed
the performance at different time nodes in the same time period (0.5 m, 1 m, 2 m and
3 m), as shown in Fig. 5.

Through the model performance test results under different time periods shown in
Fig. 5, it can be seen that for the same time period, the correlation of the model is not
the higher the closer it is to the P1 time node, from 0.5 Hm to 3 Hm also shows a kind
of Inverted U trend. In other words, for the same observation period, since the user data
was obtained at the P1 time point, the P2 node in the correlation test of the model is
the highest point under the same time period, that is to say, using the user's network
behavior to predict the depression state has hysteresis characteristics. Under the same
period of time, as the time node goes from P1 to P2, P3, and then to P4 and P5, the
prediction accuracy of the model also has a clear trend of high in the middle and low on
both sides. The drop from P2, P3 to P4, P5 may be caused by the data getting farther
and farther away from the P1 time point. From the lateral level overall data, the mining
correlation of this method is higher than 0.92, and the prediction accuracy is higher than
93%, with a good mining and prediction level.

It can be seen from the above two sets of experiments, although the best observation
period is fixed, the mining and prediction results of the present method both achieve
good levels. If you want to better predict the mental health status of social media users,
it is best to use the data of the previous month or two to make the prediction results more
accurate.

7   Conclusion

Data mining technology has been successfully applied in many fields and achieved
certain results in various fields. In this paper, data mining technology is applied to the
mental health data of social media users, and a data mining method for social media
users' mental health testing based on machine learning algorithm is proposed. Calculate
the clustering results of each data set; Innovatively extract the characteristics of social
media users' mental health status, and distinguish users' mental status; Build a data
mining model based on machine learning algorithm, design a data analysis algorithm,
and obtain the mining results of social media users' mental health. The test results show
that the mining results of social media users' mental health status obtained by this method
are highly correlated, with high prediction accuracy, and improve the effectiveness of
mental health mining. It is expected that the best prediction results will be obtained one to
two months before the time, so as to better serve the purpose of mental health. However,
due to the limitation of time and its own level, there are still some shortcomings and
deficiencies in the research on the mental health data mining of social media users in
this paper, and many previous assumptions have not been completed in the research. It is
hoped that these remaining issues can be further studied under conditions in the future.

References

1. Yang, M.: Mental prediction algorithm of college students based on internet big data mining. Inf. Technol. (11), 26–30, 36 (2021)
2. Liu, H.: Research on early warning analysis technology of mental illness based on data mining. Electron. Design Eng. **29**(15), 31–35 (2021)
3. Guo, Y.: Design of college mental health online service platform based on cloud computing technology. Mod. Electron. Tech. **44**(11), 177–181 (2021)
4. Hao, W.: Research on gray correlation algorithm of factors for college students' mental health early warning. Electron. Design Eng. **30**(11), 12–16 (2022)
5. Wen, M., Liao, W.: incremental mining algorithm for uncertain data based on machine learning. Comput. Simul. **38**(11), 290–294 (2021)
6. Wei, F.: College students' psychological management and control analysis system based on embedded data mining. Electron. Design Eng. **29**(24), 75–79 (2021)
7. Yu, M.: Prediction model of mental disorder based on historical data. Microcomput. Appl. **37**(12), 166–169 (2021)

Early Warning Method of College Students Mental Subhealth Based on Internet of Things

Xiang Li[✉]

Jingchu University of Technology Normal University, Jingmen 448000, Hubei, China
qihang7895@126.com

Abstract. Aiming at the problem that the precision of information node localization is low, which leads to the low speed of information transmission. This paper puts forward an early-warning method of college students' mental sub-health based on Internet of Things. Using sensors to build the Internet of Things network in colleges and universities to complete the college students' mental health information collection and transmission. Association rule algorithm is used to analyze the original psychological information of students. Draw radar chart and evaluate the early warning grade of college students' mental health by radar chart comparison. Design the early warning information transmission plan according to the operation requirements of the IOT. At this point, based on the Internet of Things college students mental sub-health early warning method design completed. The experimental results show that this method can improve the accuracy of information node location and speed up the transmission of mental sub-health warning information.

Keywords: Internet of Things · Information Transmission · Mental Health · College Students · Early Warning Evaluation · Local Maintenance Mapping Algorithm

1 Introduction

Health is not only the foundation of people's lives, study and work, but also the guarantee of life quality. With the development of modern science and technology and the improvement of social civilization, people's understanding of health has changed from that of biology to that of sociology and psychology. This change in understanding, so that people's understanding of human health has undergone profound changes. Based on the formation of new ideas, it is also recognized that the standards of human health for most people are not met, but in a state of "sub-health" is not a disease. Scientific research has found that many diseases are related to psychological factors, such as coronary heart disease, hypertension, angina pectoris, etc., collectively referred to as psychosomatic diseases. Mental health is not only related to the success or failure of disease, career, but also closely related to people's survival [1, 2].

Mental sub-health, which exists in all occupations and all ages, has become a social and medical problem that can not be ignored. With the development of society and

S. Wang (Ed.): IoTCare 2022, LNICST 501, pp. 49–60, 2023.
https://doi.org/10.1007/978-3-031-33545-7_4

the popularization of networks, people's quality of life and life rate have improved accordingly. Everything is more haste, less reach, fast high-quality living environment easy to cause psychological burden, leading to the psychological sub-health of this new disease began to spread to college students in this group. From the demand of scientific research and practice promotion, college students as a professional group should pay attention to their overall risk structure. Further clarification of the distance and direction between the group risk structure and the idealized zero risk state and scientific early warning to provide quantitative support for action to reduce risk [3].

Reference [4] method studies the automatic detection and classification of cognitive distortions in mental health texts. A mental health dataset was collected based on a machine learning framework. Exploratory analyzes were performed using unsupervised content-based clustering and topic modeling algorithms. This method can detect the state of mental health to a certain extent, but the transmission rate of early warning information still needs to be improved. Reference [5] uses machine learning algorithms and deep neural networks to build electronic health record data models. A final risk score for each individual is calculated and calibrated. Individual-level analyzes of risk scores were performed to help healthcare providers managing risk cohorts interpret results. This method can detect abnormal mental health states to a certain extent. The intercommunication method in the transmission of information can be further improved.

The necessity of early warning stems from the severe situation of high incidence of group sub-health and the increasingly urgent requirement of mental health improvement. From the crisis management, scientific management, dissemination of energy efficiency, information support, scientific research, groups and individuals to effectively improve the existing needs. For modern universities, many universities use advanced information management system and operation system to make students study and live more convenient, fast and efficient. However, these activities are increasing in unprecedented depth and breadth, which creates an opportunity for us to analyze and understand the mental sub-health state of college students automatically and comprehensively. In the past studies, some college students' mental sub-health warning methods were also put forward, but the overall warning effect is not good. After comparing many kinds of technologies, we choose IOT technology to accomplish the early warning of college students' mental sub-health, and design the method based on IOT.

According to the application and development direction of Internet of things, the application architecture of Internet of things can be divided into three categories: WSN, RFID and machine-to-machine. The study used the Internet of Things to transmit the collected data to the gateway nodes. After all the data are collected at the gateway node, they are transmitted to Ethernet to provide treatment basis for teachers and counselors. These data can also be analyzed and processed through the analysis and processing warning mechanism of the host computer. If it goes beyond the normal scope, it will make a prompt, warning and other decision-making and control to promote the development of college students' mental health education.

2   Collection and Transmission of Information on College Students' Mental Subhealth

In this study, sensors were used to build the Internet of Things network in colleges and universities, and to perceive the psychological state of college students. In order to ensure the accuracy of the sending of early warning information, we first complete the positioning of college students with mental sub-health status. After comparing several methods, use the local preserving mapping algorithm to complete this partial processing.

In this study, the transfer time between nodes can be expressed as:

$$t = t_a + t_b + t_n \tag{1}$$

Among them, t_a is the time needed to transmit the signal between the receiving end and the transmitting node in the LOS environment. The ratio of t_b to error is small, which represents the system measurement error. It can be expressed as a Gaussian random variable subject to $N(0, \alpha)^2$ distribution. The ratio of t_n to error is very large, which represents the time error caused by non-line-of-sight radio propagation. It can be expressed as a random variable subject to an exponential distribution. Because the Internet of things used in colleges and universities are non-line-of-sight environment. Therefore, the statistics of the signal propagation time are expressed by the actual distance between nodes, and there are:

$$A\left[t_N^n\right] = nt_1^n d^n a^{\frac{n^2\delta}{2}} \tag{2}$$

where d represents the actual distance between nodes. t_1^n is the median of signal propagation time. n^2 represents the exponent of 0.5–1. δ is the calculated Gaussian random variable. Replace sample t_N^n with first order statistics. Then, the relationship between the signal arrival time and the distance between nodes in a sensor network can be expressed as:

$$t(g, g') = \frac{d(g, g')}{v} + t_1 d(g, g') a^{\frac{n^2}{2}} \tag{3}$$

$t(g, g')$ represents the signal transmission time between nodes. $d(g, g')$ represents the actual distance between nodes. v indicates the speed of the signal. The distance-based radial basis kernel function has the following form:

$$l(g, g') = f(d(g, g')) \tag{4}$$

$f(\cdot)$ represents the function defined in the target interval.

Since there are multiple nodes in the Internet of Things, the nodes have similarity. In the process of data collection and transmission, the process can be completed according to the similarity of nodes to improve the speed of information transmission. Therefore, the similarity between computable nodes provides convenience for the follow-up research, and the similarity between nodes can be calculated by the following Gaussian kernel function, specifically in the following form:

$$\begin{aligned} h(b_i, b_j) &= \exp(-o_G \|\eta(b_i) - \eta(b_j)\|^2) \\ &= \exp(-\sum_{i=1}^{n} o_G(t_{i1} - t_{j1})^2) \end{aligned} \tag{5}$$

o_G represents the adjustable function in the calculation. $\|\cdot\|$ stands for Euclidean norm. Through the above calculation process, the college students' psychological information is collected and transmitted. At the same time, according to this part of the content of the early warning information transmission process to control.

3 Design of Early Warning Methods for College Students' Mental Sub-Health

3.1 Information Analysis of College Students' Mental Subhealth

The collected psychological state information of college students is integrated into the designated database, and the original information is analyzed by association rule algorithm [6, 7]. Set $W = \{W1, W2, W3, ..., Wn\}$ as the information set or information set. Wi is a separate information, $R = \{R1, R2, R3, ..., Rn\}$ is a set of psychological features. Ri is a single psychological feature, and Ri is a subset of W.

In a rule $A' \Rightarrow B'$, A' and B' are mental feature sets. A' sets of psychological features represent the conditions under which rules are valid. The set of B' psychological features represents the result of the rule. The confidence level of the rule can be expressed by conditional probability $p(A'|B')$, based on the knowledge of probability theory:

$$confidence(A' \Rightarrow B') = p(A'|B') = \frac{p(A'B')}{p(A')} \tag{6}$$

According to this association rule, the following association rules are obtained. In a rule $A' \Rightarrow B'$, A' and B' are mental feature sets. The A' psychological feature set represents the condition of rule validity, and the B' psychological feature set represents the result of rule validity. The support of the rule can be expressed by probability $p(A'B')$, that is:

$$\sup port(A' \Rightarrow B') = p(A'B') \tag{7}$$

Through the fusion analysis of the above two laws, the promotion of the rules in application is obtained. The specific formula is as follows:

$$life(A' \Rightarrow B') = \frac{confidence(A' \Rightarrow B')}{\sup port(B')}$$

$$= \frac{p(A'B')}{p(B')} \tag{8}$$

According to the above association rules, the confidence between the original information is calculated. The original information is preprocessed and analyzed, and it is drawn as a radar chart.

3.2 Early Warning Information Arrangement of College Students' Mental Subhealth

Based on the analysis of college students' mental sub-health state information, the radar map of college students' mental health is drawn, and the students' mental state is set as 8 dimensions. The 8-dimension offset vector is defined by the coordinate difference of eight index dimensions. Then:

$$P_i = P_{\alpha i} - P_{\beta i} \tag{9}$$

Here, P_i represents the offset of goal α from the i-dimension of goal β risk assignment. $P_{\alpha i}$ is the coordinates of the i-dimension of the target α (risk assignment). $P_{\beta i}$ is the coordinates of the i-metric dimension of goal β.

The coordinate definition of eight index dimensions of individual is clear, and the coordinate average value of each individual in group is used to define the coordinate coordinate of group radar chart. The overall risk drift is a ratio of the maximum area of two objectives. Namely:

$$S = \frac{W_c}{W_d} \tag{10}$$

Among them, S is the global offset of target c from target d risk assignment. W_c is the maximum area of the radar map for target c. W_d is the maximum area of the radar diagram for target d. From this formula, it can be seen that the overall deviation of an individual from the ideal zero risk is the risk assessment level corresponding to its own maximum risk radar area [8]. Namely:

$$S_i = H_i \tag{11}$$

Among them, the definition rule of H_i takes the concept of life model of radar area as the main content.

Using this formula, the total deviation is compared with the ideal zero risk value to obtain the arithmetic average of the maximum danger radar region for each person. For example:

$$S_j = H(E_i) \tag{12}$$

Among them, $E_i = \frac{(E_1+E_2+E_3+...+E_n)}{n}$. According to this formula, the early warning and evaluation grades of college students' mental health can be obtained, as shown in Table 1.

According to this form, the early warning information of the mental sub-health state of students can be obtained. And organize it into the form of information, and transmit and distribute it according to the design content of the first part of the text.

3.3 Design Early Warning Information Transmission Scheme

It is assumed that there are N wireless sensor nodes randomly and evenly distributed in an $M * N$ square area G. The set of nodes is represented as $\Im = \{\Im_1, \Im_2, \Im_3, ..., \Im_N\}$, which has the following properties:

(1) The network is a stationary network, and the sensor nodes and data aggregation points are both stationary nodes. That is, the positions are not moving after placement.

Table 1. Early warning and evaluation grade of college students' mental health

Level	Value result	Level content
I	0–0.5	Stablize
II	0.5–0.8	More stable
III	0.8–1.2	Convergence
IV	1.0–1.2	Warn
V	1.2–2.0	Alarm

(2) The sensor node knows its location. Nodes can rely on GPS, positioning algorithms and other auxiliary facilities or algorithms to obtain specific coordinates [4, 9].

According to the above two parts and the same energy attenuation model of LEACH protocol, the early-warning information transmission network model is constructed. The details are as follows:

$$Q_i(u, h) = Q_1(u) + Q_2(u, h)$$
$$= \begin{cases} uQ_1 + u\varpi_1 h^2, h < h_0 \\ uQ_1 + u\varpi_2 h^4, h \geq h_0 \end{cases} \tag{13}$$

$$Q_{ei}(u, h) = Q_1(u) = uQ_1 \tag{14}$$

h represents the Euclidean distance between node i and node j. Q_1 represents the energy consumption of a circuit in receiving and transmitting radio waves. ϖ_1 and ϖ_2 represent the amplifier energy consumption of the free-space model and the multiplexed attenuation model, respectively. h_0 represents the constant in the calculation. u represents the number of bits a sensor node is sending and receiving data.

According to this network model, the sending cluster of early warning information is determined. When the first stage of cluster is established, the sensor node automatically generates a random number If $Z < \aleph$ ($\aleph$ indicates the threshold generated by the network), the node automatically becomes the cluster head. The size of the threshold is determined by the following formula:

$$\aleph = \begin{cases} \dfrac{k}{\left\{1 - b*\left[t \bmod \left(\frac{1}{b}\right)\right]\right\}} & j \in G' \\ 0 & else \end{cases} \tag{15}$$

Among them, b means the proportion of the selected cluster head in the whole network. t is the number of cycles in progress for the current network. G' represents a collection of all sensor nodes that have not been selected as cluster heads in the current network cycle. After the above calculation, the fusion analysis is made with the first part. The early warning information transmission scheme is drawn as shown in Fig. 1.

The information of mental sub-health state and the result of mental state evaluation were collected. According to the structure shown in Fig. 1, it transmits and warns the information in the form of early-warning information, and completes the process of early-warning. Organize the above settings. So far, based on the Internet of Things college students mental sub-health early warning method design completed.

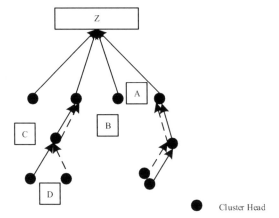

Fig. 1. Schematic Diagram of Early Warning Information Transmission for College Students'
Mental Sub-Health

4 Experiment Analysis

In this study, an early-warning method of college students' mental sub-health based
on the Internet of Things is proposed. In order to confirm the application value of this
method, the experimental link was constructed to compare the application effect of this
method with the current method.

4.1 Experimental Analysis on the Positioning Accuracy of Early Warning Nodes

In order to verify the proposed algorithm can improve the location accuracy of unknown
nodes. We use MATLAB7.0 software to do simulation experiment. Factors such as positioning accuracy are commonly used in wireless sensor networks. In this paper, the
accuracy of orientation, the accuracy of mental sub-health assessment and the transmission speed of early warning information are taken as the evaluation criteria. The
distribution of alert information nodes in this experiment is shown in Fig. 2.

As shown in Fig. 2, in the simulation experiment, the area of college students' mental
sub-health warning network is set to 50 * 50 m square area. In this region, 20 beacon
nodes and 10–20 unknown nodes are distributed evenly and randomly. Suppose the
calculated unknown node location is (x_2, y_2) and its real location is (x_1, y_1). Then the
positioning error *Error* is:

$$Error = \frac{\sqrt{(x_2 - x_1)^2 + (y_2 - y_1)^2}}{n} \tag{16}$$

n represents the number of unknown nodes in the network. In this experiment, the method,
basic method and artificial intelligence method are used to locate the receiving node of
early warning information. The positioning accuracy of different methods is compared
and the results are shown in Fig. 3.

Compared with the above experimental results, it can be seen that the positioning
accuracy of early warning information node is relatively high. In the process of early

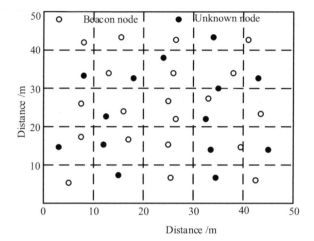

Fig. 2. Early warning network of mental sub-health state of college students

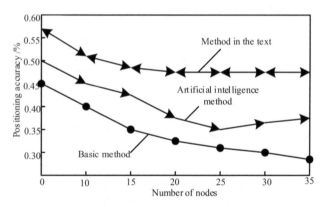

Fig. 3. Experiment results of early warning node positioning accuracy

warning information transmission, the transmission route of early warning information can be determined in the shortest time to improve the transmission speed of early warning information. Compared with the proposed method, the positioning accuracy of the basic method and the artificial intelligence method is relatively low. The results of this experiment may affect the transmission of early warning information. Therefore, the node location performance of these two methods needs to be optimized.

4.2 An Experimental Analysis on the Accuracy of Grades for Assessing Students' Mental Sub-Health State

In this experiment, 20 college students were selected as the experimental subjects, and experts in related fields were invited to evaluate the psychological sub-health status of their students after obtaining this behavioral information. The specific results are shown in Table 2.

Table 2. Student's mental sub-health state assessment results

Student number	Mental health rating	Student number	Mental health rating
D01	I	D11	III
D02	II	D12	IV
D03	I	D13	II
D04	I	D14	V
D05	I	D15	I
D06	IV	D16	II
D07	V	D17	V
D08	III	D18	II
D09	I	D19	III
D10	II	D20	IV

Using the contents of Table 2 as the control group, the mental health ratings of the subjects were evaluated by the above methods and other two methods. The accuracy of mental sub-health assessment was determined by three methods. The experimental results are shown in Table 3.

Table 3. Experimental Results of the Accuracy of Mental Sub-health Assessment of Students (unit: %)

Student number	Method in the text	Basic method	Artificial intelligence approach	Student number	Method in the text	Basic method	Artificial intelligence approach
D01	95.86	93.24	94.49	D11	95.46	94.86	94.67
D02	96.72	93.25	94.85	D12	96.08	94.21	94.18
D03	95.68	94.48	94.61	D13	96.15	94.84	94.03
D04	96.16	94.75	94.56	D14	96.61	94.01	94.52
D05	96.66	94.75	94.81	D15	96.61	93.18	94.79
D06	95.09	94.69	94.26	D16	95.42	94.17	94.91
D07	96.57	94.35	94.14	D17	96.26	94.23	94.35
D08	96.69	94.81	94.96	D18	95.26	93.46	94.65
D09	95.77	94.7	94.33	D19	96.85	94.23	94.22
D10	96.49	94.04	94.36	D20	95.55	93.58	94.58

Through the analysis of the contents in Table 3, it can be seen that the mental sub-health status of the students in the method is more accurate. The evaluation results are more close to the expert evaluation results. Using this part of information can achieve high precision early warning. Compared with the other two methods, the accuracy of mental sub-health assessment is relatively poor. In the process of early warning, some teachers and departments can not get the real warning information of students' mental sub-health and can not guide students in time. On the basis of collecting the mental health information of college students, the original psychological information is analyzed by using the association rule algorithm. The level of mental health warning of college students is evaluated by radar map, thus improving the accuracy of mental health warning.

4.3 Experimental Analysis on Transmission Speed of Early Warning Information

In order to ascertain the early warning information of mental sub-health state of college students, the information used in the experiment was sorted out. This part of the information is used to complete the experiment of early warning information transmission

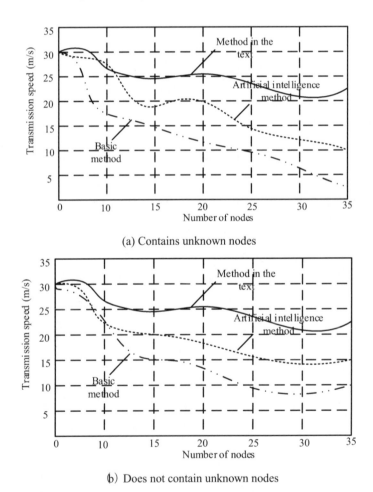

(a) Contains unknown nodes

(b) Does not contain unknown nodes

Fig. 4. Experiment results of early warning information transmission speed

speed. During this experiment, we set the environment to contain unknown nodes and not unknown nodes. The result is shown in Fig. 4.

Analysis of the experimental results in Fig. 4 shows that when there are unknown nodes in the early- warning network, the transmission speed of early- warning information is different from other two methods. The data transmission speed of this method is better than other two methods. When there are no unknown nodes in the early- warning network, the difference of transmission speed of early-warning information between the proposed method and the other two methods is obviously reduced. Under the two experimental conditions, the transmission speed of early warning information is better than that of other two methods. Because this paper method uses sensors to build the information collected by the university Internet of Things network. According to the operation requirements of IOT, the early warning information transmission scheme is designed to improve the speed of information transmission.

5 Discussion

In order to establish the psychological early-warning mechanism, we should first establish the psychological early-warning information network and organize the existing resources in a certain way. Through this system, we can get the information about the psychological state of college students in time, process the information quickly, and respond effectively when necessary. In response to this requirement, in this study proposed based on the Internet of Things college students mental sub-health early warning methods. The main contents of this study are as follows:

(1) Because the source of students' psychological data is divided into several systems, the structure of the source database is analyzed, and a large number of data are sorted out and integrated. This makes it easier to do data mining analysis and makes it possible to analyze high-quality psychological information.

(2) This paper presents localization algorithm based on kernel local preserving mapping and localization algorithm based on gene expression programming. The feasibility of the two algorithms is analyzed, and the principle and steps of the two algorithms are introduced. The reliability of the algorithm is proved by MATLAB simulation.

On the basis of this study, the future research direction is prospected. As a systematic project, college students' mental health management has the characteristics of organic, dynamic and sustainable development. With the development of mental health management to a higher level, we should deepen the research of dynamic intelligent early warning system based on continuous monitoring time variable. The research and service objects should be shifted from focusing on college students to providing quality health management services for all citizens.

6 Conclusion

Aiming at the problems of poor accuracy and poor transmission speed in the early warning of college students' mental sub-health, this paper puts forward a method based on Internet of Things. In the future research, how to maintain the positioning accuracy while reducing the amount of node positioning computation will be discussed. How to determine the optimal control parameters through the influence of genetic control parameters on the positioning accuracy is studied further.

References

1. Nie, M., Luo, W., Deng, H., et al.: Research on the influence of college students' mental health on their social network structure. J. Univ. Electron. Sci. Technol. China **50**(2), 317–320 (2021)
2. Hemavathi, S., Latha, P., Athavale, V.A., et al.: Understanding suicidal behavior by using longitudinal electronic health records system. System **6**(4), 5048–5061 (2022)
3. Zheng, S., Zeng, W., Xin, Q., et al.: Can cognition help predict suicide risk in patients with major depressive disorder? a machine learning study. BMC Psychiatry **22**(1), 1–13 (2022)
4. Shickel, B., Siegel, S., Heesacker, M., et al.: Automatic detection and classification of cognitive distortions in mental health text. In: 2020 IEEE 20th International Conference on Bioinformatics and Bioengineering (BIBE), pp. 275–280. IEEE (2020)
5. Zheng, L., Wang, O., Hao, S., et al.: Development of an early-warning system for high-risk patients for suicide attempt using deep learning and electronic health records. Transl. Psychiatry **10**(1), 1–10 (2020)
6. Ye, W., Su, C., Luo, M., et al.: Transmission line defect state prediction based on association rule mining. Power Syst. Prot. Control **49**(20), 104–111 (2021)
7. Wang, Y., Chen, H., Zhao, H., et al.: Matching networking method for carrier communication of distribution Internet of Things under network mode. Electric Power Autom. Equip. **41**(6), 59–65, 80 (2021)
8. Olthof, M., Hasselman, F., Strunk, G., et al.: Critical fluctuations as an early-warning signal for sudden gains and losses in patients receiving psychotherapy for mood disorders. Clin. Psychol. Sci. **8**(1), 25–35 (2020)
9. Shi, X., Zhao, Z..: Dynamic coordinate transformation algorithm of mobile internet of things load terminal. Comput. Simul. **38**(1), 247–250, 260 (2021)

Automatic Assessment Method of College Students Psychological Stress Based on Medical Big Data

Xiang Li[✉]

Jingchu University of Technology Normal University, Jingmen 448000, Hubei, China
qihang7895@126.com

Abstract. Students' psychological stress assessment has become an important part of college mental health management, but the current assessment methods are qualitative analysis, combined with the scale to get the assessment results. The lack of data support in the evaluation process leads to large evaluation errors. In view of the above practical problems, this paper studies the automatic evaluation method of college students' psychological stress based on medical big data. After using crawlers to obtain medical big data, it was preprocessed. Taking physiological data as the evaluation index of psychological stress, the relationship between physiological indexes and psychological stress is obtained by data mining. The HMM model improved by SVM is used to quantify the evaluation results. After testing, the relative error of the evaluation method based on medical big data is less than 10%, and the evaluation accuracy is higher.

Keywords: Medical Big Data · College Students' Psychology · Psychological Stress · Evaluation Methods

1 Introduction

The acceleration of globalization, the rapid development of information and the openness of information increase the psychological pressure of college students. Academic, social relations, employment and other kinds of pressure on college students exhausted. When people encounter stressful events in their lives, there is a sense of stress. Psychological stress is a kind of psychological stress reaction when people face difficult situations [1]. College students also face more stressful events in complex environments. Stress and other psychological factors can affect physical health, leading to poor occupational health and insomnia, anxiety, mild depression and other physical and mental disorders. Studies have shown that appropriate levels of pressure can motivate people to progress and reach their potential. For students, proper pressure can improve their learning efficiency and benefit their growth and development. However, excessive psychological pressure may bring students physical and psychological pain. When people do not know how to deal with this kind of pressure, there will be a variety of negative emotions. Students can not solve the psychological pressure when prone to psychological problems,

S. Wang (Ed.): IoTCare 2022, LNICST 501, pp. 61–72, 2023.
https://doi.org/10.1007/978-3-031-33545-7_5

leading to accidents. Psychological stress is a more obscure topic, many students may not even notice their own situation has been very serious or deliberately ignored it. Even if students are in a state of abnormal psychological stress, because of the convergence of character rarely find others to express, which caused the school to monitor students' psychological stress. College students' mental health has become the most concerned problem in colleges and universities. Effective ways are needed to regulate students' psychological pressure and negative emotions.

Students with different levels of psychological stress can choose different ways of adjustment. Therefore, evaluating students' psychological stress is the basis of dealing with college students' psychological problems. In recent years, there are many researches on mental health of college students, but few researches on mental stress assessment of college students. The traditional psychological stress assessment scheme is mainly realized by questionnaire and manual interaction. Psychological stress was assessed by daily or multiple questionnaires and manual interviews over a period of time, and by questionnaires and wearable equipment. This approach usually requires a relatively long period of time for data collection and works only for some of the students involved in the survey [2]. Using the recorded information to predict, do not need to re-operate each survey, and after the model is built, can be extended to all students with similar records, adaptable. But choosing the right features and the right models will greatly affect the assessment [3].

With the progress of the times, the problem of psychological stress of college students has attracted people's attention more and more obviously, and it has entered the public's field of vision. It belongs to the important and practical field of the branch of educational data mining. Traditional psychological stress assessment programs are mainly realized through questionnaires and human interaction. Some use daily or multiple questionnaires and manual interviews for a period of time to assess students' psychological pressure, and some use questionnaires and wearable devices. To assess the psychological stress of students, this method usually requires a relatively long period of time to collect data, and it is only effective for some students who participated in the survey. Under the background of big data era, with the development of health care and intelligent medical care, medical information is growing exponentially every day. These accumulated medical big data contain rich information and inestimable value. With the development of key technologies such as distributed storage and distributed computing, it is easy to solve the difficult problems in traditional data warehouse. Compared with questionnaire survey data, medical big data is more objective and accurate, because it records students' real medical feedback information and diagnosis and treatment behavior. According to the above analysis, this paper will study the automatic evaluation method of college students' psychological stress based on medical big data. Use crawler technology to crawl medical data related to psychology. The medical data is then preprocessed. Through data mining technology, the relationship between physiological data and psychological stress scale was established. On this basis, automatic evaluation of psychological stress of college students is carried out. Through the big data analysis technology, the paper quantitatively evaluates the psychological stress of college students, and provides empirical data support and reference.

2   Medical Big Data Acquisition and Analysis Processing

2.1   Crawlers Acquire Medical Big Data

The rapid development of medical information industry has given birth to a considerable scale of medical platform. These medical platforms are dedicated to provide convenient medical services for ordinary users, while facilitating access to medical resources, but also accumulated a large. The medical data of college students in psychological counseling or other medical behaviors are mixed with the medical data of different groups, which affects the efficiency of follow-up analysis. Therefore, crawlers were used to crawl medical data related to college students' psychological stress assessment.

Map/Reduce is used to construct intelligent web crawler for medical big data. The crawler for medical big data includes crawler strategy design, middleware design and data storage design. The design of crawler strategy mainly involves how to parse and extract web page information, incremental crawling data and data deduplication, etc. (mainly using Redis database to select efficient mode to assign captured URL through custom module. According to the priority of crawling data and ensuring the consistency of crawling order, the crawling URL order strategy is configured. The part of middleware design mainly deals with the anti-crawler setting based on Scrapy crawler framework and the design of appropriate proxy pool for IP real-time replacement [4].

Due to the wide availability of medical big data. This study uses the distributed master-slave crawler architecture shown in Fig. 1 below to obtain medical big data of college students.

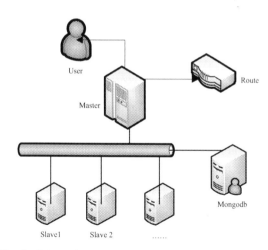

Fig. 1. Schematic diagram of distributed crawler framework

As a host, Master is responsible for scheduling crawler tasks and managing cluster resources. It also assigns crawler requests to RPC communication between Slave processing and master-slave machines for real-time monitoring of crawler tasks. Each of these Slave receives a crawler task assigned by the Master and processes the task only on its own node, storing the results in the MongoDB database. The Redis database stores the status of the crawl URL queue, which is fetched from the cache by the host and slave. The second stage mainly includes deciding whether to crawl the page. If the task is not crawled directly into Hbase for parsing, crawl the content of the page for content parsing. At the same time, the output of the parsed content is saved, and it is optional whether the parsed results should generate the next level of tasks [5]. The third stage is to store the output data, and the source data crawled after parsing the content will be stored in the mongodb database, Hbase database, and test according to different requirements. Where test is custom and optional to test the accuracy of the data.

The complete process for crawlers to obtain data on college students' psychological stress is shown in Fig. 2.

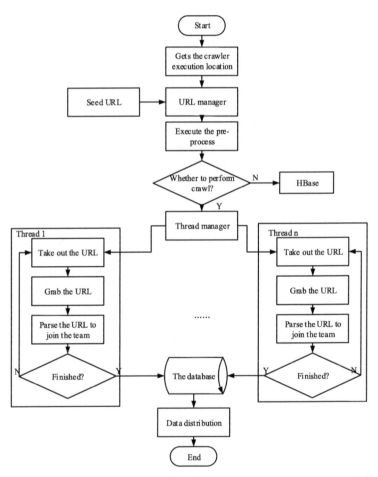

Fig. 2. Obtaining the crawler process of college students' psychological stress medical big data

Task start execution to get crawler execution configured as the first phase. This phase is the crawler task generation phase. This phase implies a timed task module that pre-generates crawler tasks based on the crawler configuration. In order to avoid the web crawler from falling into the web trap, the authoritative web pages related to medical subjects are selected as part of the seed set.

This design uses Bayesian algorithm to identify crawler crawling objects Web pages. To identify whether the text on the Web page contains medical data related to psychological stress assessment of students. Calculate Bayesian probabilities for uncategorized texts based on setting up texts for medical big data related words [6].

$$P(L_i|w) = \frac{P(w|L_i) * P(L_i)}{\sum\limits_{i=1}^{n} P(w|L_i) * P(L_i)} \tag{1}$$

In the above expression, $P(L_i|w)$ indicates the probability that the document belongs to category L_i, determined by the matching of its words with vector pattern w. Posterior probability $P(L_i|w)$ is obtained by prior probability $P(L_i)$ and conditional probability $P(w|L_i)$. By finding the maximum value of $P(L_i|w)$, you can know the classification of web pages, namely:

$$F(w) = \arg\min_{L_i \in L} P(L_i|w) \tag{2}$$

It is assumed that the medical big data texts used for classification are independent of each other. Follow the process above to categorize the URLs. According to the maximum classification results, after identifying the target web, the crawler crawls the corresponding web page. Web crawlers crawl files in a variety of formats, including Word, PDF, Excel, and so on, and the corresponding Jar packages in Java provide interfaces for processing these files. Web crawlers need to call the corresponding file parsing module based on the file extension to parse these binaries. Then the index program is used to index the analyzed web page information, and the index database is established. Finally, for user search.

2.2 Medical Big Data Preprocessing

When preparing data, be fully aware that real data is susceptible to interference, loss, and inconsistency. So the first thing to do when you get a data source is to preprocess the data to make it a high-quality data mining source. The primary function of data preprocessing is to transform raw data into a data format that can be entered into the model. It includes data cleaning, data integration, data specification and data transformation.

In medical big data processing, we often meet the problem of imbalance of positive and negative labels. If we do not deal with it, we will get a defective evaluation model. The main algorithms for dealing with imbalanced datasets are as follows: (1) Adjust the threshold value to make more samples become samples with fewer categories. (2) Cost-sensitive learning makes the category training with fewer samples get higher weight, which makes the punishment for wrong judgment greater. (3) Oversampling, copying more small categories of samples and equalizing the overall sample ratio. (4) Undersampling reduces the number of samples with a large number of categories, resulting in a balanced ratio of the overall sample. (4) Data synthesis (SMOTE), i.e., synthetic minority over-sampling technology. The algorithm will feature a small number of samples and artificially synthesize new samples to add to the dataset [7].

The value interval of data is normalized, and the projection space [0, 1] is generally taken as the projection space. Therefore, the weights of different ordinal variables are unified so as to facilitate the calculation of similarity and clustering operation. For the acquired software running dataset, the normalized formula for its data mapping is as follows:

$$S_{R-D} = \frac{R_D - 1}{\max R - 1} \tag{3}$$

In the above expression, R_D is the data whose ordinal variable attribute is k. $\max R$ is the maximum value for the data map. In order to adapt to the range of the degree of variability of different types of variables, it is necessary to transform the degree of variability of different types of data. Make their values map to the same interval [0, 1].

The LOF algorithm is used to detect outliers in the data to reduce the impact on subsequent analysis. The neighborhood point set $l_k(p)$ of data point p is the accessible distance from all points to p. Rather than the accessible distance of all points p to $l_k(p)$. The lower the data point density in the neighborhood of data point p, the more likely it is an outlier. Conversely, the higher the density, the more likely it is that the points belong to the same cluster. If the data point p and the surrounding neighbor point density is more sparse. Then the accessible distance of the point has a large probability to take a larger value, resulting in a smaller data point density in the neighborhood of data point p. If the data points p and surrounding neighborhood points are more dense. Then the accessible distance may be a smaller distance, and the density of data points in the set of data points p is higher [8].

$$LOF(p, o)_k = \frac{\sum_{q=1}^{N} q l_k(p) l_k(o)}{|l_k(p)|} \tag{4}$$

In the above formula, o is the data point in the neighbor point set $l_k(p)$ of the data point p. $l_k(o)$ is the maximum distance from the data point p in the domain set. If the value calculated by the above formula is closer to 1. Then it means that the density of point p and its neighbor set $l_k(p)$ is similar, and the more likely this point is a normal point.

3   Analysis on the Evaluation Index of College Students' Psychological Stress

College students will encounter various pressures in their daily life. When these pressures accumulate to a certain extent, it will affect students' life satisfaction level. These external pressures are objective factors, as well as subjective factors that affect an individual's attitude towards and satisfaction with life. External stressors have a direct effect on individual mental health and life satisfaction. When the individual psychological stress is too high, it will lead to changes in their physiological data. Therefore, this paper takes the physiological indexes in the big data of medical treatment as the evaluation basis, and gets more accurate evaluation results by quantification.

EEG signals are closely related to physiological and psychological information related to various parts of the body. In general, the excitation process of EEG signals increases significantly when the slow wave with high amplitude changes to the fast wave with low amplitude. Conversely, suppression occurs when a low amplitude fast wave becomes a high amplitude slow wave. When neurons in the brain are active, they exhibit nonlinear dynamics. Therefore, nonlinear dynamic analysis methods such as complexity, psychological stress index and maximum Lyapunov index (LLE) are combined. They can accurately analyze the nonlinear dynamic characteristics of EEG signals.

KC complexity is a coarse grained nonlinear dynamic method. It can judge the random degree of the sequence. When there are enough sampled data, the mean of KC complexity tends to 0 in periodic sequence and 1 in random sequence. In other sequences between 0 and 1 [9].

Let EEG sequence be $R = \{r_1, r_2, \ldots, r_n\}$. The new sequences are $R' = \{r'_1, r'_2, \ldots, r'_n\}$ and $R'' = \{r'_{m+1}, r'_{m+2}, \ldots, r'_{m+i}\}$. The KC complexity calculation steps are as follows.

(a) The sequence R' is further constructed from the sequence R, and a value greater than the average value of sequence R is replaced by 1, otherwise 0. To get the new sequence R', and then add a string of characters after the sequence R''.

(b) Compute subsequence $R'R''$ according to the sequences R' and R'' obtained from step (a). If sequence $R'' \in R'R''$, copy the sequence after R' and repeat the calculation. Otherwise, insert a "*" after $R'R''$, and repeat the process until the end of the sequence to get a new sequence.

The formula for obtaining the KC complexity from the sequence constructed by steps (a) and (b) is as follows:

$$v = \frac{R''(n)}{R'R''(n)} \tag{5}$$

The energy of EEG signals δ, θ, α, β and γ varies with the fluctuation of brain states. Therefore, this paper combines the characteristics of psychological stress in human physiological data. Based on Hilbert's marginal spectral energy, psychological stress index is defined. The calculation expression is as follows:

$$P = \frac{E\delta + E\theta}{E\alpha + E\beta} \tag{6}$$

Among them, E is the marginal spectral energy corresponding to four kinds of rhythms.

When the human body receives certain outside stimulation, will have the psychological tension or the nerve excited phenomenon, causes human body's heart to relax and the contraction speed to speed up, the heart rate will also increase accordingly. The spectral peak recognition curve calculated by the autoregressive model of heart rate variability is accurate and has high power spectral resolution. By reading the data on the spectral estimation curve, the corresponding interval of heart rate can be determined.

Respiration rate RR is calculated by means of the mean value between the peak periods of the respiration wave. Blood oxygen saturation is one of the important indexes to measure the oxygen content in human blood. Blood oxygen saturation is the amount of oxygenated hemoglobin in the blood as a percentage of the total binding hemoglobin volume. The above physiological indexes are used as the specific quantitative criteria to evaluate students' psychological stress. The relationship between physiological data and psychological stress scale was established by data mining.

4   Medical Big Data Mining

Medical big data has the characteristics of high-dimensional data. In order to simplify the processing process, a global algorithm model is used to reduce the dimensionality of the data. Given a dataset X consisting of n samples and m features. It is known that it contains C modes, and the label information B of X is known. The data is dimensionally reduced according to the principle of mutual information.

$$D = \arg\max_d \left\{ \frac{1}{|D|} \sum_{x_i \in D}^{n} I(x_i; b) - \frac{1}{|D|^2} \sum_{x_i, x_j \in D}^{n} I(x_i; x_j) \right\} \tag{7}$$

In the above formula, D is the feature selection target. Mutual information is a symmetric metric, that is, the information quantity of feature B obtained by observing feature X is equal to the information quantity of feature X obtained by observing variable $I(X; B) \equiv I(B; X)$.

This symmetry is a good attribute in feature selection. But mutual information tends to have more values. When X or B has more values, the results calculated by mutual information show that the probability of their correlation is very high. So if you compute the mutual information of the features corresponding to many tags, you can easily get a very large value [10].

Symmetric uncertainties are used to compensate for the bias of mutual information to features with more values. In order to measure the identification of feature X to tag B, the correlation evaluation matrix $V = \{DU(x_i, b_i)\}$ is constructed by using the symmetric uncertainty of feature and tag. The value of $V = \{DU(x_i, b_i)\}$ ranges between [0, 1].

The larger the value is, the more important the relevance between the representation features and the classification tasks is. Feature redundancy evaluation matrix V^* is constructed by using symmetric uncertainty between features. Combining the above evaluation matrices V and V^* to maximize the feature correlation. At the same time, the feature redundancy is minimized and the objective function is constructed as follows.

$$f = \min_W \left\{ W^T V^* W - W^T V \right\} \tag{8}$$

The process of optimizing the above objective function is mapping medical big data from high dimensional space to low dimensional space. After dimensionality reduction, k-means clustering algorithm is used to mine the relationship between data and psychological stress.

Set the densest point to the first initial cluster center point Go through it, calculate the distance from each point d_i of $C1$ in the high density region, calculate the distance between them. Set the point farthest from $C1$ as the second initial cluster center point

C2. Taking these two points as the center, two clusters are generated according to the distance between the center and other points, and the cluster centroid c_1, c_2. Find the furthest point from the two clustering centers in the high density domain. This paper sets it as the third initial clustering center point. The formula is as follows:

$$J_i = j(d_i, c_1) + j(d_i, c_2) \tag{9}$$

Among them, c_1 and c_2 represent respectively the center of mass with $C1$ and $C2$. The distance c_1 and c_2 farthest point is chosen as the third cluster center point $C3$. $j(d_i, c_i)$ is the Euclidean distance from the cluster center. Repeat the process until the number of initial cluster centers is equal to the number of predefined clusters to get the corresponding initial cluster centers. According to the process of k-means clustering algorithm, medical big data are clustered.

The following intra-cluster variation is used to evaluate the quality of clustering results.

$$e = \sum_{i=1}^{k} \sum dist\left(d_j, ce_i\right)^2 \tag{10}$$

In the above expression, e is the mean distance difference within the cluster. $dist$ is the square of Euclidean distance between clustering centers. ce_i is the cluster center. d_j is medical big data to be mined. Through cluster analysis, the data relationship between medical big data and college students' psychological stress was established. In this paper, the relational features are used as the classification basis, and the HMM model is used to analyze the data to obtain the results of psychological stress assessment.

5   Realize the Psychological Stress Assessment of College Students

This paper uses SVM algorithm to improve HMM model. In the model of college students' psychological stress assessment, SVM chooses "one-to-many" strategy, and HMM chooses continuous strategy. The input parameters in the model are dominant, which represent the probabilistic vector sequence of physiological parameters after SVM, and the output pressure emotion sequence is hidden. On this basis, the stress emotion is classified to improve the accuracy of stress emotion classification.

The training process of HMM emotion model based on SVM to optimize feature parameters is as follows:

(1) SVM training: Take the optimized feature vector sequence as the input vector of this step, rain three SVM, write down three labels, describe as A, B, C. Respectively extract A corresponding vector is positive, B, C corresponding vector is negative. B is positive and A and C is negative. C is positive, B is negative. All the samples belonging to this category are input into three SVM and the output probabilities are calculated respectively to get three probabilities.

(2) HMM training: This step involves training three HMM models $HMM = (\pi, A, B)$. Each class corresponds to a model, and the training data is three output probabilities in the previous step, that is, the output of each class is a vector (g_1, g_2, g_3). This

is done for all training samples and the vector sequence is obtained. The model parameters are then randomly initialized. BW algorithm is used to calculate the parameters of the model, and stable π, A and B are obtained, which are parametric models related to college students' psychological stress.

HMM emotion model improved by SVM is used to identify the optimized feature parameters. The corresponding parameters of SVM and HMM model are obtained after training stage. First, we input SVM to get the sequence of probabilities, then input three HMMs. The observation probability matrix of the model is estimated by using the piecewise K-means principle. After selecting the best observation probability matrix, Baum-Welch is used to reevaluate the parameters in the model and judge whether the model converges. If the model parameter is convergent, the model under the parameter is used for flutter identification, otherwise, the process is repeated until the best parameter is determined. After HMM calculation, the results of psychological stress assessment were obtained. So far, we have completed the research on the automatic assessment of college students' psychological stress based on medical big data.

6 Test Study

Above proposed based on the medical big data university student psychology pressure automatic assessment method. In order to judge the practical application value of this method, the performance of this method will be tested with data set.

6.1 Test Content

Under the same condition, the evaluation method is compared with the evaluation method based on neural network and the evaluation method based on AHP. The assessment test was carried out in A university, and the physiological data of the whole students were collected to establish a large medical database. A total of 900 students were randomly divided into 300 groups to investigate the psychological stress of all the students objectively and quantitatively. The objective investigation results are used as reference, the evaluation results of the three methods are compared with the quantized data, and the evaluation error of the method is obtained. The accuracy of evaluation is judged by analyzing the error of evaluation.

6.2 Test Result

Table 1 below is the statistical results of relative error of psychological stress assessment for students in A university by using three psychological stress assessment methods. Each group of 30 people was used to calculate the mean value of relative error in the group, and the results were compared.

Analyzing the data in Table 1, we can see that the relative error of the whole method is less than 10% when we evaluate the psychological stress of randomly grouped students. But the relative error of AHP based psychological stress assessment method fluctuates between 22–36%. The relative error of the method based on neural network fluctuates

Table 1 Comparison of relative errors of psychological stress assessment methods/%

Group	Psychological stress assessment method in this paper	Psychological stress assessment method based on neural network	Psychological stress assessment method based on AHP
1	7.46	21.31	24.38
2	9.15	20.02	23.72
3	7.23	16.24	23.20
4	5.96	19.63	33.84
5	6.58	14.46	35.55
6	9.72	20.47	23.39
7	9.07	21.59	23.27
8	8.41	15.60	25.62
9	8.74	15.28	30.58
10	9.39	15.05	29.93

between 14% and 23%. It shows that the evaluation result of this method is more close to the objective evaluation result and the evaluation result is more reliable.

To further validate the method assessing the performance of psychological stress in college students. Here, the F1 value is used as the experimental index, and the comparative experimental results are shown in Fig. 3.

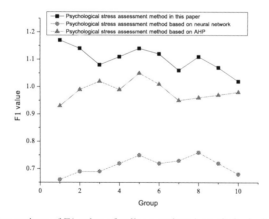

Fig. 3. Comparison of F1 value of college students' psychological assessment

From Fig. 3, the F1 value of this method is higher than the other two methods, on average, higher than 1.0. To sum up, this paper puts forward a method of college students' psychological stress automatic assessment based on medical big data, which can simplify the assessment process. And the use of big data analysis and other theories to improve the accuracy of psychological stress assessment.

7 Conclusion

The psychological pressure of students themselves is increasing, which seriously affects the normal study and life. This paper studies the automatic evaluation method of college students' psychological stress based on medical big data. First, the crawler technology was used to crawl psychologically related medical data. Then pre-process the medical data. Normalize the value interval of the data, and generally take the projection space [0, 1] as the projection space. Physiological indicators are used as specific quantitative standards to evaluate students' psychological stress state. Through data mining, the relationship between physiological data and psychological stress scale was established. So far, the automatic assessment of college students' psychological stress has been realized. Compared with other evaluation methods, the results of the proposed method are closer to the real results, and the evaluation accuracy is higher. Using this method to evaluate the psychological stress of college students can help tutors identify students who need more attention, reduce workload, and detect abnormal students early.

References

1. Li, C.: College graduate employment under the impact of COVID-19: employment pressure, psychological stress and employment choices. Educ. Res. **41**(07), 4–16 (2020)
2. Kalra, P., Sharma, V.: Mental stress assessment using PPG signal a deep neural network approach. IETE J. Res., 1–7 (2020)
3. Sun, Y., Yang, J.: Assessment of psychological pressure based on BSTL and XGDT. J. Quant. Econ. **37**(04), 148–158 (2020)
4. Yue, G.-x., Liu, J.-h., Liu, F.: Medical big data filling and classification simulation based on decision tree algorithm. Comput. Simul. **38**(01), 451–454+459 (2021)
5. Ding, Y., Chen, X., Fu, Q., et al.: A depression recognition method for college students using deep integrated support vector algorithm. IEEE Access **8**, 75616–75629 (2020)
6. Zhang, S., Ji, X.-Q., Yang, G., et al.: Research on the method of evaluating psychological stress by combination of ECG and EEG. J. Changchun Univ. Sci. Technol. **43**(02), 127–134 (2020)
7. Jia, J.: A study on the psychological pressure sources of college students and the countermeasures of psychological intervention. J. Pingdingshan Univ. **36**(06), 119–123 (2021)
8. Jin, X., Zhang, L.: Research on employment psychological pressure and coping ability improvement of college graduates from the perspective of psychological resilience. J. Qiannan Normal Univ. Nationalities **41**(04), 86–90 (2021)
9. Parthiban, K., Pandey, D., Pandey, B.K.: Impact of SARS-CoV-2 in online education, predicting and contrasting mental stress of young students: a machine learning approach. Augmented Hum. Res. **6**(1), 1–7 (2021)
10. Chenghui, B., Xinyu, W., Wenxin, G., et al.: Investigation and analysis of psychological stress of clinical medical degree postgraduates. China Continuing Med. Educ. **14**(09), 102–106 (2022)

Research on Medical Sensitive Data Protection Algorithm Based on Differential Privacy

Xiaofeng Li[1], Zhongwei Chen[1(✉)], and Zhichang Huang[2]

[1] College of Information Engineering, Guangxi University of Foreign Languages, Nanning 530222, China
top00112233@163.com
[2] Information Engineering College, Nanning University, Nanning 530200, China

Abstract. In order to avoid the wrong transmission behavior of medical data and realize the effective protection of sensitive information samples, the protection algorithm of medical sensitive data based on differential privacy is studied. According to the application principles of Laplace mechanism and index mechanism, a query control model is constructed, and then the analysis of differential privacy protection technology for medical sensitive data is realized by solving the security trust index. Based on the R-tree clustering structure, according to the sensitivity index calculation results, the search and processing of sensitive objects are completed, and the design of medical sensitive data protection algorithm based on differential privacy is completed. The experimental results show that under the effect of the principle of differential privacy, the error transmission probability of medical sensitive data will never be higher than 10%. It has strong application feasibility in solving the problem of medical data error transmission and effectively protecting sensitive information samples.

Keywords: Differential Privacy · Medical Sensitive Data · Data Protection · Query Control Model · Safety Trust Index · R-Tree Clustering Structure

1 Introduction

Since the birth and development of the Internet, it has greatly facilitated the lives of the masses. People can make mobile payments, e-shopping and surf the Internet through the Internet, but at the same time, more traces are left on the Internet. Under the circumstance of protection, relevant information will be collected and used by criminals, resulting in property damage and even life safety threats. With the development and progress of the times, various attack methods are emerging one after another. Although the traditional privacy protection technology has guaranteed sufficient protection to a certain level, it is unable to defend against background knowledge attacks. Differential privacy technology can not only analyze the data from big data to obtain effective information with unchanged statistical properties, but also protect the privacy information of users at the cost of certain loss of performance, regardless of the background attack.

© ICST Institute for Computer Sciences, Social Informatics and Telecommunications Engineering 2023
Published by Springer Nature Switzerland AG 2023. All Rights Reserved
S. Wang (Ed.): IoTCare 2022, LNICST 501, pp. 73–87, 2023.
https://doi.org/10.1007/978-3-031-33545-7_6

Through the technical disturbance and distortion of data, the balance between the effectiveness of data analysis and privacy protection is achieved [1]. With the rapid development of medical diagnostic technologies such as medical information systems and high-throughput sequencing, the medical and health field is gradually entering the "big data era". Medical big data includes basic data such as residents' behavioral health, electronic medical records, diagnosis and treatment data, detection reports, medical images, medical management, economic data, etc. It is characterized by large scale, rapid growth, diversified structure, and high application value. Therefore, medical sensitive data needs to be protected.

Reference [2] proposed a sensitive data protection algorithm based on sharding. This algorithm perturbs the data based on the idea of dynamic sharding, and completes the adjustment of data cluster size and sharded data. The isolated nodes are integrated into a set to avoid data interference. Reference [3] proposed a sensitive data protection algorithm based on Bayesian network. This algorithm uses clustering method to discretize data, and uses Bayesian model to protect data privacy. Although the above methods can complete the protection of sensitive data, there is a problem of low security factor, which makes the data easy to be stolen, intruded or tampered.

In order to improve the security of medical sensitive data, this research proposes a medical sensitive data protection algorithm based on differential privacy.

2   Differential Privacy Protection Technology for Medical Sensitive Data

The protection of medical sensitive data is based on differential privacy application technology. This chapter will study the practical methods of differential privacy protection technology from three aspects: Laplace mechanism and index mechanism, query control model, and security trust index.

2.1   Laplace Mechanism and Index Mechanism

The method of realizing the privacy protection of medical sensitive data in differential privacy protection is called "implementation mechanism". Laplace mechanism and index mechanism are the two most basic implementation mechanisms of differential privacy protection. Laplace mechanism is mainly used to protect numerical medical sensitive information results, and exponential mechanism is mainly used to protect non numerical data results, similar to geometric mechanism and Gaussian mechanism. Different noise mechanisms are suitable for different occasions, which are closely related to function sensitivity and privacy budget parameters, and provide differential privacy protection for different types of data.

Laplace Mechanism
The main method of Laplace mechanism to achieve differential privacy protection is to add random noise obeying Laplace distribution to the returned result of medical sensitive data query, so that the returned result after adding noise satisfies the differential privacy

protection constraint in formula (1).

$$
Q = \frac{1}{\chi}
\begin{cases}
\exp\left(-\dfrac{e_1 - e_2}{\dot{W}}\right), & e_2 < e_1 \\[2ex]
\exp\left(-\dfrac{e_2 - e_1}{\dot{W}}\right), & e_2 \geq e_1
\end{cases}
\tag{1}
$$

where, e_1 represents the location parameter of medical sensitive data, e_2 represents the scale parameter, $\dot{W}$ represents the sensitive eigenvalue of medical data, and χ represents the negative feedback vector.

For a given dataset $\Im$, there is a query function R, and its mean sensitivity is $\Delta\alpha$. Simultaneous formula (1) can express the differential privacy query principle of medical sensitive data based on the Laplace mechanism as:

$$
\begin{cases}
Y_R = \Delta\alpha \cdot Q + \left[\beta\left(\dfrac{\bar{r}^2}{r_1 \times r_2}\right)\right] \\[1ex]
r_1 \in \Im \\
r_2 \in \Im
\end{cases}
\tag{2}
$$

where, r_1 represents the sensitivity marking coefficient, r_2 represents the privacy query marking coefficient, $\bar{r}$ represents the average value of coefficients r_1 and r_2, and β represents the Laplace definition index.

Regardless of whether a medically sensitive data is recorded in or not in a private dataset, adding Laplace-distributed noise to the real query results has little effect on the final query results, that is to say, the attacker's same query differs between two records that differ by only one record. The probability ratio of the same outcome on the dataset is close to 1.

Index Mechanism

The index mechanism is mainly applicable to the case where the output result is non numerical. The result calculated by directly adding noise may damage the numerical characteristics. In order to select the "best" response, the index mechanism responds to any utility query (as well as any non numerical query) by designing a scoring function, while maintaining differential privacy protection. Let δ represent privacy protection parameters, ΔI represent the unit accumulation of medical sensitive data to be queried, and $\overline{U}$ represent the mean value of query vector. With the support of the above physical quantities, the simultaneous formula (2) can define the exponential mechanism expression based on differential privacy as:

$$
Q' = \exp\left(\frac{Y_R}{\delta^2}\right) \cdot \Delta I \cdot \overline{U}
\tag{3}
$$

An exponential mechanism often provides a strong utility guarantee, as its effect decreases rapidly exponentially as the score decreases. The probability of returning an option with good availability by the index mechanism is limited by the privacy protection parameter δ. When the value of δ is large, the difference between the options is large, and the option with a higher score is more likely to be output.

2.2 Query Control Model

Considering the characteristics of query trust from two aspects: the query authority and reputation value of medical sensitive data and the privacy attribute of query data, a data hierarchical query control strategy using query trust to measure the level of the inquirer is proposed. The hierarchical query control processing is carried out on the data information stored in the data collection server combined with differential privacy protection technology, so as to provide different query users with available data with different accuracy. Differential privacy protection mechanism is widely used in privacy protection data publishing, data mining and other fields, aiming to protect individual sensitive data in the database when publishing data sharing. Define the query control model as:

$$P = \frac{\left[\phi[\hat{q}]^2 - \phi'[q']^2\right]}{\varepsilon \times Q'} \tag{4}$$

where, ϕ represents the probability of medical sensitive data privacy being disclosed, $\hat{q}$ represents the disclosed data information, ϕ' represents the probability of medical sensitive data privacy being differentially processed, q' represents the differentially processed data information, and ε represents the discrimination coefficient of data information.

In the differential privacy protection mechanism, the difference of the queryer's authority and the privacy of the query data are considered, which can effectively prevent the privacy leakage threat caused by users with different authority levels querying sensitive data. In order to achieve the purpose of publishing available data information with different data accuracy rates for different levels of query users, a data hierarchical query control model based on differential privacy protection is proposed as shown in Fig. 1. Partial composition. Among them, hierarchical query control is the most important part, mainly including data preprocessing module, hierarchical query control module and usability analysis module.

In the process of publishing and sharing medical sensitive data, different query users have different needs and purposes for the published data. If they ignore the differences between the inquirers and provide data results with the same degree of privacy protection, users with low query authority will obtain information containing more sensitive data, resulting in the chain leakage of user sensitive data; Secondly, the privacy attributes of different sensitive data information are also different, and the data owners have different requirements for the degree of privacy protection of data. Each type of data will have different privacy requirements. The existing differential privacy protection research does not fully consider the impact of query user permissions, reputation values and data privacy attributes on privacy protection, which is easy to cause query users with low permissions and reputation to obtain high availability data, and then cause the indirect disclosure of user sensitive data.

The hierarchical query control module combines differential privacy protection technology and is responsible for hierarchical control of queries. Query based on data research and use needs to consider the influence of factors such as query authority and the privacy properties of query data. The solution is to perform trust quantification analysis according to the authority, reputation value of the data queryer, and privacy

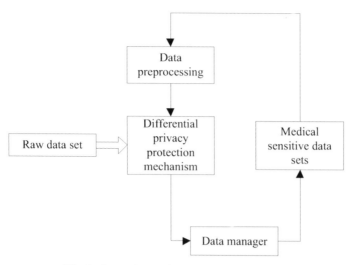

Fig. 1. Data Hierarchical Query Control Model

attributes of the data, and classify the corresponding levels to correspond to different privacy protection parameters, so as to achieve differentiated differential privacy protection effects [4]. The availability evaluation module measures the data availability after differential privacy protection processing, realizes controllable sensitive data privacy and availability protection, can effectively prevent malicious attackers from obtaining user privacy information through information query, and can greatly reduce privacy leakage. Increase the effective use of published data. Finally, the processed results are fed back to the query user.

Data asset management is to manage the data in the storage cluster according to certain rules, including data standard management, data quality detection, data operation monitoring, data resource directory, data security management and data value evaluation. Realize value realization through managed data. For example, the intelligent medical information management platform can be used for medical insurance quality control, semantic retrieval, etc., to improve medical quality. Manage the medical activities of the whole hospital through the president's cockpit, adjust the hospital resources in real time according to various reports, allocate medical resources reasonably, and solve the problem of waste of medical resources.

2.3 Calculation of Security Trust Degree

This section proposes the query security trust degree to quantify the security and trustworthiness of medical sensitive data. The query security trust degree is determined by the query subject attribute value and the query object attribute value. The larger the value, the more trustworthy. In this section, we mainly consider that the query security trust degree consists of two parts: the queryer's trust value and the data privacy attribute value. Its calculation publicity network:

$$O = \left(1 - \varphi^2\right)P + \gamma \vec{A} \tag{5}$$

where, φ represents the differential confidence index of medical sensitive data, $\vec{A}$ represents the privacy information storage vector, and γ represents the privacy query coefficient.

The weight distribution is determined by the data owner according to the data privacy protection requirements. For different privacy protection requirements, the weights of the queryer trust value and the data privacy attribute value can be adjusted to perform security trust calculation and data processing. For example, when the security trust degree does not consider the data privacy attribute, $\gamma = 0$. The queryer trust value reflects the subjective differences of data query users with different rights and reputation values, and the trust values corresponding to different query rights and reputation values are also different. The data privacy attribute value reflects the degree of privacy of different sensitive data and is usually determined by domain experts and data owners. To facilitate trust calculation, we quantify queryer authority and reputation values and data privacy attribute values as scalars between 0 and 1.

Calculation of querier trust value: the querier trust value is composed of query permission attribute and reputation value. When calculating the trust value of the inquirer, first analyze the authority value and reputation value of the inquirer according to the user attribute. The authority value and reputation value are random variables with normal distribution between 0 and 1. The specific calculation formula is as follows:

$$S = O^2 + (\lambda - 1)\frac{s_{max}^2 - s_{min}^2}{\dot{d}} \tag{6}$$

Among them, λ represents the query security item coefficient of medical sensitive data, $\dot{d}$ represents the trust measurement value, s_{min} represents the minimum value of the security confidence index of medical sensitive data, and s_{max} represents the maximum value of the security confidence index. As requests for access and public disclosure of health data continue to increase, and the line between privacy protection of personally identifiable information and aggregated data becomes increasingly blurred, laws and regulations alone cannot effectively constrain the privacy of personal information. Therefore, it is particularly important to use privacy-preserving technologies to improve information retrieval of medical big data. Privacy-preserving technologies can not only improve access management, monitoring, and control of data, but also improve the identification of personal health information, helping to assess and reduce the risk of re-identification.

Smart hospitals use intelligent technology, Internet technology and some AI technologies in the field of medical services, making it a new trend of modern medical development in China. Smart hospitals help hospitals integrate resources, optimize processes, reduce hospital operating costs, and improve service quality, management level, and work efficiency. Patients use the hospital introduction in the palm hospital to understand the hospital before seeing a doctor, and then directly locate the hospital location according to the navigation [5]. Learn about doctors through specialized consultation and introduction of famous doctors in palm hospital, and select appropriate doctors for registration and appointment according to their actual situation. After making an appointment, you can use real-time query to understand the treatment situation of experts, and arrange an appropriate time for medical treatment according to the current treatment situation, so as to save the waiting time of patients.

The security trust degree is a key indicator to judge the differential privacy performance of medical sensitive data, and the interaction is based on whether it meets a certain trust level. The division of trust levels mainly reflects the relationship between the level of trust in the inquirer, and it is not necessary to be too precise in specific applications. By analyzing the difference of the queryer's authority attribute and the dynamic change of the data privacy attribute, the query security trust degree is calculated and corresponding to different trust levels and different privacy protection parameters, so that when the sensitive data privacy attribute changes, the query users of different levels can obtain different results. Availability of privacy-preserving data to achieve hierarchical control of the accuracy of sensitive data information in query responses under the premise of protecting privacy.

3　Medical Sensitive Data Protection Methods

Based on the application principle of differential privacy, according to the processing flow of R-tree clustering structure construction, sensitivity calculation and sensitive point search, the design of medical sensitive data protection algorithm based on differential privacy is completed.

3.1　R-tree Clustering Structure

In order to achieve effective access to medical sensitive data, a clustering model based on R-tree index is used for data retrieval of intelligent medical information system. When constructing the R-tree clustering model, if the distribution law of data is unknown, setting the clustering center in advance will make the final clustering result deviate from the reality, thus affecting the efficiency of the constructed R-tree model index [6]. In order to effectively determine the clustering center, DCC algorithm is introduced to construct R-tree model. The R-tree model can accurately calculate the distance between medical sensitive data, improve the clustering accuracy of medical sensitive data, and help improve the integrity and security of medical sensitive data protection.

Set the distance index of measuring adjacent sensitive data as l, which is expressed as:

$$l = \frac{S}{\sqrt{\frac{f}{G}}} \tag{7}$$

In the formula, f is the quantity of medically sensitive data, and G is the range of a given spatial area. Using the dynamic R-tree generation algorithm, reasonable leaf nodes are inserted into the target object, and the above-mentioned dynamic determination of the cluster center algorithm is used to construct the large-scale dynamic optimization of the R-tree. The R-tree generation for either spatial dataset is shown in Fig. 2. The main process of its establishment is as follows: First, establish the minimum bounding rectangle for all spatial objects. Then the base rectangles are grouped according to the algorithm of dynamically determining the cluster center. For example, in Fig. 2, the R12 closest to the mean point is first selected as the initial cluster center. Then select R19 farthest from R12 and R8 farthest from R19 as the cluster center and start clustering. Among them, R13, R14, R17 and R18 are divided into R19, R9, R10, R11, R12, R15 and R16 are divided into R8. At this time, two clusters are formed, and the cluster center and cluster measurement function are calculated. Select the cluster with the largest radius and its cluster center R12 from the two clusters, select R15 with the farthest distance from R12 and R11 and R18 with the farthest distance from R15 as the cluster center to re-cluster, and then calculate its cluster center and the clustering measure function. The loop repeats until the clustering function is known to converge.

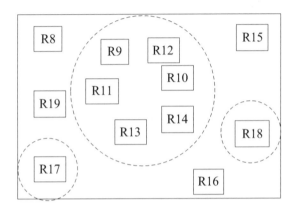

Fig. 2. R-tree structure clustering center

Although using big data can improve medical quality and solve current problems, its unique characteristics also bring challenges to technology and management. For example, big data has many sources and formats, from early images and text to video, audio, graphics and even GPS data from mobile phones. Complex data forms greatly increase the difficulty of storing, mining and analyzing data. Because many hospitals have digitized their administrative and treatment procedures, the speed and quantity of data generation exceed the limitations of traditional data processing software. In the database system, when the stored objects are very large, the efficiency of data query and retrieval is an important bottleneck that restricts the application of medical information. Therefore, improving the information retrieval ability in the context of medical big data is of great significance to improve the level of medical services and promote the construction of medical informatization.

With the development of medical informatization, the traditional paper medical records are gradually replaced by electronic medical records. However, for special medical records, paper medical records still have an irreplaceable position. Users can access real-time through personal computers or mobile phones, providing users with convenient and fast information query services. When the medical record room manages these paper medical records, they can quickly query relevant information through the smart hospital system to complete the management of paper medical records [7]. Medical institutions are responsible for the management and protection of personal information, and bear the corresponding legal responsibilities and risks when processing these information. In the face of increasingly complex data processing needs, it is very important to establish and improve relevant laws to meet the reasonable requirements for data processing.

3.2 Sensitivity

Differential privacy protects the user's private information by adding noise to the query results. The amount of noise added is the key. It is required that the added noise can not only protect the user's privacy, but also prevent the data from being added too much. The noise makes the data unavailable. Function sensitivity is an important parameter to control noise. By controlling the amount of noise generated by global sensitivity, a privacy protection mechanism that meets the requirements of differential privacy can be implemented.

The global sensitivity for a query data h is defined as follows:

$$K(h) = \max_{\iota=1} \iota \times [F(h) - X(h)] \tag{8}$$

where, ι represents the tuple definition coefficient, $F(h)$ represents the privacy query function based on coefficient h, and $X(h)$ represents the differential definition function based on coefficient h. Global sensitivity reflects the upper limit of the output that can be disturbed when protecting privacy. It is independent of the data set and is determined by the query function itself.

When solving the sensitivity index of medical data information, the cooperation of the following equipment structures is also required.

(1) Information perception layer: It is a physical layer that includes sensor networks, sensors, data collectors, etc., which are used to store parameters or identifiers in object events. Its task is to complete the acquisition, communication and coordination of data.

(2) Network Cognitive Layer: Provides connection and transmission between objects, network devices, wireless or wired and cloud systems, and sends and processes data obtained locally; it also includes data received from the perception layer. Gateway component [8]. Starting from the information perception layer, processing hosts can obtain a large amount of heterogeneous perception information, and use the interconnection mechanism between networks to distribute and share these perception information.

(3) Intelligent application layer: responsible for providing applications and services to human or non-human users. It can specify and locate various application processes, programs and application software in the Internet of things. For example, intelligent medical record management system, medical image management system, etc.

Then the geometric data table and related attribute data table are designed for the hierarchical geometric object set. The geometry table consists of the unique identifier of the geometry object and two binary coordinate fields (strings). Accordingly, the unique identifier of the object and several attribute fields are designed in the attribute data table, and the connection between the geometric data table and the attribute data table is realized through the unique identifier.

Although privacy-preserving schemes emerge in an endless stream, they all have a common disadvantage, all relying on the background knowledge of the attacker and not making reasonable assumptions about the attack model. The emergence of the differential privacy model effectively solves this problem. The concept of differential privacy comes from cryptography and aims to maximize the accuracy of data queries and minimize the chances of records being identified when querying from statistical databases. The differential privacy model ensures that the public results will not change significantly because of whether an individual is in the data set by adding random noise to the data set, and provides a quantitative model for the degree of privacy leakage [9]. Because the change of an individual will not have a significant impact on the data query results, the attacker cannot infer the private information of individual samples from the public results based on their own background knowledge. Differential privacy model does not depend on the background knowledge possessed by attackers and provides a higher level of semantic security for private information, so it is widely used as a new type of privacy protection model.

3.3 Sensitive Point Search

Because the data collected by the medical Bracelet changes in real time, its data usually remains almost constant or increases (or decreases). For example, when collecting and monitoring the vital signs of patients, their ECG and blood pressure are almost unchanged in general, but they will increase or decrease in unstable periods. Therefore, the goal of the first stage of collecting such health data is to search for sensitive points when the trend begins to change.

In order to better protect the privacy information in medical and health data, after analyzing the data, we further develop an anonymous privacy publishing model suitable for medical and health data. Due to the correlation between the attributes of medical and health data, publishing all attributes in the same data table and then surfacing this data to all users will increase the risk of privacy disclosure [10]. One of the principles of privacy protection is to reduce the number of people who have access to privacy. According to the data characteristics of medical and health data, two different publishing methods are proposed:

1. For some data users with lower authority, only data tables consisting of quasi-identifiers and main sensitive attributes, such as gender, age, and disease, are released, thereby reducing the probability of information leakage. Only disease is a sensitive attribute in the medical and health data table released at this time, so it is necessary to formulate a single-sensitive attribute privacy protection scheme suitable for medical and health data. The released single-sensitive attribute data sheet can not only reduce the probability of link attack and homogenization attack, but also have good performance against background knowledge attack and similarity attack.
2. For another part of data users with high authority, the data table includes not only multiple quasi identifiers and primary sensitive attributes, but also some secondary sensitive attributes, such as the attending doctor and the treatment method adopted. At the same time, we also need to consider the sensitivity of the main sensitive attributes of disease and the correlation between the attributes. For this kind of data, it is

necessary to formulate an appropriate privacy protection scheme for multi sensitive attribute medical and health data, so that the published data can not only deal with the semantic attacks that single sensitive attribute data may face, but also have the ability to resist sensitivity and association attacks.

Let J represent the assignment coefficient of medical sensitive data, ΔZ represent the unit accumulation of the data text to be processed, and ϖ represent the sensitivity feature measurement index. With the support of the above physical quantities, formula (8) can be combined to express the sensitive point screening index M as:

$$M = K(h) + J\left(\frac{\Delta Z}{\varpi^2}\right) \tag{9}$$

The similarity or dissimilarity between the values of each sensitive attribute can be calculated according to the position of the disease in the semantic hierarchy tree. For a given disease value, if the distance between other diseases and it is calculated, first find the specific positions of the two disease values in the semantic hierarchy tree, and traverse the hierarchy tree upwards according to their positions until the minimum of the two disease values is found. Common parent node, and then calculate the distance from the leaf node where the disease value is located to its smallest common parent node. On the basis of formula (9), let c_1, c_2, $\cdots$, and c_n E represent the definition coefficients of n different medical sensitive data cotyledon nodes, ϑ represents the sensitivity measurement index, $\tilde{b}$ represents the fluctuating transmission characteristics of medical sensitive data, and σ represents data processing vector.

The search results of medical data sensitive points based on differential privacy are:

$$V = (c_1 + c_2 + \cdots + c_n)\frac{\vartheta \cdot M}{1 + \left|\tilde{b}\right|^{-\sigma}} \tag{10}$$

Combining the concept of differential privacy to develop a reasonable and available medical sensitive data protection algorithm is the research focus. In the process of processing, the research on the privacy protection scheme of single sensitive attribute and multi sensitive attribute medical health data will be carried out respectively, in order to reduce the attack vulnerability of the published medical health data table. The effectiveness of the scheme is proved by experiments. In addition, on the basis of privacy protection, how to minimize the loss of information in the process of anonymity is also one of the issues that need to be considered in the formulation of privacy protection schemes.

4 Case Analysis

In order to verify the practicability of the differential privacy-based medical sensitive data protection algorithm, the following comparative experiments are designed.

Step 1: Implant a sensitive data protection algorithm based on differential privacy in a medical operation system, use the system to normally store daily medical information, analyze the changes of relevant index parameters, and record the obtained data as the variable index of the experimental group;

Step 2: Implant the conventional data protection algorithm in the medical operation system, use the system to normally store daily medical information, analyze the changes of relevant index parameters, and record the obtained data as the variable index of the control group;

Step 3: Compare the variable indicators of the experimental group and the control group, and summarize the experimental rules.

The layout of the complete medical operation system is shown in Fig. 3.

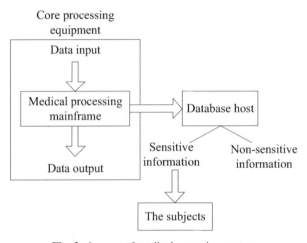

Fig. 3. Layout of medical operation system

In the medical operation system, the transmission effectiveness of sensitive information samples can be used to describe the processing ability of the medical host for data objects. Without considering other interference conditions, the stronger the transmission effectiveness of sensitive information samples, the stronger the processing ability of the medical host for data objects. During this experiment, if the sensitive information sample can be successfully transmitted to the target location, the coding result will be recorded as "1"; If the sensitive information sample cannot be successfully transmitted to the target location, the coding result will be recorded as "0". The specific experimental results are shown in Table 1.

Analysis of Table 1 shows that the algorithm in the experimental group has relatively weak coding ability for equipment usage indicators. Among the 10 variable indicators, only the coding result of this type of medical sensitive data is "0"; The algorithm in the control group has department information, drug information, the coding ability of the three types of indicators of treatment duration is weak. Among the 10 variable indicators, the encoding result of the above three types of medically sensitive data is "0".

Table 1. Encoding results of medically sensitive data

Data classification	The experimental group	The control group
The patient information	1	1
Department of information	1	0
Medical information	1	1
The fee information	1	1
The doctor's advice information	1	1
Return information	1	1
Drug information	1	0
Equipment usage	0	1
Drug dosage	1	1
The treatment time	1	0

The ability of the selected protection algorithm to transmit medical sensitive data can be expressed as:

$$\begin{cases} \eta_1 = \dfrac{M_1}{M_0} \times 100\% \\ \eta_2 = \dfrac{M_2}{M_0} \times 100\% \end{cases} \tag{11}$$

where, η_1 represents the effectiveness index of the experimental group, M_1 represents the total amount of sensitive data with the coding result of "1" in the experimental group, η_2 represents the effectiveness index of the control group, M_2 represents the total amount of sensitive data with the coding result of "1" in the control group, and M_0 represents the total amount of medical sensitive data samples.

Combine Table 1 and formula (11) to calculate the η_1 and η_2 indicators. Without considering other interference conditions, it can be seen that $\eta_1 = 90\%$ and $\eta_2 = 70\%$, the effectiveness of the experimental group is significantly greater than that of the control group.

After the above experiments are completed, in order to further verify the performance of the algorithm in this paper, the security factor is taken as the indicator to test the protection security of the algorithm in this paper. Set the maximum safety factor to 1.0. The higher the safety factor, the stronger the protection performance of the algorithm. The algorithm in this paper is compared with the algorithm in reference [2] and the algorithm in reference [3]. The comparison results of the safety factors of the three algorithms are shown in Table 2.

It can be seen from the comparison results of the safety factors shown in Table 2 that, with the increase of the number of experiments, the safety factor of the algorithm in this paper is significantly higher than that of the two literature comparison algorithms. The maximum safety factor of the algorithm in this paper reaches 0.98, while the maximum

Table 2. Safety factors

Number of experiments	Safety factor		
	Algorithm in this paper	Reference [2] algorithm	Reference [3] algorithm
10	0.95	0.72	0.83
20	0.98	0.56	0.84
30	0.96	0.78	0.80
40	0.94	0.69	0.74
50	0.96	0.71	0.71
60	0.97	0.83	0.64
70	0.98	0.73	0.62
80	0.95	0.76	0.68
90	0.96	0.68	0.64
100	0.98	0.65	0.69

safety zone coefficient of the algorithm in reference [2] and the algorithm in reference [3] reaches 0.9. Therefore, the data protection security of this algorithm is high.

5   Conclusion

In order to improve the security of medical sensitive data, a medical sensitive data protection algorithm based on differential privacy is proposed. The performance of the algorithm is verified from both theoretical and experimental aspects. The algorithm has high coding and transmission performance when protecting medical sensitive data, and improves the security of medical sensitive data. The experimental results show that, compared with the protection algorithm based on fragmentation and Bayesian network, the algorithm in this paper can improve the security factor of medical sensitive data and improve the security of medical sensitive data.

Aknowledgement. 2020 Guangxi College and University Young and Middle aged Teachers' Basic Scientific Research Ability Improvement Project "Research and Development of Panoramic Campus Roaming System Cross platform" (2020KY63022).

References

1. Kou, L., Liu, N., Huang, H., et al.: Data aggregation privacy protection algorithm based on distributed compressive sensing and hash function. Appl. Res. Comput. **37**(01), 239–244 (2020)
2. Jun, W., Xu, Y., Li, L.: Lightweight data fusion privacy protection algorithm based on sharding. Comput. Eng. Des. **43**(05), 1207–1213 (2022)

3. Xiao, B., Yan, H., Luo, H., et al.: Research on improvement of Bayesian network privacy protection algorithm based on differential privacy. Netinfo Security **20**(11), 75–86 (2020)
4. Kshetri, N., Voas, J.: Thoughts on general data protection regulation and online human surveillance. Computer **53**(1), 86–90 (2020)
5. Qaisar, S.M., Alsharif, F., Subasi, A., et al.: Appliance identification based on smart meter data and event-driven processing in the 5G framework. Procedia Comput. Sci. **182**(3), 103–108 (2021)
6. March, R.D., Leuzzi, C., Deffacis, M., et al.: Innovative approach for PMM data processing and analytics. IEEE Trans. Big Data **6**(3), 452–459 (2020)
7. Silva, M., Kaesler, J.M., Reemtsma, T., et al.: Absorption mode spectral processing improves data quality of natural organic matter analysis by Fourier-transform ion cyclotron resonance mass spectrometry. J. Am. Soc. Mass Spectrom. **31**(7), 1615–1618 (2020)
8. Ttsch, K., Fjeldsted, J.C., Stow, S.M., et al.: Effect of sampling rate and data pretreatment for targeted and nontargeted analysis by means of liquid chromatography coupled to drift time ion mobility quadruple time-of-flight mass spectrometry. J. Am. Soc. Mass Spectrom. **32**(10), 2592–2603 (2021)
9. Wielgat, R., Jdryka, R., Lorenc, A., et al.: POLEMAD–A database for the multimodal analysis of Polish pronunciation. Speech Commun. **2020**(127), 29–42 (2021)
10. Zhou, A.I.: Research on weighted social network deep differential privacy data protection algorithm. Comput. Simul. **37**(10), 282–285+373 (2020)

Classification and Storage Method of Medical Health Monitoring Data Based on Bayesian Algorithm

Xiaofeng Li and Zhongwei Chen[✉]

College of Information Engineering, Guangxi University of Foreign Languages,
Nanning 530222, China
top00112233@163.com

Abstract. In the storage of medical health monitoring data, the overall storage is chaotic and takes up more backup space. A classified storage method of medical health monitoring data based on Bayesian algorithm is designed. Collect and integrate medical health monitoring data. Data collection is realized by relying on the unified data exchange platform in the big data platform. Each collection node uploads the required data by accessing the data exchange platform. Data integration is mainly about data preprocessing of collected medical and health big data. Based on Bayesian algorithm, an integrated naive Bayesian algorithm based on knowledge transfer is designed to implement the classification and processing of medical health monitoring data. A hybrid storage model is designed to implement the classified storage of medical health monitoring data. Test the data classification and storage performance of the design method. The test results show that the method has less startup nodes, less computing power requirements as a whole, can realize the sharing of medical and health monitoring data, and the data classification time is relatively short as a whole, which proves that the method has a broad application space.

Keywords: Bayesian Algorithm · Medical Health · Monitoring Data · Data Classification Storage

1 Introduction

With the improvement of people's material living standards, the trend of population aging in many countries is gradually obvious. With that comes a rise in the number of people with geriatric and chronic diseases. According to the "Report on Nutrition and Chronic Disease Status of Chinese Residents" released in 2015, the prevalence of hypertension and diabetes among adults aged 18 and over in my country in 2012 was on the rise compared with 2002, and the number of deaths from chronic diseases in the country that year accounted for It accounts for 86.6% of the total number of deaths, which has attracted much attention [1]. Chronic disease treatment is a process that requires long-term monitoring. In order to save medical resources, it is a good solution to use the mobile medical method to monitor the human body for a long time and in real time by the health monitoring terminal.

S. Wang (Ed.): IoTCare 2022, LNICST 501, pp. 88–101, 2023.
https://doi.org/10.1007/978-3-031-33545-7_7

In recent years, the development of medical informatization has promoted the integration of medical and mobile communication technology, and gave birth to the concept of mobile medicine. Mobile medicine generally refers to the provision of medical services and information through mobile communication tools, such as PDA, mobile phone, etc., including remote patient monitoring, online consultation, online consultation, wireless access to electronic medical records, etc. [2]. It provides an effective way to solve the problem of shortage and uneven distribution of high-quality medical resources. It not only changes the traditional treatment mode, but also enables patients to perform simple operations on the mobile medical service platform established by medical institutions, so that they can complete the appointment for treatment and avoid the toil of queuing up for registration in the hospital. At the same time, it also realizes telemedicine monitoring with the help of mobile communication technology, and effectively manages the health information of patients.

Reference [3] proposed a method to build a safe storage model of health data based on the alliance blockchain. This method divides medical institutions based on the distribution of medical resources, and uses the share authorization certification mechanism and the practical Byzantine mechanism to achieve the safe transmission of health data. According to the characteristics of the blockchain, such as decentralization, security and trustworthiness, and tamper prevention, health data is stored on the blockchain to improve the security of health data. Reference [4] proposed a method to build a safe storage model of health data based on the blockchain. This method designs a safe storage model of health data based on the blockchain storage structure to improve the practicality of the storage model. And optimize the storage process of the blockchain, and improve the storage efficiency through the consensus mechanism of random number election. Although the above methods can complete the classification and safe storage of health data, there is still a high intrusion rate and it is difficult to resist external attacks. Therefore, in this study, a classification storage method of medical health monitoring data based on Bayesian algorithm is proposed.

2 Classification and Storage of Medical Health Monitoring Data

2.1 Data Collection and Integration

Collect and integrate medical health monitoring data. Data collection is realized by relying on the unified data exchange platform in the big data platform. Each collection node uploads the required data by accessing the data exchange platform. Data acquisition and exchange include a variety of access methods, including but not limited to data tables, front-end libraries, real-time communication, documents, data distribution, etc. when accessing the new system, the appropriate and best access method should be selected according to the exchange requirements and characteristics of the new system. Data collection methods are divided into document based and intermediate library based forms [5]. Based on document collection, nodes can upload documents directly, or convert and upload the original library through the document conversion tool. Based on the collection of the intermediate library, the node writes the data to the front-end computer and uploads it. Combine two ways to collect.

Document-based collection means that each data collection node collects according to the document format specified in the data collection specification, and directly uploads the exchanged document to the big data platform by calling Web service; the platform reviews the document format and quality information and feeds it back to the collection node. Document-based data collection is suitable for the collection of unstructured data or structured data whose update frequency is relatively slow. Document-based data collection has the following characteristics: high real-time data collection and scalability, no need to adjust the service interface due to the increase of collection services; Lower maintenance costs, more conducive to management; If the collected data content is large, the pressure on the network and the exchange server will be very large.

The access node takes the document as the carrier and can upload data by calling the Web service. However, due to the different data storage forms of the collection node, the process of data uploading will be different, which can be uploaded in three ways:

(1) Access nodes upload documents directly: for data in the form of documents, access nodes can directly call web services to upload documents;
(2) The access node uploads the data in the document library: the local data stored in the document library in the form of documents. The platform can directly call the service interface of the platform to upload the data of the local document library;
(3) Data is converted into document format and uploaded: local data stored in relational database can be converted into documents and uploaded through document conversion tools.

The document library includes documents in any format, such as XML, CDA, XLS, PDF, DOC, TXT, etc.

In the process of data exchange based on the intermediate library, the intermediate library will be used as the intermediate link of the exchange between the platform and the access node. Database table exchange is a sharing method of medical and health big data based on database table structure. The front-end database table is used as the interface for data acquisition and push between the data exchange system and the access node. The data exchange system exchanges data through the front-end database, and the access node obtains the data of the front-end database or pushes it to the front-end database through bridging. The data and database exchange method has the following characteristics: It is relatively safe not to access the business database; Simple configuration and less operation and maintenance workload; Clear boundaries, clear responsibilities and rights; The data transmission efficiency is high, the real-time performance is high, the exchange mode is flexible, and it can adapt to many scenarios [6].

Data integration is mainly to preprocess the collected medical and health big data. Medical and health big data has the characteristics of large data volume, heterogeneity, asynchronous (sequential) and incompleteness. Therefore, it is undoubtedly difficult to analyze and apply the original data of medical and health data. In order to provide higher quality for the data analysis stage Generally, data preprocessing operation is required for the target data set of the data processing. There are generally four methods for data preprocessing: data cleaning, data integration, data reduction and data transformation.

(1) Data cleaning: Data cleaning is to serve the high-quality data requirements of subsequent data analysis. The tasks of data cleaning mainly include:

① Fill in missing data values.
Fill in data values that are vacant in the record.
② Noise data smoothing.
Noise refers to random errors in the data. A common way to remove noisy data is to divide the noisy data equally into nearby data.

(2) Data integration: data integration refers to the process of merging data from multiple data sources into one data set. According to different data conditions, the conversion work of data integration is different, such as null value filling, standardized and unified data format, data splitting, data correctness verification, etc.

(3) Data specification refers to the compression of data sets, but the integrity of data must be maintained. There are three types of data protocols:

① Quantity specification: replace the original data with smaller data. Simple original data can be replaced by sampling data. For complex data, the cluster center in cluster analysis needs to replace the original data first.

② Data compression: transform the original data into a compressed form through the compression algorithm, which can keep the content and characteristics of the data unchanged, mainly for image and video data.

③ Dimension reduction: extract the dimensions from the original data, remove those dimensions that have no use value, and only retain the main dimensions, so as to reduce the size of the data set [7].

(4) Data transformation: The purpose of data transformation is to eliminate the difference in the data type and data format of the original data. The specific operation methods are as follows:

① Data normalization: Reducing the attributes with huge differences between the maximum value and the minimum value in the original data according to an appropriate ratio can effectively improve the performance of the data algorithm.

② Data aggregation: Aggregate raw data according to the granularity required for data analysis, such as aggregating daily data into annual data.

③ Attribute construction: Combine several attribute constructions in the original data into a new attribute.

④ Discretization: Replace the data type values in the original data with interval labels, such as the eastern, western, and central regions for regional distribution, and divide the ages into children, youth, middle-aged, and elderly.

2.2 Data Classification

Bayesian classification algorithm is a classification method of statistics, which is a kind of classification algorithm using probability and statistics knowledge. In many occasions, Naïve Bayes (NB) classification algorithm can be comparable to decision tree and neural network classification algorithm. This algorithm can be applied to large databases, and the method is simple, the classification accuracy is high, and the speed is fast.

Based on Bayesian algorithm, an integrated naive Bayesian algorithm based on knowledge transfer is designed to implement the classification and processing of medical health monitoring data. Ensemble learning is an effective strategy to deal with concept drift in streaming data classification. In ensemble learning, the historical model can be updated and reorganized to meet the current distribution of the latest data blocks. However, there will be a disadvantage when using this method only to deal with the concept drift problem, that is, when the new data block arrives, it only filters the historical model and integrates it in some way, without making corresponding adjustments to the historical model to make it more suitable for the current data. Although this method is simple and easy to understand and implement, it can not fully mine the useful knowledge for learning the latest data distribution only by simply combining the historical models. Therefore, the combination of ensemble learning method and knowledge transfer makes the model more effective in dealing with the problem of concept drift in data flow classification. That is, knowledge transfer is introduced into FWNB algorithm and combined with naive Bayesian algorithm based on forgetting mechanism weighting. In transfer learning, the source domain and the target domain belong to the same learning task, so they are interrelated. It can also use the knowledge of the historical model after knowledge migration to assist in the learning of the latest data. Therefore, an integrated learning algorithm FTENB based on knowledge migration is proposed, which takes the historical model as the initial solution, and then migrates it based on the latest data to make it more suitable for the latest data distribution after concept drift.

The model usage strategy based on knowledge transfer is as follows: The existing ensemble learning models in the classification of data flow have a same characteristic. Whenever the newly arrived data block is classified, the historical model is only analyzed by integrating various methods, without taking into account that the historical model is adjusted according to the latest data and then integrated. So these approaches differ mainly in the various integration and combination approaches to the preserved historical models. While these methods are less complex and easier to implement, doing so alone may not fully exploit the knowledge that is most useful for classification learning on current state-of-the-art data.

Suppose there are two data distributions, P1 and P2, respectively. P1 represents some historical data distribution in the data stream, and P2 represents the current latest data distribution. P1 is different from P2, which means that concept drift has occurred [8]. The classification performance of the historical model learned from the historical data distribution P1 may not be high on the latest data, so in the ensemble model, the importance of this historical model should be reduced, that is, give it a lower weight, some extreme case may be zero, then all the knowledge in the model will not be used. If P1 and P2 are regarded as the source domain and target domain of transfer learning, respectively, then P1 and P2 belong to the same classification learning task, and there is a certain connection between the two. Based on this, after knowledge transfer, the knowledge of the transferred historical model can be used to assist the learning of the latest data. Therefore, it is very advantageous to use transfer learning in ensemble models.

The classification learning algorithm is different, and the learning method is also different, so the method of transferring the historical model according to the new data is also different. In this paper, naive Bayesian algorithm is used as the basic learning algorithm, and a method based on Naive Bayesian model is designed and proposed to adjust the historical model, aiming to adjust the retained historical naive Bayesian model to adapt to new data.

The specific migration process is divided into the following two steps:

Step 1: Combine all the data in the newly arrived data block B_a with the historical data B_i respectively. At this time, the data in the new data block is marked, and the newly generated data block contains both historical knowledge and current knowledge, and does not belong to a specific real data distribution;

Step 2: Build a classifier E_i^a for the new data block B_i^a, obtain new class probability and conditional probability, and generate a new Naive Bayesian model.

After performing knowledge transfer on historical models based on new data, the newly generated models not only contain previous knowledge, but also current latest knowledge. Therefore, the newly generated model E_i^a is a new distribution that mixes various data, and does not really belong to the real distribution of a certain piece of data in the dataset. The naive Bayesian model after knowledge transfer can be more adapted to the latest data B_i^a, but it will also reduce the model difference between E_i^a, so these transferred models will be discarded after use, just for the classification of the current data block service without being retained by the system.

In FTENB algorithm, selecting N historical model can be defined as selecting n storage from a model. Take the stored n models as the starting model, and then implement knowledge migration based on the latest data. The migrated model will be used as the base model in the subsequent integration algorithm.

The integration strategy of models in streaming data classification is actually an effective combination of multiple models. In order to have a better combination effect, it is bound to choose the best base model for integration [9]. Based on this, FTENB algorithm uses the classification effect of historical model on the latest data block as the screening criterion of historical model. Following this criterion, the FTENB algorithm selects the historical model for knowledge migration as follows.

Suppose FTENB can hold n historical models. After receiving B_a, test all saved historical models based on B_a, and at the same time, build FWNB model E_a based on this data. Then check whether the number of models saved in the current system reaches the threshold n. If not, save E_a, otherwise, add E_a to the ensemble model first, and then select the worst model according to the performance of each model on the current data, and remove it from the system. In addition, the removed model is selected from all models in the current system, so both E_i and E_a may be removed.

Each data block $B_1, B_2, \cdots, B_a$ arrives sequentially in the form of a stream. The FTENB algorithm first establishes a naive Bayesian model E_1 on the data block B_1 and saves it in the system. When B_a arrives, based on the latest data block B_a, the knowledge migration is performed on all the stored historical models E_i, and the migrated model E_i^a is obtained. At the same time, a weighted model based on the forgetting mechanism is established on B_a as a new base model E_a. After integrating the historical model with knowledge transfer and E_a, the integrated model at time a can be obtained. At the same time, the FTENB algorithm also needs to update the historical model in the system in time to ensure that the ensemble model uses the optimal base model.

When integrating classification models, we also need to consider the weight calculation of each model. AUE2 algorithm has the best classification learning ability among the current integration algorithms, so we refer to the integration method of AUE2 algorithm. For all migrated historical models, formula (1) is used to calculate the weight of the model. For the base model E_a trained by Weighted Naive Bayes based on forgetting mechanism on the latest data block B_a, it is the most "perfect" model based on B_a, and formula (2) is used to calculate the weight of E_a.

$$\omega_i^a = \frac{1}{M_i^a + M_i^{a'} + \chi} \tag{1}$$

In formula (1), M_i^a refers to the classification error of E_i^a on B_a; $M_i^{a'}$ refers to the mean square error of the random classification model; χ refers to the positive value.

$$\omega_a = \frac{1}{M_i^{a'} + \chi} \tag{2}$$

The formula for calculating M_i^a is as follows:

$$M_i^a = \frac{1}{|B_a|} \sum_{\{c,d\} \in B_a} \left(1 - l_i^a(d|c)\right)^2 \tag{3}$$

In formula (3), $l_i^a(d|c)$ refers to the posterior probability of model E_i^a after migration; c and d refer to the medical and health monitoring data flow in B_a.

The formula for calculating $M_i^{a'}$ is as follows:

$$M_i^{a'} = \sum_d l^a(d)\left(1 - l^a(d)\right)^2 \tag{4}$$

In Eq. (4), $l^a(d)$ refers to the prior probability of data stream d in B_a.

Complete the classification of medical health monitoring data.

2.3 Data Classification Storage

Design a hybrid storage model to implement classified storage of medical health monitoring data after classification. The hybrid storage model is introduced in three parts. The first part is the related implementation in the Linux kernel, the second part is the implementation of metadata distinction, and the third part is the implementation of logical block mapping.

In the hybrid storage model, the relevant implementations in the Linux kernel are as follows: The Device Mapper mechanism in the Linux kernel exists in the kernel in the form of modules, which did not appear until the kernel version 2.6, and is mainly used to implement the mapping mechanism for logical volume management. It implements a modular kernel architecture for creating virtual logical devices and managing multiple underlying storage resources. If developers want to use the Device Mapper mechanism to develop, it must be included in the kernel, and a management tool for users to be installed. The current management tool of Device Mapper uses dmsetup, which mainly includes related configuration and interface library functions. In fact, the role of Device Mapper can be regarded as combining multiple underlying storage devices into a logical device, so that users cannot feel the existence of the underlying device, but can only see the created virtual logical device. In addition, Device Mapper is a "stack" structure, and its underlying device can be composed of Device Mapper. It is mainly composed of 3 kinds of objects: (1) Mapper Device: the logical device displayed to the outside world; (2) Mapping Table: custom rules to link different underlying devices; (3) Target Device: the actual physical device.

Several mapping rules have been defined under the Device Mapper architecture of the kernel to implement different logical devices. First of all, the target driver module is inserted into the Linux kernel in the form of a module. The main function of this module is to redirect or modify the I/O requests of the upper layer. At present, there are many different types of mapping rules in the kernel, including linear rules, soft raid, et al.The data request sent by the user is passed to the block layer, which will be converted into a request of bio structure, and then the bio request will be processed by the unified processing method of the Device Mapper mechanism. Corresponding processing, the algorithm will modify the corresponding address contained in the bio request, and the device pointed to in the bio structure also specifies the underlying physical device corresponding to the physical address. The bio request processed by the mapping rule will still be put into the request queue owned by the block device, and then the method generic_make_request will be used again to submit the request that has been redirected by the Device Mapper mechanism. Therefore, it can be considered that the Device Mapper mechanism just performs a simple redirection operation on the received request, and converts the I/O request to the logical device into a request to the underlying device. The Device Mapper mechanism has an interface that can accept the submission and processing of the upper general block layer and re-initiate the bio request. Therefore, developers can easily implement their own mapping rules according to their own needs, and only need to follow the Device Mapper architecture definition. Rules to write modules, and then insert the module into the kernel, do not need to worry about the interaction with other modules in the kernel, so it has good generality.

In the process of implementing the hybrid storage model, it is not only necessary to distinguish all metadata requests, but also to reduce the movement of the head when accessing the disk, it is also necessary to aggregate all scattered metadata and data requests in the disk, so that different kinds of data are gathered in different areas of each block group. Therefore, the active identification method is used, but on the basis of active identification, Make a few modifications to the model to distinguish all metadata [10].

The layout of the model disk can distinguish some static metadata requests. However, since the directory item is a dynamically allocated data block, the allocation function of the data block needs to be modified (for example, ext2_get_block function, et al.) to make the dynamically allocated metadata block and the statically allocated metadata block together. First, select to reserve some data blocks after the fixed metadata blocks of each block group for allocation to the dynamically allocated directory, so that all statically allocated metadata blocks will be stored after the dynamically allocated metadata blocks, so that the former part of each block group stores all metadata, while the ordinary files are allocated to the latter part outside the reserved area of the block group. In this way, Aggregate all metadata and data in each block group in the file system.

The metadata in the Ext2 file model mainly exists in two ways, one is fixedly allocated metadata, and the other is dynamically allocated metadata. For fixed allocation metadata, such as superblock, group descriptor table, and inode table, disk blocks are allocated at fixed positions in each block group of the device when mkfs formats the file model. For example, when the Ext2/Ext3 file model divides the disk storage space into 128 MB block groups, at this time, the disk blocks at the beginning of each group are reserved for storing metadata as data blocks of statically allocated metadata, but For a directory (the disk block of which is used to store directory items, which is also a kind of metadata), the disk block is dynamically allocated in the corresponding block group when the user creates it, which is a kind of dynamically allocated metadata.

For statically allocated metadata blocks, the number and storage location of disk blocks occupied can be calculated from the relevant information recorded in the superblock when creating the file system. However, for dynamically allocated metadata, in order to put it together with statically allocated metadata blocks, it is necessary to reserve a certain area of data blocks after fixing the disk blocks reserved for metadata during file model formatting to store these dynamically allocated metadata.

The data blocks allocated to the directory are uncertain, because directories, like regular files, are created according to the needs of users, so the creation of directories is related to application scenarios. Under different load scenarios, the number of data blocks occupied by directories will be very different. For example, for deep directory loads, many directories will be created. By testing different loads, estimate the number of directories created under different conditions, and then reserve almost the same data blocks to store the directory items of the directory, and the number of data blocks reserved here to store the directory can also be dynamically adjusted.

Each driver type (target_type) of Device Mapper has a target type name as an identifier, which also corresponds to a module in the kernel. There are multiple callback functions for each driver type, including some necessary and non-essential callback functions, such as constructors, destructors, and mapping functions that must be implemented. The callback function is optional. The Device Mapper mechanism is used in the hybrid storage model, a target device type called raid_target is defined as the identifier, and four callback functions are implemented as required. The name of the callback function and the introduction of related functions are shown in Table 1.

Table 1. Names and related functions of callback functions

Serial number	Function name	Callback function
1	Constructor	raid_ctr()
2	Destroy function	raid_dtr()
3	Mapping function	raid_map()
4	State function	raid_status()

Constructor raid_ctr(). This function is mainly used to allocate the required memory and data structure, parse the target rules configured by the user, and use the various parameters obtained by parsing to initialize each field in the data structure.

The destruction function raid_dtr() is just the opposite of raid_ctr(), so this function will release the data structure and memory allocated in raid_ctr(). So when the user exits, this function will release the memory space and various resources allocated by the constructor and return it to the model.

Mapping function raid_ map () is a very important function. It is the interface for the whole model to obtain the bio request from the upper layer and process the bio request to the lower layer. In the constructor, the received bio request needs to be segmented according to the required size, and then the segmented request is submitted to the mapping function for filtering and redirection. Finally, the processed bio request is submitted to the underlying device for further processing.

Status function raid_ status () is provided for the user to call, so that the user can obtain various states of the current device from the recorded information.

The function dm_register_target registers the defined target_typ. This method will be called when inserting target_type using insmod. After calling this function, a corresponding descriptor target_type will exist in the kernel, which can then be used for some of the above functions.

The function dm_unregister_target unregisters the target_type that has been registered in the kernel. Each target type of the kernel is unregistered when the module rmmod is used, and this function is used at this time.

The implementation process of model initialization is as follows: The hybrid storage model logical device is described by a data structure raid_c.

The process of reading and writing is mainly controlled by raid_ map () function implementation. First of all, the requests sent from the user space will be processed by the modified file system. After processing, the requests will be handed over to the general block layer. In the general block layer, the user requests on the upper layer will be converted into bio structure for description, and then processed by the unified processing module of the Device Mapper mechanism to divide the bio requests. After pre-processing by Device Mapper, the bio is handed over to raid_ map function, and then use the configuration you have created to map bio to the underlying device disk. Among them, the most important process is to modify the sector number field Bi corresponding to the bio request_ sector and the underlying storage device Bi corresponding to the bio request_ bdev, in this way, can retransmit the bio redirected using the mapping rules to the block layer for processing.

In the callback method raid_map of map, the bio request that has been divided and modified by Device Mapper will be received. First, the corresponding logical block device number (LBN) will be calculated through the bi_sector field of the record in the request bio structure, because the file model Modify so that in each block group of the file model, the first half of the blocks are used to store metadata and the second half of the data blocks are used to store data. All the currently requested LBNs that can be obtained are in each block group. The first half or the second half, so as to judge whether the current bio request is a metadata request or a data request, and decide to redirect the bio request to the SSD or HDD according to the judgment result. At the same time, modify the bi_bdev and bi_sector fields to point to the corresponding underlying device. And the corresponding physical address. For example, after the request sent by the user is modified in the Linux kernel I/O stack, the bio will eventually be sent to the created logical device, and the redirection algorithm will check the LBN requested by the bio. If the number is less than EXT2_METADATA_COUNT, the request will be redirected to RAID1 consisting of high-speed solid state disks (SSD). If the requested LBN number is greater than or equal to EXT2_METADATA_COUNT, it will be redirected to RAID5 consisting of ordinary disks (HDD).

3   Storage Test

3.1   Experimental Data and Test Environment

For the designed classification and storage method of medical health monitoring data based on Bayesian algorithm, its classification and storage performance is tested through experimental data. In a hospital, some medical health monitoring data were collected as experimental data, a total of 1000000 pieces, which were divided into five types: blood pressure data, blood oxygen data, ECG data, blood glucose data, body fat data. The performance format of each type of data is shown in Table 2.

Table 2. Scope and basic data types of various types of medical data

Serial number	Data type	Basic data type	Company	Medical data range
1	Blood pressure	Integer	mmHg	80–140
2	Blood oxygen	Float	%	88–100
3	Electrocardiogram	Double	Times/minute	62–105
4	Blood sugar	Integer	Bomol/L	3.2–7.0
5	Body fat	Integer	index	15.2–45.0

The test environment in the experiment is as follows: both Target and Initiator use centos 6.5 system, Target kernel version uses 2.6.34.1, and Initiator uses kernel version 2.6.32.26. On the Target side, two 120 G SSDs are used to form RAID1 to store metadata, and three 1T HDDs are used to form RAID5 to store data. The initiator uses the discovery command to mount the devices in the Target node to the local. Then, the mapped logical device is formatted as an Ext2 file model on the initiator side. In order to eliminate the impact of network bandwidth, 10 Gigabit network cards are used on both the initiator and target sides.

The basic information of the configuration environment in the test is shown in Table 3.

Test the classified storage performance of the design method in this environment. The testing tools used mainly include Postmark, Filebench and fio.

After setting the experimental data and environment, set the experimental process: verify the classification performance of the text method by taking the number of starting nodes, computing power requirements, and data classification time as indicators; Taking

Table 3. Basic information of the configuration environment in the test

Serial number	Project	Specific information
1	Memory	Kingston 32GB DDR
2	Operating system	CentOS 8.2
3	Linux kernel version	Linux 2.6. 22
4	HDD	6TB
5	SDD	240G
6	Network card	Intel 8 Gigabit

the intrusion rate as the indicator, and the reference [3] method and the reference [4] method as the comparative experimental method, the security of the method in this paper is verified.

3.2   Test Results

First, test the number of start-up nodes and computing power requirements of the design method, and the test results are shown in Table 4.

Table 4. Number of startup nodes and computing power requirements for the design method

Data volume (GB)	Number of startup nodes (PCs.)	Computing power demand	Whether to realize data sharing
5	5	Small	Yes
10	8	Small	Yes
15	11	Small	Yes
20	15	Small	Yes
25	17	Small	Yes
30	19	Small	Yes
35	21	in	Yes

The test results in Table 4 show that the number of startup nodes of the design method is small, and the overall demand for computing power is small. At the same time, it can realize the sharing of medical and health monitoring data.

Then test the classification time of medical health monitoring data of the design method, and the specific test results are shown in Fig. 1.

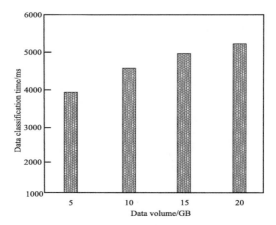

Fig. 1. Classification time of medical health monitoring data

According to the test results in Fig. 1, the classification time of the medical health monitoring data of the design method is relatively short as a whole. With the increase of the amount of data, the classification time also increases, but the overall increase is low.

In order to further verify the security storage performance of the method in this paper, the intrusion rate is taken as the comparison index, and the method in this paper is compared with the method in reference [3] and the method in reference [4]. The intrusion rate comparison results of the three methods are shown in Fig. 2.

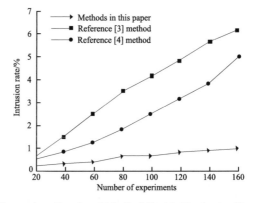

Fig. 2. Comparison Results of Medical Health Monitoring Data Security

It can be seen from the test results shown in Fig. 2 that, under many comparative experiments, the intrusion rate of the method in this paper is always lower than that of the two literature comparison methods. The maximum intrusion rate of the method in this paper is only about 1%, while the maximum intrusion rate of the method in Reference [3] and Reference [4] is more than 6% and 5% respectively. Therefore, this method can reduce the intrusion rate of health monitoring and improve the security of storage.

4   Conclusion

With the increasing emphasis on chronic diseases and the development of health monitoring terminals, medical and health big data and precision medicine have become the current development direction. Therefore, it is necessary to realize the integration and sharing of medical and health data. Therefore, a classification storage method of medical health monitoring data based on Bayesian algorithm is designed to realize the rapid classification and classification storage of medical health monitoring data. The experimental results show that this method can shorten the time of medical health monitoring data classification, reduce the intrusion rate of medical health monitoring data, improve the security of health monitoring data storage, and has great significance for the integration and sharing of medical health data. In the future research work, targeted encryption measures should be taken for different intrusion modes to effectively ensure the storage security of medical health monitoring data.

Acknowledgement. 2020 Guangxi College and University Young and Middle aged Teachers' Basic Scientific Research Ability Improvement Project "Research and Development of Panoramic Campus Roaming System Cross platform" (2020KY63022).

References

1. Nguyen, T.T., Cai, K., Immink, K., et al.: Capacity-approaching constrained codes with error correction for DNA-based data storage. IEEE Trans. Inf. Theory **67**(8), 5602–5613 (2021)
2. Cai, K., Chee, Y.M., Gabrys, R., et al.: Correcting a single Indel/Edit for DNA-based data storage: linear-time encoders and order-optimality. IEEE Trans. Inf. Theory **67**, 3438–3451 (2021)
3. Feng, T., Jiao, Y., Fang, J., et al.: Medical health data security model based on alliance blockchain. Comput. Sci. **47**(04), 305–311 (2020)
4. Bai, Y., Man, J., Zhang, H.: Secure storage model of electronic health records based on blockchain. J. Comput. Appl. **40**(04), 961–965 (2020)
5. Liu, H., Ye, L.: Implementation of health data sharing based on distributed storage and computing technology. Chin. J. Health Inf. Manag. **18**(01), 143–146 (2021)
6. Hu, Y.C., Lokhandwala, M., Te, I., et al.: Varifocal storage: dynamic multi-resolution data storage. IEEE Micro **40**(3), 47–55 (2020)
7. Zheng, D., Xue, L., Yu, C., et al.: Toward assured data deletion in cloud storage. IEEE Network **34**(3), 101–107 (2020)
8. Cheng, L., Qi, Z., Shi, J.: Blockchain based secure storage and sharing scheme for EHR data. J. Nanjing University Posts Telecommun. (Nat. Sci. Ed.) **40**(04), 96–102 (2020)
9. Chang, J., Shao, B., Ji, Y., et al.: Efficient identity-based provable multi-copy data possession in multi-cloud storage, revisited. IEEE Commun. Lett. **24**(12), 1 (2020)
10. Yue, G., Liu, J., Liu, F.: Medical big data filling and classification simulation based on decision tree algorithm. Comput. Simul. **38**(01), 451–454+459 (2021)

Analysis on the Balance of Health Care Resource Allocation Based on Improved Machine Learning

Ying Wang[1](✉) and Helin Li[2]

[1] Xiamen Institute Of Technology, Xiamen 361000, China
wangying1102@126.com
[2] Sanmenxia Polytechnic, Sanmenxia 472000, China

Abstract. Health resource planning is an important means for the government to adjust resource allocation and achieve fair and efficient development of health. Its core is the balanced allocation of health resources. In order to solve the problem of low accuracy of health resource demand prediction, an analysis method of health resource allocation equilibrium based on improved machine learning was designed. Using the two-step mobile search method, combined with the Gaussian distance attenuation function and the search threshold set according to the classification of medical facilities, the spatial accessibility of weekday medical services is calculated. Based on the improved machine learning, the demand for health resources is predicted, and the change of resource characteristics and relevant policy variables leads to the change of health resource demand. According to the prediction results of the demand for health care resources, a supply-demand coordination model is constructed to measure the degree of coupling and coordination and the level of hierarchy. Lorentz curve was used to quantify the accessibility distribution of medical resources, Gini coefficient and global Moran index were calculated, and the equilibrium of health resource allocation was analyzed. The results show that this method can accurately predict the demand for health resources, and get the analysis results of allocation balance, which is conducive to the overall integration of medical resources.

Keywords: Improving Machine Learning · Medical Care · Health Resources · Allocation Balance

1 Introduction

Under the background of the basic establishment of the public health service system, the basic improvement of the national medical security system, and the deepening reform of the national health care system, the people's health level has significantly improved. The contradiction between residents' demand for healthy life and the current insufficient and unbalanced supply of medical facilities resources has become increasingly prominent, resulting in social phenomena such as "it is difficult and expensive to see a doctor". Health

S. Wang (Ed.): IoTCare 2022, LNICST 501, pp. 102–116, 2023.
https://doi.org/10.1007/978-3-031-33545-7_8

resource planning is an important means for the government to adjust resource allocation and achieve fair and efficient development of health. The core of health resource planning is to optimize the allocation of health resources. China's central and local governments have carried out a lot of health resource planning work, which has played an important role in optimizing the allocation of health resources [1]. The comprehensive promotion of the equalization of regional health services has brought about a significant improvement in people's health. The analysis of the supply and demand framework of basic public services shows that China is about to enter a period of consolidation and improvement of the equalization of basic public services characterized by "comprehensive coverage, fairness and equality, and balanced burden". Objectively, there is an imbalance in the development of economic and social levels between regions, resulting in great supply differences in medical facilities between regions and between urban and rural areas, which has a negative impact on the health level of residents in some backward areas. Due to the lack of reasonable theoretical framework and model in the existing health resource planning, the allocation of health resources follows the feeling of health managers and is divorced from the actual needs of residents. The quality of health services is increasingly prominent, the supply of public health services is fragmented and other problems are prominent, health resources are divided into blocks, unreasonable structure and layout, shortage and waste of health resources coexist, and there is a lack of overall and comprehensive planning within and between regions [2]. This also leads to the unbalanced allocation of health resources in the health service system and the provision of health services cannot meet the health needs and other problems. The current medical and health management mechanism still has shortcomings, resulting in prominent problems such as the quality of medical and health services, unreasonable structure and layout, which are specifically manifested as the lack of medical means in hospitals in some areas and the lack of customers, while some hospitals are overcrowded, resulting in the coexistence of shortage and waste of medical resources [3]. How to use health resource planning to better deepen the reform of the medical and health system and promote the construction of "healthy China" still needs to make greater efforts in the scientificity of planning and the effectiveness of planning implementation. Based on improved machine learning, this paper analyzes the balance of the allocation of health care resources, which is of great significance for the overall planning of the distribution of health care resources within and between regions, and to solve the current imbalance and unfairness of distribution.

2 Space Accessibility Calculation of Health Care Services

The research on the balance of medical resources involved in this study emphasizes the rational allocation of resources at the macro level, that is, using scientific planning means to enable residents in different locations to enjoy efficient and fair medical and health services, which should be reflected not only in geographical space, but also in quantity and quality. In this paper, the two-step mobile search method, combined with the Gaussian distance attenuation function and the search threshold set according to the classification of medical facilities, is used to study the spatial accessibility of weekday medical services. Accessibility impact mainly involves three factors: the attributes of medical service institutions (facility scale, grade, number of health technicians, financial and material resources of institutions, etc.), the attributes of medical service demand points (population, consumption level, population composition, medical preference, etc.), and travel costs (traffic network direction, road grade, speed limit, time spent, etc.). The two-step mobile search method and the gravity model method are most widely used in the evaluation of spatial accessibility, but the two-step mobile search method is easier to understand, has strong operability, and takes comprehensive consideration of both supply and demand sides. Because of its scale, personnel, equipment, capital and other advantages, hospitals are actually the most important subject of medical and health facilities and the most important research object in related fields [4]. The first step of the two-step mobile search method is to calculate the supply-demand ratio. The specific method is to divide the opportunity quantity or supply quantity of each facility by the demand quantity within the respective search threshold in the defined search threshold. The formula is:

$$p_x = \sum_{x=1}^{m_1} \frac{\alpha_x d_{xy}^2}{\sum\limits_{z=1}^{m_2} \beta_z d_{xy}} \tag{1}$$

In Eq. (1), p_x represents the ratio of the supply capacity α_x of the supply point x to the number of demanders served within the search threshold; d_{xy} is the distance cost between the supply point y and the supply point x; m_1 and m_2 represent the total number of supply points and demand points; β_z refers to the demand quantity; z indicates the demand point. The second step of the two-step mobile search method is medical accessibility. Its concept is a decisive factor affecting the fairness of medical and health services. As an important indicator to judge the shortage area of medical services, it plays an extremely important role in the scientific layout and planning of medical services. Supply capacity α_x can be calculated by substituting the number of beds, licensed doctors, registered nurses, daily outpatient volume and other data in the study. When considering accessibility, only the medical institution points within the threshold range are considered, and the points beyond the threshold range are not considered, and for the points within the threshold, regardless of distance, each medical point has the same impact on the accessibility of demand points [5]. In real life, the travel distance and time cost of medical facilities with different travel distances are very different for residents, so simple summation fails to take into account the distance attenuation between supply points and demand points. According to the attenuation characteristics and actual needs of the distance attenuation function, this paper selects the Gaussian function as the distance attenuation function, and the formula is:

$$d_{xy} = \frac{e^{-\frac{1}{2}\left(\frac{d_{xy}}{d_0}\right)^2} - e^{-\frac{1}{2}}}{1 - e^{-\frac{1}{2}}} \tag{2}$$

In Eq. (2), e is the natural constant; d_0 indicates the search threshold. Then calculate the sum of the supply-demand ratio of all facilities in each demand area within the search threshold. According to the accessibility score of the demand point x calculated by the two-step mobile search method, the actual meaning is the average facility resources that each demander can reach at the demand point x. Different from the original two-step mobile search method, the accessibility decay rate in the Gaussian distance decay function first accelerates and then slows down with the increase of distance, which is similar to people's expectations for the choice of medical facilities with the increase of travel distance or travel time in real life, and can more truly simulate the real decision-making state. The search scope selects the linear distance between the supply point and the demand point, Manhattan distance, great circle distance, or the actual road network distance according to the researchers' research purpose. The purpose of this paper is to study the medical accessibility of the actual situation, so the actual road network distance is selected for analysis. Associate the calculated spatial accessibility value to the residential population point data layer, use the point grid tool, select the spatial accessibility value as the generated value, turn the residential population point into a grid, and draw the spatial accessibility distribution diagram through the natural discontinuity method. Residents' access to ideal medical services is basically concentrated in urban areas or counties, and residents in areas with general spatial accessibility and below are mostly distributed in suburban or rural areas. The spatial accessibility is similar to the distribution characteristics of the traffic network. The regional accessibility of the dense traffic network also shows a high law. On the contrary, the regional accessibility of the sparse traffic network is also low.

3 Prediction of Health Resource Demand Based on Improved Machine Learning

Accurate prediction of demand is the basis of health resource planning, and the core of health resource planning is the optimal allocation of health resources. Therefore, accurate prediction of demand is the basis of health resource allocation. Health needs are affected by many factors, including personal factors, such as age, gender, occupation, education level, behavior style, etc. at the same time, they are also affected by many macro factors, such as economic level, health-related policies, etc. [6]. Medical service facilities can be divided into four categories: hospitals, basic medical service facilities, special public health facilities and other facilities. Among them, hospitals are divided into three levels, namely, tertiary hospitals, secondary hospitals and primary hospitals. The basic medical system includes urban and township parts. The township system consists of village health stations and township health centers, and the urban part consists of outpatient clinics and community health service centers (stations). This paper predicts the demand for health care resources based on improved machine learning. The basic idea of health resource demand prediction is shown in Fig. 1.

First, according to the characteristics of people's health needs, the micro units were sampled to obtain data to form a data file. According to the real health needs of the population, build a model to simulate the changes in the parameters of demand influencing factors. The residential population point data is the center point of the pixel converted from the 1-km spatial resolution grid. Crop worldpop 100 m spatial resolution grid data using administrative boundaries. Resample the grid and resample the original data into 1km spatial resolution grid data. When resampling, select the superposition method to process the value of the grid. Use the administrative boundary to crop the 1km spatial

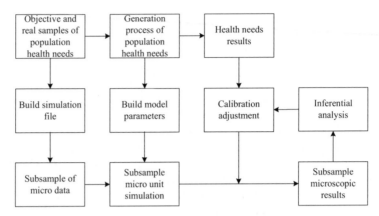

Fig. 1. Basic idea of health resource demand prediction

resolution grid, and then convert the grid data into the pixel center as the residential population point to participate in the calculation [7]. The kernel function of SVM can map low dimensional space to high dimensional space. In nonlinear problems, kernel functions can be used to add dimensions to the original data, thus transforming it into a linear problem in a higher dimensional space. The main function of Gaussian kernel function is composed of Euclidean distance equation, which is expressed as:

$$\vartheta(a, b) = \|a - b\| \tag{3}$$

In Eq. (3), ϑ represents Gaussian kernel function; a, b is the sample point. The traditional Gaussian kernel function can be expressed as:

$$\vartheta(a, b) = \exp\left(-\frac{\|a - b\|^2}{2\varepsilon^2}\right) \tag{4}$$

In Eq. (4), exp refers to exponential function; ε represents the width parameter. Computer programs are used to realize the changes of eigenvalues related to micro units due to the characteristics of micro units and the changes of relevant policy variables. Through the statistics, analysis, inference and synthesis of characteristic variables, the impact of policy changes on micro units can be obtained, and the implementation effects of policies at macro and all levels can be obtained. The population ratio is obtained by dividing the specific population allocated to each medical facility by the total service population of the corresponding medical facility, and then multiplying the population ratio by the number of resources of medical institutions within each range to calculate the number of medical resources of each medical facility occupied by each residential population. The main indicators in the database are individual health needs, needs and related influencing factors, including gender, age, marriage, education, urban and rural areas, healthy lifestyle factors, income, medical insurance, patient visits and hospitalization flow and other indicators. For the sample data of this study, each sample point is dense. When it is mapped to the high-dimensional space through the Gaussian kernel function, the sample points will become sparse. The way to alleviate this problem is to attenuate the Gaussian kernel function to a certain extent when it is far away from the test point, so as to enhance the learning ability. According to this condition, this study deforms the Gaussian kernel function by adding two displacement parameters φ_1 and φ_2 on the basis of the traditional Gaussian kernel function. The improved Gaussian kernel function is as follows:

$$\vartheta(a, b) = \exp\left(-\frac{\|a - b\|^2 + \varphi_1}{2\varepsilon^2} + \varphi_2\right) \tag{5}$$

In Eq. (5), φ_1 is the parameter that adjusts the amplitude of the function; φ_2 is the displacement bias of the adjustment kernel function. The improved SVM establishes a dynamic model of abstract system changes from discrete medical resource data to predict the demand for health care resources. After the model construction and test, the prediction results are analyzed and the fitting grade of the model is judged, and the prediction results of the original data are obtained. Reasonable allocation of community health service resources and Realization of the balance between supply and demand of community health services are the basic requirements for the optimal allocation of community health resources. The ultimate goal of the optimal allocation of health resources is to maximize the efficiency and benefits of community health services.

4   Build a Supply-Demand Coordination Model

In the process of using public medical resources, there may be inconsistencies between patients' personal needs and actual needs. When medicine believes that there is no need for medical services, but the actual utilization of medical services occurs, that is, there is "no need for demand", which will lead to the waste of medical resources. According to the prediction results of the demand for health care resources, a supply-demand coordination model is constructed, as shown in Fig. 2.

The essence of supply-demand coordination is to achieve dynamic balance between total supply and total demand, and to coordinate the proportion of supply and demand organically. Consistent with the actual needs, and based on this, we can obtain the expectation of effective medical services in medicine, that is, the reasonable expectation of public medical resources. The key factor is whether the individual on the demand side can obtain enough effective information. The supply system of medical and health facilities is divided into three primary indicators and six secondary indicators. The three primary indicators are economic input, facility allocation and medical efficiency. Among them, economic investment mainly reflects the strength of government capital investment and the level of regional economic development through medical financial investment and regional GDP; The facility allocation mainly reflects the facility scale, equipment scale and personnel scale through the building area, the number of beds and the number of health technicians; Medical efficiency mainly reflects the benefit efficiency of medical resources through the average number of daily diagnosis and treatment. The mismatch between supply and demand of public medical resources and the failure of graded diagnosis and treatment will cause great harm to patients and society. From the perspective of demand, the medical demand of outpatient services is calculated by

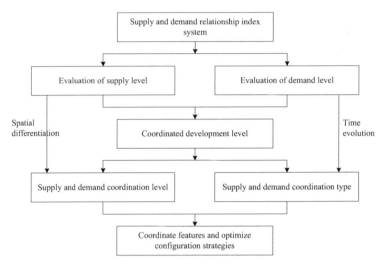

Fig. 2. Supply and demand coordination model

multiplying the number of people allocated to each medical facility by the annual per capita outpatient visits, and the resource supply is obtained by multiplying the number of health technicians by the medical ratio by the per capita daily visits of doctors by the number of doctor visits [8]. The residents' medical demand system is divided into three primary indicators and six secondary indicators. The three first-class indicators are population structure, economic level and traffic accessibility. Among them, the population structure mainly reflects the characteristics of population structure through the total population of each community, the proportion of floating population, the proportion of elderly population, and the proportion of population with high school education or above; The economic level is mainly reflected by the per capita income of residents; Traffic accessibility mainly selects the regional medical accessibility obtained from the previous analysis. After obtaining the supply-demand ratio between each residential population point and each medical facility, the Gauss distance attenuation function is used to modify the supply-demand ratio according to the time cost, and then the total number of residential population points on the assigned population ratio is multiplied by the supply-demand ratio to obtain the supply-demand ratio of each part of the population contribution. Finally, the probability of residents in each residential population point to obtain outpatient services is obtained by summarizing these supply-demand ratios according to the residential population points, Take this as the basis for evaluating the relationship between supply and demand. When it is considered that there is a need for medical services in medicine, but due to the high cost of medical treatment, inconvenient medical treatment, no corresponding medical resource supply or poor quality of medical resources and other conditions, the medical needs cannot be transformed into real needs, and the patients' diseases cannot be treated in a timely and effective manner. In order to quantitatively evaluate the coordinated development level of medical and health facilities, this paper constructs a coupling coordination degree model to judge its coupling coordination degree and level. The coupling coordination degree model involves the calculation of three index values, namely, the coupling degree S value, the coordination index γ value, and the coupling coordination degree χ value. The coupling degree is calculated as follows:

$$S = \left[(\beta_1\beta_2) \frac{(\beta_1 + \beta_2)^{-2}}{2} \right]^{\mu} \tag{6}$$

In Eq. (6), β_1 and β_2 are the comprehensive evaluation indexes of the supply and demand of medical and health facilities in the community respectively; μ refers to the adjustment coefficient, and the value is 2. The value of coupling degree S is used to reflect the relationship between supply and demand. The coordination index γ is used to reflect the overall synergy between facility supply and demand, and the formula is:

$$\gamma = \varpi_1\beta_1 + \varpi_2\beta_2 \tag{7}$$

In Eq. (7), ϖ_1 and ϖ_2 represent undetermined coefficients, both of which are taken as 0.5. The coupling coordination degree χ is an important index to evaluate the degree of supply-demand coordination. The formula is:

$$\chi = \sqrt{S\gamma} \tag{8}$$

When the value of coupling coordinated development degree is between 0–0.49, it is in the stage of supply and demand imbalance, and when the value of coupling coordinated development degree is between 0.50–1.00, it is in the stage of supply and demand imbalance. It is difficult for individual patients to do so because of information asymmetry; And in order to ensure good treatment effect, we often take adverse selection behavior according to our own cognition, giving priority to medical treatment with medical resources that we think are good brand, strong medical power, excellent equipment, good drugs, low risk and excellent quality, resulting in overcrowding in large hospitals and idle resources in small hospitals, which is mainly manifested in cross regional medical treatment. The current policies and allocation standards mostly take the service population and service radius as indicators to allocate medical and health facilities in the area. However, in the actual use process of residents, due to the different input-output ratio and use efficiency of various facilities, the supply level is also different; Even if the supply level is the same, residents' demand for medical and health facilities is different due to their own situation differences and external factors, indicating that the same supply can not meet the differentiated needs of residents.

5   Analysis on the Balance of Health Resources Allocation

The concept of health services is to serve citizens and ensure that residents in different areas of economic development and people of different income groups can enjoy equal health care services. In this study, Lorentz curve is used to quantify the accessibility distribution of medical resources. Lorentz curve refers to the curve formed by the point where the percentage of population "from the poorest population to the richest population" corresponds to the income percentage of each population percentage in a whole (country, region). The drawing method is that the horizontal axis is the percentage of population and the vertical axis is the cumulative percentage of accessibility. The drawing is completed by connecting the corresponding points. The fairness of medical resource allocation between urban regions is an important goal that must be considered. The economic, geographical, demographic and traffic conditions of different regions of a city are different, so the fairness of resource allocation must be guaranteed, and spatial accessibility is also the key to urban medical resource allocation from a spatial perspective. The Lorentz curve accumulates the population data of social wealth and wealth from small to large, and connects the data points corresponding to the percentage of population and its percentage of social wealth [9, 10]. Assuming that the closer the gap between the allocated resources of each region and the population percentage (or geographical area percentage) of its city, the fairer the hospital medical resources allocated by each region will be. Draw the absolute fair line on the basis of Lorentz curve. The area between the curve and the absolute fair line is A_1, and the area below the actual Lorentz curve is A_2. Using $A_1(A_1 + A_2)$ can reflect the degree of unfair distribution. This calculated value is called Gini coefficient. The Gini coefficient is the percentage of all residents' income used for uneven distribution. The minimum Gini coefficient is equal to 0, representing the absolute average of income distribution; The maximum is equal to 1, indicating that the income distribution is absolutely uneven. The actual Gini coefficient is between 0 and 1. If the difference between the resource allocation of each region and its percentage in the city's population (or the percentage of geographical area) is closer, the more equitable the resource allocation will be considered. The calculation formula of Gini coefficient is:

$$g = 1 - \frac{\frac{1}{2}\sum_{i=1}^{n}(q_i + q_{i+1})\psi_{i+1}}{5000} \tag{9}$$

In Eq. (9), g represents Gini coefficient; i and n respectively represent the sequence number and collection sequence of residential areas; q represents the cumulative proportion of resources and represents the accessibility value of medical resources in this study; ψ represents the corresponding proportion of population, which is calculated based on the population data of residential areas in this study. The absolute fairness between regions that only pay attention to resource allocation will ignore the accessibility of residents at the regional boundary, and will also lead to the problem of allocation efficiency, while paying attention to the spatial accessibility of resource allocation will ignore the balance of development between regions, and lack of consideration for the coordinated development between different regions of the city in the future. The global Moran index is used to judge the aggregation state of accessibility data distribution and the degree of correlation between data, the global Moran index is the most commonly used spatial autocorrelation index, which is an important research index to study the potential interdependence between the observation data of variables in the same distribution area. In short, it is to determine whether there is a correlation between spatial entities within a certain range, and its calculation expression is:

$$M = \frac{n}{\sum\limits_{i=1}^{n} q_i} \frac{\sum\limits_{i=1}^{n} \theta(q_i - \overline{q})}{\sum\limits_{i=1}^{n} (q_i - \overline{q})^2} \tag{10}$$

In Eq. (10), M represents the global Moran index; θ represents the spatial weight matrix; $\overline{q}$ represents the average of all study area data. For the specific model planning formula, the functional positioning of different levels of medical institutions, residents' medical behavior, regional balance, medical needs and other factors should be considered, and can be dynamically adjusted according to the future development of the city. Using the global Moran index, we can effectively obtain its spatial distribution equilibrium, and identify the corresponding data aggregation and dispersion state. For areas lacking medical resources or areas with waste and overflow of medical resources supply, it is also more accurate to identify, and then put forward planning suggestions for the scientific and reasonable allocation of medical resources and health facilities [11, 12]. If we want to achieve the goal of fairness of community health services, we need to have adequate protection in human resources, material resources and financial resources, eliminate the unfair factors of health services caused by geographical environment and economic conditions as far as possible, fully reflect the public interests of residents in the allocation of community health service resources, and ensure that residents can have fair access to community health services. Through continuous improvement, we will finally achieve a fair, reasonable and optimized allocation of community health service resources.

6 Experimental Study

6.1 Overview of the Study Area

Taking the allocation of health care resources in a city as the research object, the data of population distribution and medical resource distribution in the region were collected, and the balance of resource allocation was analyzed. The total population of the city is 2036528, and the regional population distribution is uneven. There are 43 medical and health institutions in the city, including 16 first-class hospitals, 14 s-class hospitals and 13 third-class hospitals. There are 58 township health centers and community health service centers. The distribution of medical and health institutions is relatively concentrated and mostly distributed in urban areas, with less distribution in township areas. Township health centers and community health service centers are evenly distributed, and each township and street has at least one health center or community health service center. On the whole, the spatial accessibility level of the southern region is higher than that of the northern region, and the spatial accessibility level of the central region is higher than that of the eastern and western regions. More than 85% of the residents are located in areas with good spatial accessibility and excellent grade, which shows that most of the population can enjoy better medical services. After the data collection in the study area is completed, the data are statistically analyzed and sorted out, and the obtained data are visually expressed by using Excel chart tools. And the final visualization is reflected in the demand forecast of health resources and the equilibrium analysis of health resource allocation. Combined with the data published in the statistical yearbook of the city, the general situation of medical resource allocation in each administrative region in the study area is summarized.

6.2   Prediction and Analysis of Health Resource Demand

In order to verify the prediction effect of this method on the demand for health care resources, the prediction accuracy is calculated. The test results are compared with the resource allocation equilibrium analysis method based on GM (1,1) grey prediction model and ARIMA model. The test results of the accuracy of demand forecast results are shown in Table 1.

Table 1.   Accuracy of demand forecast results

Number of tests	An improved machine learning based equilibrium analysis method for health care resource allocation	Analysis method based on GM (1,1) grey prediction model	Analysis method based on ARIMA model
1	0.692	0.584	0.524
2	0.755	0.561	0.511
3	0.693	0.542	0.582
4	0.756	0.575	0.595
5	0.742	0.526	0.597
6	0.781	0.513	0.614
7	0.724	0.502	0.601
8	0.748	0.551	0.625
9	0.765	0.584	0.642
10	0.782	0.567	0.616

According to the results in Table 1, this paper predicts the demand for health resources based on improved machine learning, with an accuracy of 0.744, which is 0.193 and 0.153 higher than the analysis methods based on GM (1,1) grey prediction model and ARIMA model. Therefore, the data prediction effect of this method is good, and it can effectively evaluate the demand for health care resources. The number of health institutions, licensed (Assistant) doctors, registered nurses and beds were analyzed by using the prediction results of improved machine learning.

5.3   Analysis of Resource Allocation Balance

The equilibrium of health resource allocation was analyzed from two aspects: Gini coefficient and global Moran index. The Gini coefficient of health resources is calculated according to population distribution and regional area distribution, and the results are shown in Table 2 and Table 3.

Table 2. Gini coefficient of health resources by population distribution

Particular year	Health institutions	Practicing (Assistant) doctor	Registered nurse	Bed
2012	0.2920	0.1832	0.2051	0.1788
2013	0.2762	0.1915	0.1934	0.1550
2014	0.2878	0.1858	0.1862	0.1632
2015	0.2853	0.1627	0.1825	0.1563
2016	0.2745	0.1546	0.1707	0.1449
2017	0.2686	0.1783	0.1618	0.1355
2018	0.2631	0.1455	0.1556	0.1256
2019	0.2360	0.1624	0.1585	0.1262
2020	0.2164	0.1567	0.1149	0.1036
2021	0.2412	0.1564	0.1426	0.1154

If the Gini coefficient is less than 0.2, it means that the degree of unfairness is very low, and the height in the region is average; If the value is 0.2–0.29, it means that the degree of unfairness is low and the region is relatively average; If the value is 0.3–0.39, it means that the degree of unfairness is moderate and the region is relatively reasonable; If the value is 0.4–0.59, it means that the degree of unfairness is high and the regional gap is large; If the value is above 0.6, it means that the degree of unfairness is very high, and the gap within the region is wide. According to the results in Table 2, from 2012 to 2021, the average Gini coefficients of health institutions, licensed (Assistant) doctors, registered nurses and beds were 0.2641, 0.1677, 0.1671 and 0.1405 respectively. The Gini coefficient of health institutions does not exceed 0.29, indicating that the imbalance of resource allocation is low; The Gini coefficient of the number of licensed (Assistant) doctors, registered nurses and beds is less than 0.2, and its resource allocation has a very low imbalance and is in a fair state. When the health resources are distributed according to the population, the Gini coefficient shows a downward trend with the increase of years, indicating that the balance is improving, and the allocation of health resources is becoming more and more equitable.

According to the results in Table 3, when medical and health resources are distributed by regional area, the average Gini coefficients of health institutions, licensed (Assistant) doctors, registered nurses and beds during 2012–2021 are 0.3792, 0.3344, 0.3090 and 0.2998 respectively. The number of health institutions, licensed (Assistant) doctors and registered nurses is between 0.3–0.39, indicating that the imbalance of the above three

Table 3. Gini coefficient of health resources distribution by regional area

Particular year	Health institutions	Practicing (Assistant) doctor	Registered nurse	Bed
2012	0.4133	0.3651	0.3425	0.3292
2013	0.4026	0.3586	0.3215	0.3145
2014	0.3895	0.3548	0.3288	0.3025
2015	0.3974	0.3434	0.3146	0.3186
2016	0.3826	0.3359	0.3143	0.3058
2017	0.3768	0.3285	0.3058	0.2954
2018	0.3648	0.3215	0.3072	0.2835
2019	0.3615	0.3176	0.2964	0.2902
2020	0.3521	0.3167	0.2837	0.2811
2021	0.3516	0.3023	0.2751	0.2772

medical resources is moderate, relatively reasonable in the region, and generally fair. The Gini coefficient of the number of beds is less than 0.3, indicating that the imbalance of resource allocation is low, which shows a relatively fair state. With the change of time, the Gini coefficient of the distribution of health resources by regional area shows a downward trend, indicating that the balance of resource allocation is improving year by year. Compared with the Gini coefficient of population distribution, the resource allocation balance of geographical distribution is relatively poor. There are certain differences between the two, which is relatively unfair. The global Moran index of various health care resources is calculated according to the population distribution, and the results are shown in Table 4.

Table 4. Global Moran index of health resources by population distribution

Particular year	Health institutions	Practicing (Assistant) doctor	Registered nurse	Bed
2012	0.0814	0.1406	0.1863	0.0935
2013	0.0951	0.1512	0.1752	0.0867
2014	0.1135	0.1455	0.1628	0.0854
2015	0.1268	0.1334	0.1586	0.0781
2016	0.1126	0.1268	0.1465	0.0748
2017	0.0953	0.1451	0.1554	0.0925
2018	0.0842	0.1243	0.1377	0.0856
2019	0.0984	0.1372	0.1441	0.0663
2020	0.0827	0.1285	0.1313	0.0792
2021	0.0865	0.1256	0.1292	0.0634

According to the results in Table 4, the global Moran index mean values of the number of health institutions, licensed (Assistant) doctors, registered nurses and beds are 0.0977, 0.1358, 0.1527 and 0.0806 respectively, indicating a high balance of resources. With the growth of time, the overall Moran index shows a downward trend, so the allocation equilibrium is also improving year by year.

In conclusion, the data prediction effect of the method presented in this paper is good, and it can effectively evaluate the demand for health care resources. The balance is improved and the allocation of health resources is more and more fair. Compared with the Gini coefficient of population distribution, the balance of resource allocation of geographical distribution is relatively poor, and there are some differences between the two, showing a more unfair performance. With the increase of time, the global Moreland index decreased, and the allocation balance also improved year by year.

7 Conclusion

At present, the spatial service scope defined by the 3000 m medical service circle used in the planning of medical facilities in China is often difficult to meet the actual medical needs of residents in reality. In order to match the actual medical needs, we need to give priority to policy guidance and further expand the medical service circle. Expand the service scope of various medical service resources, integrate various medical resources and facilities at all levels, and promote the establishment of medical consortia. Based on improved machine learning, this paper proposes an analysis method for the balance of health care resource allocation. This method can accurately predict and evaluate the resource demand, and is helpful to improve the accessibility and balance level of high-quality medical services. In this paper, the supply of medical services only considers the number of licensed (Assistant) doctors and registered nurses, without a comprehensive evaluation of the overall service capacity of the hospital, which can be considered in future research.

Fund Project. Xiamen Institute of Technology 2021 School-level Young and Middle-aged Scientific Research Fund Project: Binhai Nuclear Power Plant Disaster-Causing Organisms—Detection and Identification of Haitigua, Project No. 6

References

1. Li, X.-w, Zhu, W.: Equity evaluation of health resource allocation in Traditional Chinese Medicine hospitals in Henan. Mod. Preventive Med. **48**(17), 3157–3161 (2021)
2. Jiang, Y.-c., Yang, Y.-q., Wang, Z.-z.: Equilibrium of resource allocation in local health standardization in China: a cross-sectional survey among provincial level CDCs. Chinese J. Public Health **38**(6), 730–733 (2022)
3. Rodrigues, T.F., Nogueira, K., Chiarello, A.G.: Noninvasive low-cost method to identify armadillos' burrows: a machine learning approach. Wildl. Soc. Bull. **45**(3), 396–401 (2021)
4. Dang, A.T., Tsujimura, M., Ha, N.T., et al.: Evaluating the predictive power of different machine learning algorithms for groundwater salinity prediction of multi-layer coastal aquifers in the Mekong Delta, Vietnam. Ecol. Ind. **127**(1), 107–120 (2021)

5. Hou, J., Zhang, G.-y.: Dynamic scheduling simulation of massive fragment resources based on cloud computing. Comput. Simulation **37**(1), 360–364 (2020)
6. Tian, H., Zhu, J., He, X., et al.: Using machine learning algorithms to estimate stand volume growth of Larix and Quercus forests based on national-scale Forest Inventory data in China. Forest Ecosystems **9**(3), 396–406 (2022)
7. Huang, W., Tian, K.: Current status and equity of regional health care resource allocation in Jiangsu Province. China Med. Administration Sci. **12**(2), 23–27 (2022)
8. Jain, D.K., Kalyanapusrinivas, A., Srinivasu, S., et al.: Machine learning based monitoring system with IoT using wearable sensors and Pre-convoluted Fast Recurrent Neural Networks (P-FRNN). IEEE Sens. J. **21**(22), 25517–25524 (2021)
9. Zhou, T.: Analysis of the characteristics of spatial and hierarchical differentiation and its driving mechanism of urban and rural medical resources in Chongqing. Chin. Health Service Manag. 39(4), 275–279,300 (2022)
10. Wang, H., Luo, L., Yu, C.: Research on the planning completion rate and disequilibrium of health resource allocation in Guangxi in 2015–2019. Chinese Hospitals **25**(11), 20–23 (2021)
11. Penido, E.K., Paixa, R.C.F.D., Costa, L.C.B., et al.: Predicting the compressive strength of steelmaking slag concrete with machine learning - Considerations on developing a mix design tool. Constr. Build. Mater. **341**(25), 1–10 (2022)
12. Huang, M.C., Xu, H.Y., Yu, H.: Fast prediction of methane adsorption in shale nanopores using kinetic theory and machine learning algorithm. Chem. Eng. J. **446**(3), 1–12 (2022)

Data Acquisition Method of Human Injury in Sports Based on Internet of Things

Helin Li[1(✉)] and Ying Wang[2]

[1] Sanmenxia Polytechnic, Sanmenxia 472000, China
lihelin674h0@163.com
[2] Xiamen Institute of Technology, Xiamen 361000, China

Abstract. Traditional data acquisition methods usually collect and upload data at a fixed time interval, which is easy to generate a large number of redundant data, leading to large acquisition errors. To solve this problem, this study designed a new method of human injury data collection in sports based on the Internet of things. First of all, select the strong representative features such as the mean value and peak mean value of human injury data, and detect the human motion state according to the resultant acceleration, signal intensity region and tilt angle. Then, set up multiple sensors. Capture multi angle information of human motion data. Finally, using the adaptive strategy, the ratio of the residual energy and the total energy of the Internet of Things collection node is used to characterize the overall energy state of the node, reduce data redundancy, and then send the data to the data sink node through wireless transmission to confirm the current human motion injury state. Test results show that the average acquisition error of this method is relatively small, and it can collect human injury data more accurately in long-term sports.

Keywords: Internet of things · Athletic sports · Human body injury · Data collection · Movement characteristics · Adaptive acquisition

1 Introduction

Good health not only helps us to maintain a positive and optimistic mood and attitude towards life, but also helps to enhance happiness and self-confidence. Having a strong physique is the fundamental guarantee for our study, work and life. At present, regular sports have been proved to be helpful in slowing down and preventing the development of chronic diseases, and have important significance in sub-health intervention and promoting human health. But in sports, we need to follow a certain scientific way, otherwise, it will not only be difficult to achieve the purpose of strengthening the body and curing diseases, but even counterproductive, causing secondary damage to the body.

In sports, it is necessary to monitor the sports state of athletes, and understand the exercise situation of sports participants according to their state, including whether the action category is correct, the number of actions, the amount of exercise and the period

S. Wang (Ed.): IoTCare 2022, LNICST 501, pp. 117–130, 2023.
https://doi.org/10.1007/978-3-031-33545-7_9

are appropriate. In this process, it is an important link to collect and analyze the injury data of sports participants, which can help people track their own health at the sports fitness level [1].

At present, the wireless body area network (WBAN) composed of multi-sensor is usually used to assist instructors to monitor the movement of sports participants, determine the movement status of participants by collecting human injury data, and make timely corrections and guidance, adjust their exercise intensity in a timely manner, give early warning to individual sports fatigue, and give an alarm at the first time when abnormal conditions occur in the participants' bodies, The medical staff shall be informed to carry out timely rescue and realize continuous dynamic monitoring of important parts of the human body [2].

On the basis of traditional research, this paper proposes a method of collecting human injury data in sports based on the Internet of Things, which makes it possible to monitor user oriented sports, and makes it easier for people to obtain professional sports guidance when participating in sports exercises, so as to improve the professionalism of sports and exercise participants, effectively avoid the occurrence of sports injuries, and improve the effect of sports exercises.

2   Analysis of Human Motion Characteristics

The movements of the lower limbs of the human body are achieved by driving the bones through the relevant skeletal muscles to complete the rotation of the corresponding joints. The main muscles of the lower limbs are the hip muscles, thigh muscles, calf muscles and foot muscles. The human body has different exclusive characteristics in different movement modes such as standing, walking, and running. The travel speed, ups and downs of the center of gravity, height and posture in different movement modes will all affect the gait of the movement. A general multi-sensor human posture data acquisition system needs to configure 11 sensors, which are located in 11 parts of the human body's head, upper arm, lower arm, chest, abdomen, thigh and calf, and the sensor binding position is between the two joints on body parts. However, due to the large number of sensors used in this process, the system has high requirements for data aggregation and fusion, which easily leads to low effective recognition rate of the final information.

In order to improve the operation and recognition efficiency of the system, the sensor nodes of the head, chest and lower arm are removed in this paper, because the pose data of the head and lower arm have little impact on the pose recognition, which is relatively redundant. The motion of the chest and abdomen are basically similar, so one is taken as the node. When the human body remains standing, there is no obvious movement sign except for the normal natural weak shaking of the human body. The characteristic data with strong representativeness such as the mean value, peak mean value, standard deviation, covariance and skewness of the data are selected as the characteristic values of motion pattern recognition.

The standard deviation of human injury data in sports is calculated as follows:

$$\varepsilon = \sqrt{\frac{1}{u} \sum_{i=1}^{u} \left(A_i - \overline{A}\right)^2} \tag{1}$$

In formula (1), ε is the standard deviation; u is the number of data samples; i is the data serial number; A_i is the data sample; $\overline{A}$ is the mean. The standard deviation reflects the volatility of the action range. The standard deviation can reflect the range of human motion in sports. The larger the range of motion, the greater the standard deviation. The smaller the range of motion, the smaller the standard deviation.

Seven sensors were used in the study, which were bound to seven parts of the human body, including the left upper arm, right upper arm, abdomen, left thigh, left calf, right thigh and right calf. The coordinate system that specifies the initial binding position of each sensor is consistent, the X axis points to the left side of the human body, the Y axis points to the top of the human body, and the Z axis points to the front of the human body [3]. Because the muscles of the lower limbs need to maintain the balance of the human body, stand stably, and walk frequently, they are more developed and powerful than the muscles of the upper limbs of the human body. The complete time from the heel of a lower extremity touching the ground to the heel of the lower extremity touching the ground again is the gait cycle. In this time period, the gait cycle can be effectively divided into a support period and a swing period according to whether the foot of the lower limb touches the bottom. Covariance is often used to calculate and evaluate the overall error between two sets of variables. Therefore, calculate the covariance difference between the acceleration and angular velocity at the upper and lower limbs of the human body, and identify the motion state according to the calculation results. The covariance is calculated as follows:

$$c = \frac{\sum\limits_{i=1}^{u} \left(b_i - \overline{b}\right)(\gamma_i - \overline{\gamma})}{u - 1} \tag{2}$$

In formula (2), c is covariance; b_i and $\overline{b}$ represent acceleration samples and combined values; γ_i and $\overline{\gamma}$ represent the sum of angular velocity samples. The covariance feature of the standard matrix of the static attitude is roughly distributed between 0.09 and 0.011, and the variance feature of the standard matrix of the moving attitude is highly distinguishable from the static attitude. Therefore, the static attitude and the moving attitude can be distinguished by this feature. The data point distribution dispersion, peak valley value difference and numerical point distribution ratio have characteristics similar to acceleration. The respective kurtosis of the data represents the slope of the data fluctuation peak, which can reflect the maximum amplitude of human movement. The calculation formula is:

$$\varphi = \frac{\sum\limits_{i=1}^{u} \left(A_i - \overline{A}\right)^4 h}{u\varepsilon^4} \tag{3}$$

In formula (3), φ is the kurtosis; h is the sample interval of the data. Different from the slow walking mode, the running speed in the running mode is faster, and the frequency of changes in the center of gravity of the human body increases. It is necessary to increase the frequency, speed up, and increase the range of motion and elbow curvature to maintain the stability of the human body. The phase division of the gait cycle presents periodic changes in time and space [4]. And according to the phase change of the corresponding gait cycle, the data characteristics of the surface EMG signal of the lower limbs of the human body also have corresponding periodic changes, and at the same time have a high correlation with the gait cycle.

3 Motion State Description

In order to describe the motion state of human body, it is necessary to introduce several motion features, including acceleration, signal intensity region and inclination angle. The principle of the accelerometer is to calculate the acceleration value of the block at this moment through the force generated by the inertia of a block in motion. The accelerometer can not only measure the acceleration of the block, but also the gravity value of the block. The resultant acceleration represents the arithmetic square root of the vector sum of squares of triaxial accelerations in space. The calculation formula of resultant acceleration $v(t)$ at time t is as follows:

$$v(t) = \sqrt{v_x^2(t) + v_y^2(t) + v_z^2(t)} \tag{4}$$

In formula (4), $v_x(t)$, $v_y(t)$, $v_z(t)$ represents the output value of the acceleration sensor in the three directions of X, Y, and Z, respectively. $v(t)$ is a general description of the acceleration value changes in all directions, which can reflect the intensity of the human body's motion state.

Compared with the standing state, when the human body is in the slow walking state, the acceleration in the X, Y and Z directions increases with the increase of the swing arm speed and frequency. The resultant acceleration fluctuates between 5.285–17.391 m/s2. The angular velocity changes with the action amplitude and the curvature of the axis joint, the peak valley value difference increases, and the resultant angular velocity fluctuates between 0.125–2.847 rad / s.

Due to the abnormal jitter in the movement process and the influence of the measurement environment, it is inevitable to produce noise. The frequency of human motion is generally concentrated in 0-20Hz, and the change is more obvious in 0-5Hz, and the frequency of noise is certainly greater than this frequency. Therefore, low-pass filter can be selected to suppress noise [5].

When a fall occurs, the change of the $v(t)$ curve increases significantly, so the fall behavior can be preliminarily judged by setting the threshold value of the resultant acceleration. The SMV curve changes of falls are similar to those of strenuous exercise and running. This paper uses a 4th-order Butterworth low-pass filter to denoise the triaxial acceleration and triaxial angular velocity data. Filter parameters: the pass-band cut-off frequency is 20 Hz, the stop-band cut-off frequency is 23.5 Hz; the minimum pass-band attenuation is 3 dB; the stop-band maximum attenuation is 20 dB. Use the signal strength area to make up for the lack of $v(t)$-curve threshold detection. The signal strength area W can be used to analyze the amplitude of dynamic motion, and its expression is:

$$W = \frac{1}{t} \left(\int_0^1 \left| v_x(t) \right| dt + \int_0^1 \left| v_y(t) \right| dt + \int_0^1 \left| v_z(t) \right| dt \right) \tag{5}$$

For some movements, the limbs always move in the horizontal plane during the movement, so the average acceleration along the axis of the limb direction is always near zero. For other movements, the limbs always move in the vertical plane, so the average acceleration along the axis of the limb direction is around 1g. Because there are some similarities in the behavior of human activities, such as the acceleration changes of falling and rapid sitting are relatively similar, the tilt angle is used to judge the posture. The inclination angle represents the angle between the body and the vertical direction, and the formula is:

$$\beta = ar\cos\left(\frac{l(t)}{g}\right)\left(\frac{180}{\pi}\right) \tag{6}$$

In formula (6), β is the inclination angle; $l(t)$ is the height of the body torso; g is the acceleration of gravity. In the whole process of falling, the human body will be in different states over time during the fall, and the change of the posture of the human body from $0°$ to $90°$ during the fall process can be reflected by the inclination angle. In the static state, the three-axis angular velocity data should be zero, the X, Y axis acceleration should be zero, and the Z axis acceleration should be $+1g$ or $-1g$, but the data measured by the sensor will drift during the actual measurement process. Data to compensate. After compensation, the acceleration measurement value of the sensor is stable at 0.001g, and the angular velocity measurement value is stable at 0.05°/s, which corrects the error.

4 Multi-sensor Data Fusion in Human Motion

The motion data collected by the sensor will be uniformly encrypted and stored in the database, and the identification result is only the motion status information and the number of the safety device worn. Therefore, it can effectively avoid adverse effects caused by personal data leakage [6].

Before entering the designated area, the person being tested should enter personal characteristic information, that is, personal movement characteristic data, so as to ensure that all safety device wearers can be accurately identified. The terminal locations in the area are similar, and the collected environmental parameters have strong coupling, that is, there is a spatial correlation between the sensing data of each terminal in the monitoring area. The time synchronization server is the timing center of the system, which can provide millisecond-level time synchronization for all distributed positioning devices. The sensing data of a single collection terminal can form a time series, and through the analysis of the time series, it can be found that the sensing data within a certain period of time has a strong temporal correlation [7]. Each pressure sensor can actually provide complementary information. That is to say, each sensor in complementary fusion captures different aspects of the monitored object, which is used to improve the accuracy and reliability of the system. Therefore, the sensing data collected by the terminals in the adjacent monitoring area have strong spatial and temporal correlation. The data fusion process is shown in Fig. 1.

The time synchronization server is equipped with a microcontroller and a RF transceiver, which periodically broadcasts the relative time value to all distributed positioning devices in the space field through wireless communication. Each distributed position device maintains time synchronization with the time synchronization server,

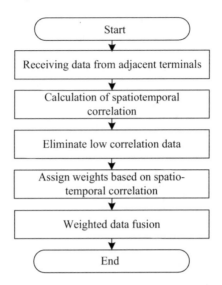

Fig. 1. Schematic diagram of isomorphic data fusion

thereby realizing time synchronization between all distributed positioning devices [8]. Firstly, the dynamic time planning distance method is used to calculate the spatial distance of terminal data at each time point in a period of time. In the window time, the time data series of terminals E_1 and E_2 are $\zeta(E_1)$ and $\zeta(E_2)$ respectively, and the distance D between terminal perceived data is expressed as:

$$D=f[\zeta(E_1), \zeta(E_2)] + \min f\left[\zeta'(E_1), \zeta'(E_2)\right] \tag{7}$$

In formula (7), f is the Euclidean distance between the corresponding data points in the sequence; ζ' is the sequence of the previous data sampling period. The main function of the time synchronization server is to send time information regularly to ensure the time synchronization of the entire network. The distance between data points is calculated recursively. By calculating the distance of each terminal data, the median absolute dispersion method is used to set the correlation threshold, and the low correlation terminal data exceeding the threshold will not participate in this data fusion.

Generally, for statistical data, the number of digits is reserved to 6 significant digits at most. Therefore, for the data extracted by different sensors, the data digits are unified respectively to avoid the error impact on the subsequent eigenvalue extraction. Take the median of the calculated space-time distance and calculate the absolute difference with each distance, and then take the median of all the obtained absolute values as MAD. Calculate the correlation degree between the terminal data according to the calculated dynamic time planning distance, and use the exponential function to quantify the spatiotemporal correlation degree between the terminal data, which is expressed as:

$$R = e^{-\frac{D^2}{2}} \tag{8}$$

In formula (8), R is the spatiotemporal correlation degree; e is an exponential function. The weight is allocated according to the strength of the correlation degree, wherein the higher the correlation degree between the terminal perception data, the greater the allocated weight. According to the size of the weights, weighted data fusion is performed on the currently collected sensing data to achieve the purpose of improving the accuracy of the sensing data.

In order to directly import relevant data into MATLAB for eigenvalue calculation, the sensor category name and time node information are eliminated, and only the human motion dynamic data detected by the sensor is retained. Even if the information provided by multiple pressure sensors is used, it is still unable to obtain gait spatial measures such as stride length and pace. When multiple kinds of sensor signals are needed to obtain information that cannot be obtained by observing these signals independently, collaborative fusion plays a role. According to the assigned weights, the isomorphic perceptual data with strong spatial-temporal correlation is weighted for data fusion, and the fusion results will be reported to the server as the final measured data value of the terminal.

5 Establishing a Sports Injury Data Collection Model Based on the Internet of Things

The above contents analyze the human motion characteristics, describe the motion state, and implement the fusion of multi-sensor data in the human motion process. On this basis, take the fused multi-sensor data as the basic data, and establish the sports injury data acquisition model based on the Internet of Things.

Large-scale data acquisition and transmission requires the acquisition system to support long-distance communication and support a large number of sensor nodes to work at the same time. The data acquisition model proposed in this paper is shown in Fig. 2.

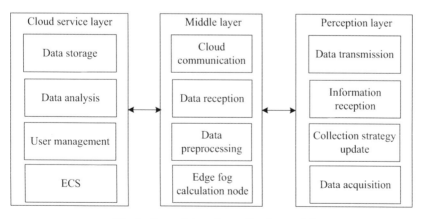

Fig. 2. Sports injury data collection model

Collection setting is a necessary configuration module for data collection, mainly an interface management module that needs to be configured for a collection task. In this part, the interface design of configurable collection, analysis and conversion will be realized. It includes task ID, DTU enable, acquisition command, acquisition cycle, task mode, matching rules, data segmentation, data conversion, filtering rules, incremental threshold, maximum and minimum value (optional), adaptive switch, etc. The data acquisition of human sports injury is located in the perception layer, and the adaptive adjustment of data acquisition interval is completed according to the set adaptive acquisition strategy.

In traditional data collection methods, data are generally collected at fixed time intervals and uploaded. The data interaction is carried out in the CBI mode, and all the information in the system interface will be saved through the configuration file, which is logically the corresponding relationship between nodes and sub-nodes [9]. The fixed acquisition interval requires consideration of energy consumption and data sensitivity. When the human body motion is in a stable state, performing data collection at fixed intervals will generate a large amount of redundant data and waste energy. When sports are in a state of rapid change, if the set collection time interval is too large, it will inevitably lead to less data collected. The information display method of each check box in the configuration interface is the node name and the node field name consists of two important parts. The precondition for data transmission is to establish a connection between the two parties. This part is transmitted using the TCP protocol, and the data transmission is performed by establishing a socket channel.

When the acquisition system adopts fixed interval for data acquisition, there will be problems if the acquisition interval is set too short or too long. Therefore, the acquisition system needs to be able to reasonably set the acquisition frequency according to the demand, so as to maximize the contradiction between data perception and energy consumption [10]. In this paper, an adaptive strategy is proposed to select the ratio of residual energy and total energy of nodes to represent the overall energy state of nodes. After initializing the acquisition, start to adjust the acquisition interval. When the collected data changes frequently, the collection interval will be dynamically reduced. Assuming that the value of the data currently collected by the system is Z_0 and Z is the data reference threshold, there are:

$$Z = \begin{cases} Z_{min}, Z_0 < Z_{min} \\ Z_{max}, Z_0 > Z_{max} \end{cases} \tag{9}$$

In formula (9), Z_{min} and Z_{max} are the minimum and maximum thresholds of sports injury data, respectively. After obtaining the reference threshold, it is necessary to calculate the degree of deviation of the data. At this time, the following method is used to calculate:

$$\begin{cases} \eta_1 = |Z_0 - Z| \\ \eta_2 = Z_{max} - Z_{min} \end{cases} \tag{10}$$

In Eq. (10), η_1 is the difference between the collected data and the reference threshold; η_2 is the difference between the maximum threshold and the minimum threshold. On this basis, the adaptive acquisition strategy can be expressed as:

$$\kappa = \begin{cases} \kappa_0 \left(1 - \dfrac{\eta_1}{\eta_2}\right)\left(1 - \dfrac{\delta}{\delta_0}\right), \eta_1 \le \eta_2 \\ \kappa_{min}, \eta_1 > \eta_2 \end{cases} \tag{11}$$

In formula (11), κ represents the updated acquisition interval; κ_0 and κ_{min} represent the initial acquisition interval and the set minimum motion injury data acquisition interval, respectively; δ and δ_0 represent the current state and initial energy of the acquisition node, respectively. The entire transmission process includes initializing the connection of the device, obtaining the mac address for data MD5 verification, obtaining the node data of the configuration file, establishing the channel and authenticating, and waiting for the data packet to be sent. When the data is in a normal state, the system tends not to update the collection interval, but uses the initial collection interval for data collection; when the data fluctuation exceeds the normal range, the system needs to update the collection interval. After the transmission channel is established, the gateway sends a collection command to the gateway through the Modbus TCP protocol. After receiving the collection command, the collection end will immediately feed back the information data stream. After the gateway receives the data, the data will be analyzed, matched and filtered. Operation, and send the collection result package to the cloud. Data needs to be formatted and preprocessed after collection.

In the txt text file, in addition to the real-time sensor data in the X, Y and Z directions, the data information collected by the sensor also includes the category annotation and coordinate axis annotation of each sensor. In addition, the digital digits recorded and saved by each category of data are lack of consistency, so it is necessary to sort out all data contents according to categories. Considering the extreme situation that the data deviates too much, and when the new acquisition cycle calculated is less than the sleep time supported by the hardware, this acquisition interval will be set as the minimum acquisition interval. Control the relevant sensors and obtain the readings of the equipment to obtain the data of the motion state; Send data to the data convergence node by wireless way; Receive the information of the data convergence node to confirm the current motion state. Before data analysis, it is necessary to import the contents of txt file recording motion data into the Excel table of Office, and classify the contents and set the digits of the imported information.

6 Experimental Studies

In order to verify the practical application effect of the data collection method of human injury in sports based on the Internet of Things, a comparative experiment was designed to compare the method in this paper with the traditional data collection method based on association rule algorithm and the data collection method based on edge computing.

6.1 Experiment Preparation

The data processing program in this paper is based on the GUI module in MATLAB as the development platform, and the upper computer software system is built. In the experimental test, 10 volunteers (aged 25–45 years old, height 160cm-180cm, 5 males and 5 females) were invited to conduct sports data collection experiments.

The acquisition experiment requires the subjects to perform the data acquisition experiment of the exercise process in a state of no muscle fatigue and a good mental state. The purpose of the action counting and cycle calculation experiments is to verify the accuracy of data collection. For this experiment, the objectiveness of the experimental results is largely affected by the number of trials. Especially for action counting, the validity of the analysis method can only be demonstrated if the results are still accurate when the number of times is sufficient. The experiment set the data collection time as 60 min, and repeated 50 movements during this time. This value is higher than the number of times required for a single exercise, which can verify the accuracy of the method.

During the experiment, in addition to using sensors to collect and record motion data, a stopwatch was also used to time the cycle of each action as the actual standard.

6.2   Results and Analysis

For the movement of limbs rotating around joints, the sensitive axis is generally angular velocity, while for the vertical movement of limbs such as shoulder pushing and heel lifting, the sensitive axis is acceleration. Therefore, the angular velocity and acceleration of motion are selected as the collected data for the experiment.

Due to the different structure of the crowd and the different physical characteristics of individual pedestrians, the statistical distribution of stride length and stride frequency is often relatively discrete, because for individual pedestrians, the size of their stride length is largely subject to their physical characteristics. In motion, the amplitude and frequency of motion fluctuations fluctuate in varying degrees with the intensity of motion changes. Therefore, it is of practical significance to select stride and stride frequency data to analyze the effect of injury data collection.

The average error of data acquisition is obtained by comparing the motion data acquisition value with the actual value. In the 60 min test time, the results of motion angular velocity, acceleration, stride and step frequency data acquisition error obtained by different methods are shown in Table 1, 2, 3 and 4.

In the angular velocity data acquisition, the average acquisition error of the human injury data acquisition method in sports based on the Internet of things designed in this paper is 2.34%, which is 1.32% and 2.11% lower than the comparison acquisition method based on association rule algorithm and edge calculation.

In the sports acceleration data acquisition, the average acquisition error of the human injury data acquisition method in sports based on the Internet of things designed in this paper is 2.02%, which is 1.81% and 2.45% lower than the comparison acquisition method based on association rule algorithm and edge calculation.

In the movement stride data acquisition, the average acquisition error of the human injury data acquisition method in sports based on the Internet of things designed in this paper is 2.17%, which is 1.49% and 1.95% lower than the comparison acquisition method based on association rule algorithm and edge calculation.

In the step frequency data acquisition, the average acquisition error of the human injury data acquisition method in sports based on the Internet of things designed in this paper is 2.27%, which is 1.00% and 1.64% lower than the comparison acquisition method

Table 1. Motion angular velocity data acquisition error (%)

Acquisition time (min)	Data collection method of human body injury in sports based on Internet of Things	Data collection method of human body injury in sports based on association rule algorithm	Data collection method of human body injury in sports based on edge computing
5	1.84	3.59	4.16
10	1.91	3.66	5.52
15	2.55	3.45	3.46
20	2.60	3.14	5.36
25	2.52	4.57	4.95
30	1.86	2.31	3.85
35	2.78	3.68	5.47
40	2.25	4.52	4.52
45	2.54	5.26	5.58
50	2.82	3.23	3.36
55	1.96	2.65	3.49
60	2.43	3.88	3.63

Table 2. Motion acceleration data acquisition error (%)

Acquisition time (min)	Data collection method of human body injury in sports based on Internet of Things	Data collection method of human body injury in sports based on association rule algorithm	Data collection method of human body injury in sports based on edge computing
5	1.34	4.43	4.26
10	1.61	3.16	5.28
15	2.25	4.05	5.59
20	1.92	2.52	4.96
25	1.83	3.28	3.37
30	2.76	5.86	3.41
35	2.65	3.93	4.86
40	2.78	4.61	5.50
45	2.09	3.34	4.29
50	1.66	3.57	3.63
55	1.52	3.72	4.14
60	1.84	3.45	4.35

Table 3. Movement stride data collection error (%)

Acquisition time (min)	Data collection method of human body injury in sports based on Internet of Things	Data collection method of human body injury in sports based on association rule algorithm	Data collection method of human body injury in sports based on edge computing
5	2.54	3.16	3.26
10	2.41	3.25	3.48
15	2.95	3.48	4.47
20	1.82	3.96	2.95
25	1.66	2.52	3.63
30	1.43	2.74	4.48
35	1.72	4.96	5.96
40	1.55	4.35	4.58
45	2.28	3.35	4.47
50	2.36	3.48	5.11
55	2.43	4.62	3.35
60	2.84	4.08	3.68

Table 4. Movement cadence data collection error (%)

Acquisition time (min)	Data collection method of human body injury in sports based on Internet of Things	Data collection method of human body injury in sports based on association rule algorithm	Data collection method of human body injury in sports based on edge computing
5	2.66	2.48	2.86
10	1.85	2.62	3.74
15	1.44	3.59	4.98
20	2.57	4.47	5.61
25	2.61	2.58	2.95
30	2.75	2.63	2.90
35	2.48	3.12	3.39
40	1.82	3.15	3.65
45	1.96	2.41	4.58
50	2.53	4.86	4.46
55	2.34	3.59	4.73
60	2.28	3.75	3.12

based on association rule algorithm and edge calculation. The data acquisition interval of the design method in this paper will be adjusted adaptively with the deviation of the collected data and the change of energy. Therefore, the average error of the acquisition is relatively small, and the data acquisition of human injury can be realized more accurately in long-term sports.

7 Conclusion

In sports training, it is necessary to monitor the movement state of the athlete. A network composed of multi-sensors can assist the instructor to monitor the body movements of the sports participants, and by collecting the data of the human body injury, it is possible to know whether the number and cycle of the athlete's movements are appropriate.

In the traditional data collection method, data is generally collected and uploaded at fixed time intervals, which will generate a large amount of redundant data and cause a waste of energy. Aiming at this problem, this paper designs a data collection method for human injury in sports based on the Internet of Things. After the acquisition is initialized, the adjustment of the acquisition interval begins. When the collected data changes frequently, the collection interval will be dynamically reduced. Control the relevant sensors and obtain the readings of the equipment to obtain the motion data, and send the data to the data aggregation node wirelessly to collect the current motion state data. The average error of the collector in this paper is relatively small, which can achieve accurate collection of long-term motion data.

Although the method designed in this paper improves the ability of environmental perception, the overall energy consumption of the proposed strategy is still large in the case of drastic changes in the environment. Therefore, the next step is to study a more reasonable node sleep strategy to further reduce the energy consumption of data collection.

References

1. Shi, L., Xu, C.: Construction and application of sports monitoring big data platform. Contemporary Sports Technol. **12**(12), 9–13,18 (2022)
2. Sun, J., Zhou, Z.: Design of human movement data acquisition system based on wearable devices. Developm. Innovat. Mach. Electrical Products **35**(1), 38–41 (2022)
3. Hu, C., Zhao, H.: Human motion pattern recognition based on wrist imu data collection. J. Ningxia Univ. (Nat. Sci. Ed.) **42**(1), 45–50+57 (2021)
4. Ren, K., Wang, C.: Indoor data acquisition and monitoring system based on Internet of things. Chin. J. Liquid Crystals Displays **35**(2), 136–142 (2020)
5. Zhu, C., Ren, J.: Heterogeneous Data fusion method of internet of things based on intelligent optimization agorithm. J. Jilin Univ. (Sci. Ed.) **57**(03), 627–632 (2019)
6. Tong, X.: Multi channel communication network data cross layer acquisition timing control. Comput. Simulat. **38**(12), 341–344+419 (2021)
7. Huang, Y., Zeng, P.: Study on all-day intelligent motion assistant system. Intell. Comput. Appli. **17**(7), 120–123 (2021)
8. Deng, F., Fan, Y.: Intelligent sport-health management system based on big data mining and internet of things.Henan Sci. Technol. **40**(07), 14–17 (2021)

9. Liu, C., WEI, S., Jia, J., et al.: Research of respiratory motion monitoring using microsoft Kinect v2 sensor. Foreign Electronic Measure. Technol. **39**(12), 6–10 (2020)
10. Liu, Y., Wang, S., Jia, Y., et al.: Design and implementation of human motion data acquisition system. Internet of Things Technol. **12**(08), 130–132 (2022)

Big Data Technologies for e-Care

The Psychosocial Therapy Mode Intervened in the Emotion Management of Property Management Staff

Qianyi Wan[1](✉) and Changyan Liu[2]

[1] Institute of Health and Industry, Sichuan College of Arts and Sciences, Dazhou 635002, China
dgsgs7882@163.com

[2] Sichuan University of Arts and Sciences, Chengdu 610110, China

Abstract. With the continuous growth of our country's economy and people's happiness, people's improvement of the living environment and competition in the real estate industry have become increasingly fierce. The emotions of property employees at work will have a direct impact on the owners, and the construction of a harmonious living environment will have a significant impact on the improvement of the human resource management level of the property's capabilities and the impact of the company's brand. The purpose of this article is to study the psychosocial therapy model involved in the emotional management of property management employees. This article first introduces the basic theory of emotional management, and then elaborates on the current situation of the property management staff, and analyzes the problems existing in the work of the staff. On this basis, combined with the psychosocial therapy model to carry out emotional management research on the employees of property management. This article systematically expounds the process of psychosocial therapy for employees to carry out emotional management treatment, and uses questionnaire surveys, field surveys and other research methods to study the themes of this article. Experimental research shows that after psychosocial treatment, property managers learn to perceive emotions and consciously perceive negative emotions, which improves their insight into self-emotion and self-emotion management ability.

Keywords: Psychosocial Therapy · Estate Management · Emotional Management · Research Analysis

1 Introduction

With the continuous improvement of people's living standards, people's desire to pursue a high-quality life is becoming more and more urgent [1, 2]. High-quality property services have become one of the first choices that people consider when buying a house [3, 4]. Research on property companies and improve the management level of property companies, to improve the service level of property companies, has attracted more and more attention [5, 6].

S. Wang (Ed.): IoTCare 2022, LNICST 501, pp. 133–142, 2023.
https://doi.org/10.1007/978-3-031-33545-7_10

In the research on property employee relationship management, many scholars have achieved good results. For example, Zhang Xiaohua pointed out that emotional management is an indispensable part of employee relationship management in his research on emotional management of property employees; regulating emotions by establishing communication channels can improve work efficiency [7]. In his research on real estate human resource management, Chen Murong concluded that companies must be strategically oriented, consolidate the foundation of human resource management, reform the salary system, and improve the performance management system in order to improve employee relationship management more effectively [8]. ZOU Yanchun et al. studied the specific strategies of leaders' interpersonal emotional management from the perspective of overall emotional management, negative emotional management and emotional management efficacy, and summarized them as constructive strategies, neutral strategies and destructive strategies. The above strategies have different effects on employees' attitudes, behaviors and performance through different mechanisms. Social exchange theory, resource conservation theory, threat regulation theory, emotional event theory, emotion namely social information theory and attribution theory are the main theoretical mechanisms to explain the impact of leaders' interpersonal emotion management [9]. LAN Jijun et al. studied the influencing factors of mental health of subway employees. The typical sampling method was used to investigate their mental health, mental capital and job investment. The research analysis shows that there is a close relationship between the mental health of subway employees and their work involvement [10].

This article aims to improve the efficiency of property services. Combining the psychotherapy model to study the emotional management of property managers, the feasibility of the content of this article is judged by comparing and analyzing the emotional management status of property managers before and after receiving psychosocial treatment. The experimental results demonstrate that the contribution of this method is that property managers learn to perceive emotions and consciously perceive negative emotions if not only for employees, and improve their insight into self-emotion and self-emotion management, which is application-wise feasible.

2 Psychosocial Therapy Model Involved in the Application of Emotional Management of Property Management Employees

2.1 Emotion Management

This article divides emotional management into three dimensions. First, with the help of social workers, employees can correctly understand their own emotional state and realize that they have a certain degree of emotional problems; second, employees can judge themselves rationally whether their emotions are positive or negative, and can accurately express their emotions; finally, employees can find suitable methods and strategies for coping with emotions, so as to adjust and change their own bad emotions. Effectively enhance personal positive emotions and balance their internal and external emotions, thereby helping employees achieve their career planning and life goals with a positive attitude [11, 12].

2.2   Analysis of the Causes of Emotional Problems of Property Management Employees

2.2.1   External Reasons

Immature owners' assembly system
The owners' meeting system has not yet matured. The owners' meeting of some projects has not only failed to act as a "barrier", but has aggravated the conflict between the owners and the property company, and finally led to a substantial increase in the workload of the property company. According to the survey, the most psychologically stressed positions for property employees are related to customer service relationship management positions responsible for coordinating and handling owners' complaints. This also shows that there is a correlation between the maturity of the owners' assembly system and the company's employee relationship management.

It is difficult to use and renew the expenses such as property management expenses and special maintenance funds
The difficulty in the use and renewal of expenses such as property management fees and special maintenance funds has led to increased pressure on the income of the property management company, which has also affected the increase in employee salaries. With the ultra-fast development of the real estate market in recent years, people enjoy services from old-style management communities to modern management mode properties. The necessity of paying property management fees has not been universally recognized, and the payment of property management fees is delayed or not. The situation is still more serious.

The market for qualification training and certification for property practitioners is chaotic
The market for qualification training and certification for property practitioners is chaotic. Various types of property practitioner qualification certificates are inadequate and the training of practitioners is insufficient, which adds to the cost of training practitioners for property companies. The role of property management professionals in employee relationship management goes without saying. Excellent property management professionals not only need to have professional skills to serve owners, but also to have human resource skills to manage employees. For example, in the training and examination of registered property managers, it is necessary to conduct systematic inspections on human resource management, psychology and public relations management.

2.2.2   Reasons for Organizational Characteristics

Formula values and company culture
The company highly emphasizes the obedience of employees, and emphasizes the contributions of employees to the company and the unconditional execution of work tasks. The militarized corporate culture ensures that the company's various tasks can be completed to the greatest extent, it also objectively limits the exercise of the employees' subjective initiative and increases the psychological pressure of employees at work. In addition, the militarized management style and corporate culture also bring about unconditional obedience to the leader. There is no more equal interpersonal relationship between the

leader and the employee, which objectively hinders the bottom-up communication in the communication, especially the reflection This is particularly evident in terms of leadership issues.

Company organizational structure
There are also different levels within the project, such as living properties, high-rise properties, villas, and marketing areas. These differences will place higher requirements on the management of the company's employee relations, but the company is only in the headquarters. There are human resources related positions, and the employee relationship management lacks professional staff management in the project.

Company human resource management
First, the coverage of employee promotion is small. Only regular employees in the company can enjoy the qualifications of "public job bidding", and labor dispatch employees cannot become the company's management-level personnel included in the performance appraisal category; second, there is a serious shortage of management positions. The ratio of management personnel to the total number of employees is about 79:1000, and the number of management positions cannot meet the actual needs of the company's management; third, the company's "public promotion and competition" system has many unreasonable points, which discourage employees from competing for management positions.

2.3 Analysis of the Application of Psychotherapy Model to Emotional Management Methods of Property Employees

2.3.1 Direct Treatment Services Intervene in the Emotional Management of Property Management Employees

Direct treatment services are based on the communication between social workers and employees, as well as reflecting the internal thoughts and feelings of employees. It can be divided into non-reflective direct treatment services and reflective direct treatment services.

Non-reflective direct treatment services are all kinds of necessary services directly provided by social workers to employees, and employees are only passively obeyed counseling services. This kind of service often does not pay attention to whether it reflects the feelings and thoughts of employees. Non-reflective direct treatment mainly includes support, direct influence, exploration-description-catharsis. Support is to reduce the anxiety of the client through the understanding, acceptance and empathy of social workers, and to give the client the necessary affirmation and recognition. Direct influence refers to the direct expression of their own ideas through social workers to promote changes in service targets. Exploration-description-catharsis refers to the process by which social workers allow employees to explain and describe the causes and development of their own dilemmas, to provide employees with opportunities to vent their emotions, to reduce their inner impulses, and to change their bad behaviors.

2.3.2 Indirect Treatment Services Intervene in the Emotional Management of Property Management Employees

In addition to the direct treatment model, the psychotherapy model also emphasizes indirect treatment methods that indirectly affect employees by improving the surrounding environment or counseling a third party. Indirect treatment does not directly affect employees, the impact on employees is also very important. Including support, direct influence, exploration-description-catharsis and reflection on reality. These four indirect intervention methods are the same as direct intervention, but the target clients are different. The clients of indirect treatment mainly include parents, friends, colleagues, etc.

2.4 The Psychotherapy Model is Applied to the Analysis of Countermeasures for the Emotional Management of Property Employees

2.4.1 Improve Employees' Awareness of Emotional Management

Increasing the importance of company management on emotional management
To improve the awareness of emotional management of all property employees in the enterprise, first, we must let the managers of the enterprise realize the importance of emotional management to the enterprise. Because the senior management of a company is the implementer of this corporate culture and system, if you want to form a new culture and system in the company, the most direct and effective way is to let the company's managers pay attention to this new culture first. When managers recognize the importance of corporate emotional management, they will find ways to implement this new culture into the corporate system, or provide a beneficial enterprise for the effective implementation of this system and the penetration of this culture. The environment is conducive to the establishment of new systems and new cultures. When enterprise managers have a comprehensive and profound understanding of emotions and emotional management, they will not only have a beneficial effect and influence on the managers themselves, but also will be beneficial to the establishment of corporate emotion management systems.

Enabling all employees to correctly understand emotions
For employees to master effective emotional management methods, they must first increase the awareness of the entire company's employees on emotions. Only by correctly and scientifically understanding emotions can employees actively participate in the learning and mastery of emotional management methods. Only then can I effectively manage my emotions and improve my happiness.

Specific ways to change employees' perceptions of emotional management
Expert lectures: through hiring experts, conducting lectures, through lectures to understand and understand emotions to popularize the knowledge of emotional management. Or use online video resources to popularize emotions and emotional knowledge.

Parallel exhibition group: The group work of the three major professional methods of social work can be applied to the popularization of employee emotional management knowledge and the mastery of emotional management methods.

Case: For employees who have encountered relatively serious emotional disorders and problems, such as the above cases, they can achieve emotional awareness through individual cases, and guide her out of emotions through professional methods.

2.4.2   Improve the Company's Natural Environment

A good company's natural environment will bring joy to the work of employees. If employees work in a better mood, their work efficiency will naturally increase. Working in a happy mood will also increase employees' interest in work, and produce a good emotional experience for their own work.

2.4.3   Regularly Carry Out Activities that Benefit Employees' Emotional Health

After employee's work, the company can carry out some activities. These activities can be designed for positive purposes, such as activities to enhance the relationship between employees and activities to relieve employee pressure. The organization of these activities should give full play to the employees' own ingenuity allows employees to design themselves, and the company only gives some support when appropriate, to increase the enthusiasm and sense of value of employees.

3   Psychosocial Treatment Model Involved in the Experimental Study of the Emotions of Property Management Employees

3.1   Experimental Protocol

In order to make this experiment more scientific and effective, this experiment went to a property company in a certain place, and carried out a questionnaire test on its emotional management and carried out psychosocial treatment. In this experiment, a total of 15 members were selected for testing, and the ratio of men to women was roughly equal to ensure the validity of the experimental data.

This experiment conducted a questionnaire survey on the overall situation of the property management staff's emotional management and their understanding of emotional management. The pre-test part is based on the self-evaluation statistics of the questionnaire filled out by the property management staff before joining the group, and the post-test is the follow-up evaluation made by the property management staff two weeks after participating in the group activities.

3.2   Research Methods

3.2.1   Questionnaire Survey Method

In this experiment, based on asking relevant experts, a targeted questionnaire was set up. The questionnaire survey is conducted in a semi-closed manner, the purpose of which is to promote the correct filling of the surveyed persons.

3.2.2 Field Research Method

This research investigated on the emotional management of property managers and collected data by going deep into the interior of a property company in a certain place. These data provide a reliable reference for the final research results of this article.

3.2.3 Interview Method

In this study, through face-to-face interviews with property management personnel and recording data, the recorded data was sorted and counted. These data not only provide theoretical support for the topic selection of this article, but also provide data support for the final research results of this article.

3.2.4 Mathematical Statistics

Use related software to make statistics and analysis on the research results of this article.

4 Psychosocial Treatment Model Involved in the Emotional Experiment Analysis of Property Management Staff

4.1 Analysis of the Overall Situation of Emotional Management of Property Personnel

In order to make this experiment more scientific and effective, this experiment conducted a survey on the overall situation of the property management staff's emotional management through a questionnaire survey (Table 1).

Table 1. Analysis on the Overall Situation of Emotion Management of Property Staff

	Pre-test	Post-test
First-class	13.3%	26.7%
Good	53.3%	53.3%
General	33.4%	20.0%
Not good	0	0
very bad	0	0

It can be seen from Fig. 1 that in the pre-test, there were 2, 8, and 5 group members who rated themselves as "very good", "good", and "fair" respectively; while in the post-test, the selection of each group member was as follows: Obvious change: There are 4 members who choose "very good", which is 2 more than before; the members who choose "good" are still 8 and remain unchanged; the members who choose "normal" are 3, 2 digits less than before. This result shows that the overall situation of the group members' emotional management is as expected by the group's goals, and the emotional management training that the group members perceive and learn in the group is helpful for the group members' improvement in emotional management.

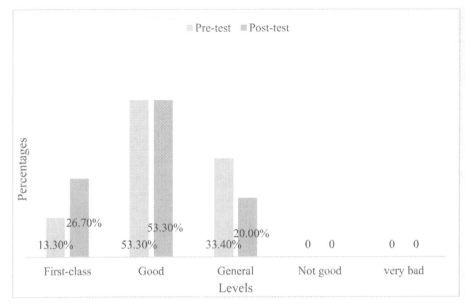

Fig. 1. Analysis on the Overall Situation of Emotion Management of Property Staff

4.2 Analysis of Property Management STaff's Awareness of Emotional Management

In order to further study and analyze the practical effects of the current psychosocial treatment model, including the reference [7] strategy, the reference [8] scheme, the three psychosocial treatment models were applied, and the results are shown in Table 2.

Table 2. Analysis of Property Management Staff's Awareness of Emotion Management

	This model		The reference [7] strategy		The reference [8] scheme	
	Pre-test	Post-test	Pre-test	Post-test	Pre-test	Post-test
Know very well	0	20%	0	13%	0	11%
Understand	20.0%	46.6%	20.0%	31.8%	20.0%	30.9%
General	53.3%	33.4%	53.3%	42.6%	53.3%	43.4%
Don't understand	26.7%	0	26.7%	12.6%	26.7%	14.7%
Don't know	0	0	0	085.3	0	0

It can be seen from Table 2 that before participating in the group activities, only 3 group members "understood" the related knowledge of emotion management in the test, accounting for 20.0% of the total number of property management personnel, and the remaining 13 property management personnel were mostly correct Emotion management is not well understood. After participating in the group activities, the group members' awareness of emotional management related knowledge has changed significantly: 3 group members chose "excellent understanding" after participating in the group, and 7 group members chose "understanding". The number of people who understand has reached 2/3 of the total number of people in the group, and no group member is "not aware" or "very little understanding". However, there is still "incomprehension" after other methods are applied. The above data shows that the actual effect of the psychosocial treatment mode of this method is better. Property management personnel have learned to perceive emotions and consciously perceive negative emotions, thus improving their insight into self emotions and self emotion management capabilities.

5 Conclusion

Through the research on the theories and methods of emotion and emotion management and psychosocial therapy in emotion management, this paper combines these with the actual situation of the property management personnel of the property company, and understands the related factors that mainly affect the emotions of the employees of the company's logistics company, and the company lack of emotional management of employees. Put forward countermeasures and suggestions in response to the problems found in the investigation. And recognize that whether for the social work of property companies or property companies, the use of emotional management in companies to improve the happiness of property management employees is a long-term and arduous task, and psychosocial treatment should be a long-term and difficult task. To make contributions to management, it is not enough to understand social work theories and methods.

Fund Project. Property management, An applied normal major of Sichuan University of Arts and Science.

References

1. Little, L.M., Gooty, J., Williams, M.: The role of leader emotion management in leader–member exchange and follower outcomes. Leadersh. Q. **27**(1), 85–97 (2016)
2. Lee, K.M.: Understanding perception of algorithmic decisions: fairness, trust, and emotion in response to algorithmic management. Big Data Soc. **5**(1), 205 (2018)
3. Chou, D., Hary, N., Naqshbandi, M.M., Philip, P.J., et al.: Employee job performance: the interplay of leaders' emotion management ability and employee perception of job characteristics. J. Manag. Dev. **36**(8), 1087–1098 (2017)
4. Peterson, G.: Developing an awareness of emotion management strategies to support athlete success. Strength Cond. J. **41**(2), 3–7 (2019)
5. Richard, E.M.: Developing employee resilience: the role of leader-facilitated emotion management. Adv. Dev. Hum. Resour. **22**(4), 387–403 (2020)
6. Tucker, M.K., Jimmieson, N.L.: Supervisors' ability to manage their own emotions influences the effectiveness of their support-giving. J. Pers. Psychol. **16**(4), 195 (2017)
7. Zhang, X.: Enhancing emotional performance and customer service through human resources practices: a systems perspective. Hum. Res. Manag. Rev. **26**(1), 14–24 (2016)

8. Murong, C.: Times property staff activity center. MARU **9**, 84–93 (2016)
9. Zou, Y., Zhang, H., Chen, X., et al.: How to manage subordinates' emotions? the strategies and influences of leader interpersonal emotion management. Human Res. Dev. China **39**(7), 88–106 (2022)
10. Lan, J., Guo, X., Jia, Z.: Mediating effect of mental health on psychological capital and work engagement in subway employees. China Occup. Med. **47**(6), 656–659 (2020)
11. Wang, H.: Research on predicament and countermeasure of property management in Chinese public rental housing: taking Chongqing as an example. **037**(001), 71–74
12. Daniel, D.I., Ojo, O., Augustina, O.: An examination of the tenancy agreement as a shield in property management in Nigeria. Int. J. Bus. Adm. **3**(4), 343–353 (2016)
13. Yau, Y., Lau, W.K.: Property management, disability awareness and inclusive built environment. Prop. Manag. **34**(5), 434–447 (2016)
14. Jiachen, Z., Yun, Z.: Research on the service quality of residential property management based on analytic hierarchy process. Value Eng. **038**(016), 51–54 (2019)

Personalized Recommendation Method of Maternal and Child Health Education Resources Based on Association Rule Mining Algorithm

Changyan Liu[1(✉)], Yu Wang[2], and QianYi Wan[3]

[1] Sichuan University of Arts and Sciences, Chengdu 610110, China
bbuah8@163.com

[2] Dazhou Hospital of Integrated Traditional Chinese and Western Medicine, Dazhou 635002, China

[3] Sichuan College of Arts and Sciences, Institute of Health and Industry, Dazhou 635002, China

Abstract. Some personalized recommendation methods of maternal and child health education resources have the problem of long response time of resource recommendation. A personalized recommendation method of maternal and child health education resources based on association rule mining algorithm is designed to improve the above defects. Automatically obtain the text content within the marking range, obtain the characteristics of digital teaching resources, use the session log to record various behaviors of users, build the user interest preference model, extract the core language concept knowledge in the language concept lattice, establish the maternal and child health knowledge base, calculate the maximum likelihood function of the ability parameter, and design the personalized recommendation method based on the association rule mining algorithm. Experimental results: the response times of the personalized recommendation method of maternal and child health education resources in this paper and the other two personalized recommendation methods of maternal and child health education resources are 5.055s, 7.119s and 7.508s respectively, which shows that the personalized recommendation method of maternal and child health education resources in this paper is more feasible after fully combining the association rule mining algorithm.

Keywords: Association rules · Mining algorithm · Maternal and child health care · Teaching resources · Personalized recommendation · Article characteristics

1 Introduction

With the progress of science and technology, the network and education inevitably collide. Especially in recent years, the number of educational websites has increased geometrically, and the educational resources in the network are also growing rapidly. Therefore, a lot of human and material resources have been invested in all aspects of

S. Wang (Ed.): IoTCare 2022, LNICST 501, pp. 143–158, 2023.
https://doi.org/10.1007/978-3-031-33545-7_11

online education at home and abroad, aiming to use computer technology and educational data to improve learning efficiency or teachers' educational quality. However, a large number of maternal and child health care teaching resources are published on the network, which leads to the rapid growth of the number of teaching resources. It is difficult for students to find suitable learning resources in the massive maternal and child health care teaching resources, resulting in problems such as learning loss and information overload. Nowadays, information technology in the field of maternal and child health care teaching has developed rapidly, and a lot of experience has been accumulated in daily life and production. Summing up these experiences has produced a large number of data texts in the field of maternal and child health education. Among them, personalized learning through the analysis of students' learning behavior is one of the current research hotspots. Knowledge-based recommendation depends on the knowledge of item characteristics and user knowledge. The user knowledge here is not necessarily the browsing records and scoring information of users, but the search information of users or the description information of items. By making full use of these data texts through existing science and technology, it can play a huge medical guiding value, effectively assist doctors in diagnosis, and effectively improve the efficiency of clinicians and patients in obtaining high-quality reference resources. Therefore, some researchers have introduced relevant technologies in the recommendation field into online teaching to recommend maternal and child health care teaching resources, which can automatically recommend teaching resources for students that meet their learning characteristics, knowledge level, cognitive ability and other traits according to students' historical learning and historical response records. In the knowledge base system, acquiring knowledge is a major difficulty in the knowledge base. In the field of maternal and child health care, the characteristics of obvious differences in the distribution of knowledge structure, unclear concepts, wide sources of resources, complexity and strong subjectivity make it very difficult to build the knowledge base in the field of maternal and child health care. Combined with the machine learning technology of artificial intelligence, we can achieve the structured storage of multi-source knowledge in the field of personalized recommendation of maternal and child health care teaching resources, achieve the goal of reuse and sharing between the fields of maternal and child health care, and lay the foundation for the construction of maternal and child health care knowledge base system. Recommendation based on association rule mining algorithm must clarify user needs, and then the system matches whether the characteristics of items meet user needs, and establishes the association between recommended items and user needs. Compared with information retrieval technology, maternal and child health care teaching resource recommendation can better meet the personalized needs of students, greatly save students' time to find suitable teaching resources, and effectively alleviate the problems of information overload and learning loss caused by massive teaching resources. Just like pesonallogic, it allows users to describe the characteristics of items they need through conversation. In addition, it also adopts decision support or case-based recommendation methods. Teaching resource recommendation service is gradually becoming an important research topic and hot spot in the fields of online education and artificial intelligence, and has attracted more and more researchers' attention. Reference [1] proposed a recommendation model of educational resources based on collaborative filtering algorithm, incorporating the attribute feature information of learning users, and constructed a learning user model and a resource model; The learning user learning resource scoring matrix is constructed, and the modified cosine similarity algorithm is used to calculate the behavior information similarity of learning users, so as to achieve personalized recommendation of resources. Reference [2] proposed a personalized educational resource recommendation algorithm based on high-dimensional tensor decomposition. Preserve the information integrity of high-dimensional space and realize personalized learning resource recommendation. Reference [3] proposed a multi task feature recommendation algorithm that integrates knowledge maps. Using multi task feature learning tools to embed knowledge maps into tasks; Through the cross compression unit, the high-level relationship between potential features and entities is established, and the recommendation model is constructed to realize the recommendation of curriculum resources. However, the above educational resource recommendation method has the problem of long recommendation and response time. In order to solve this problem, a personalized maternal and child health education resource recommendation method based on the association rule mining algorithm is designed.

2   Get the Characteristics of Digital Teaching Resources

With the development of educational informatization, teaching resource platforms are also increasing, which promotes the wide dissemination and sharing of high-quality resources. Different from commodities in e-commerce, digital teaching resources in the platform have their inherent characteristics. In the past, in traditional teaching methods, teachers mostly wrote test questions by hand, which is not only difficult to share, but also inefficient, and difficult to save. Although there are many ways to classify resources: according to the teaching level, they can be divided into basic teaching resources and higher teaching resources. According to disciplines and majors, it can be divided into science and engineering teaching resources, Reference and history teaching resources, etc. [4]. Nowadays, although teachers have entered the era of electronic information. Usually, teachers use computer office word software to edit test questions, but due to the powerful function of office software, many teachers are not proficient in using it, which leads to low efficiency. At the same time, most of the storage of test questions is in the form of documents, which is too large to be flexible, and usually requires manual test paper generation. However, no matter which classification, teaching resources are used to teach knowledge. Each teaching resource has its own knowledge and skill points, which constitute the core of this resource and represent the essential attributes of digital teaching resources. This leads to the characteristics of digital teaching resources, as shown in Fig. 1:

It can be seen from Fig. 1 that the characteristics of digital teaching resources include: linear progressive characteristics, real-time characteristics, diversity characteristics and interactive characteristics. In addition, in order to meet the various needs of teachers for the generation of test questions, facilitate teachers' operation, improve the efficiency of question production, and reduce the granularity of resource storage, this paper studies and implements a variety of ways to generate test questions resources, so that the test questions resources can be stored in the unit of small questions. Moreover, the knowledge point information of each teaching resource is marked by experts and scholars,

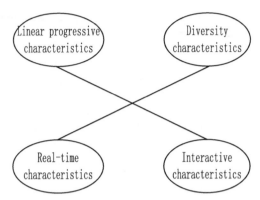

Fig. 1. Characteristics of digital teaching resources

which has a certain authority. For example, if you log on to the China University open course website, each course in the resource sharing course lists the course knowledge point information. After automatically obtaining the start and end positions of the test book, for a test document downloaded from the Internet or edited by the teacher, mark the test text, and then automatically obtain the text content within the marked range, and automatically analyze the questions, options, answers and analysis. Knowledge point information among resources may overlap, so resources can be linked through knowledge points. At the same time, users' preferences for resources also represent users' preferences for the attributes of knowledge points contained in resources to a certain extent [5, 6]. In addition, in order to improve the traditional test paper generation process, it is difficult for teachers to grasp the difficulty of the test paper and the comprehensiveness of the knowledge points examined by the test paper. Users share digital resources through the teaching platform, learn relevant knowledge, and are users of teaching resources. Personalization is the most important feature of digital education resources. Many digital education resources are selective and can effectively meet the personalized needs of learners. In order to ensure the independence of personal teaching resources among teachers and facilitate the effective sharing and reuse of teaching resources. Specifically, each teacher corresponds to a personal storage space, that is, each teacher has a personal resource library, and the test question resources and teaching courseware in the personal storage space are only used by teachers or users authorized by the owner of the library. Users generally have certain pertinence when learning, and the classification is relatively clear. For example, a science and engineering student is more inclined to learn science and engineering knowledge and choose science and engineering resources, while a Reference and history student is more inclined to choose Reference and history resources, that is, the user's own characteristic information has a certain connection with the selected resources. Resource providers provide learners with accurately pushed digital education resources through diversified service methods to meet learners' preferences, work and life, give full play to learners' potential, form learners' independent personality, and realize the personalization and customization of universal education and lifelong education. Therefore, students can be granted the right to upload their homework by teachers, which is convenient to upload it to teachers' personal space for teachers to download and review. At the same time, Teachers can also upload personal information and other teaching resources that are inconvenient to share to the personal resource library. Therefore, the similarity of choosing users of similar resources is much higher than that of choosing users of different resources. At the same time, big data technology is used to collect learners' learning tracks and data, build behavior models, match with knowledge maps, and accurately recommend digital education resources for learners.

3 Build a User Interest Preference Model

The data used in the recommended methods are generally divided into two categories. One is the attribute information of the user or the item itself, and the other is the interaction information between the user and the item. Personalized recommendation for users requires interactive information between users and items. When selecting resources, users' interests and preferences are usually concentrated in one or several types of resources, and the knowledge point attribute information of similar resources is also relatively similar. The knowledge point attribute connects different maternal and child health care teaching resources. Therefore, users' preference for resources also represents users' preference for the attributes contained in resources to a certain extent. This is the only way for users to have a relationship with items. However, most recommendation algorithms only use interactive information. When a new user just enters a new system, there is no interaction temporarily. Naturally, there is no interactive information. At this time, the user's attribute information can play a key role. Using the user model learned from the attribute information provided by the newly registered user to design the recommendation algorithm, it is easier to meet the needs of personalized recommendation [7, 8]. At the same time, the number of resource attributes in the method is far less than the number of resources. Transforming the user's preference for resources into the user's preference for resource attributes can map the high-dimensional scoring matrix to a relatively low dimensional space, which improves the response speed and reduces the sparsity of data. User's attribute information refers to the information that users need to provide when they visit the new platform for the first time, including gender, age, occupation, geographical location, etc. The platform can infer users' interests and preferences by analyzing these attribute information provided by users. Under the condition that the data of the user feature layer and the interest characteristics based on time series information are known, the data obtained from the user portrait layer is the combination of user attribute characteristics and user interest characteristics. The mathematical expression formula is as follows:

$$G_\delta = h_\delta + \frac{(1-h)}{2}\phi \tag{1}$$

In formula (1), h represents the weight of the user feature model, ϕ represents the data of the user feature layer, δ represents the set of user interest features.

Therefore, the scoring and resource attributes are fused to calculate the user similarity. In the process of user clustering, this model is used to calculate the similarity between users, which not only excavates the potential interests of users, but also alleviates the problem of data sparsity, making the clustering effect better. The discrete feature corresponds to each position of the coding vector, that is, how many discrete features there are, the number of bits of the coding vector will take value, and the value on the vector position is determined by the characteristic value corresponding to this position, so the value corresponding to this characteristic position will be set to 1, and the value not belonging to this characteristic position will be set to 0. When calculating users' preferences for resource attributes, users' specific ratings should be taken into account. The larger the proportion of the sum of users' ratings of resources with a certain attribute to the total of all their ratings, the more users prefer this attribute. Because the user clustering method belongs to unsupervised clustering, using the clustering method based on the peak density can determine the number of clusters according to the size of the density, so as to obtain the optimal number of clusters. For each user in the user model, the local density and distance should be calculated. Based on formula (1), the calculation formula of local density is obtained:

$$g = \sum_{i=1} \gamma |\gamma_i - \eta| \tag{2}$$

In formula (2), γ represents the truncated distance, η represents the number of data points smaller than the truncated distance, i represents the weight of all the scoring resources.

This determines that the coding vectors corresponding to each feature are orthogonal to each other and the distance is equal. The interaction information between users and items is the most important data in the recommendation method. This data mainly includes two forms: explicit interaction and implicit interaction. However, users' preferences cannot be comprehensively measured only by their ratings, because each resource has different attributes and the number of attributes, and the ratings are easily affected by other factors such as resource quality, evaluation scale and so on. Explicit interactive information refers to the information that can clearly see the user's preference for items, such as scoring, collection, attention, likes, purchases, etc. This type of data is easy to obtain, but it is also prone to dirty data. Implicit interaction is the user's objective operation of the object, such as user login, click, browse, search and other behaviors. Generally speaking, the more users prefer a certain attribute, the more they evaluate it. For example, if users prefer science fiction books, the number of science fiction books accounts for a large proportion of all evaluated books. At present, the more popular way to use implicit interaction is the mining of session log data. Various user behaviors are recorded in the session log, from which specific information can be extracted. Under comprehensive consideration, the expression formula of users' preference for resource attributes is:

$$K = \frac{|r - \mu_j|}{|\mu|} \times \sum_{j=1} |\gamma_i - \eta| \tag{3}$$

In formula (3), r represents the entire resource space, μ represents the set of resources scored by the user, j represents the resource attribute.

Therefore, the greater the weight of the resource containing a certain attribute in the user's scoring resource set, the more users prefer the attribute of the resource. Considering the dynamic relationship between the popularity of items and time. When calculating the user's interest in the item, add the weight parameter of the item over time:

$$Q = V^{\frac{y_\varepsilon - w_{\varepsilon-1}}{y}} \tag{4}$$

In formula (4), V represents the total amount of items, w is the time when the item is scored the first time, y is the total length of the item online, ε is the time complexity.

Due to the various types of operations of users, the types of implicit interactive information of users are more complex and diverse than the explicit interactive information. The advantage of implicit interaction is that it can avoid directly asking users for data of others' preferences and improve the goodwill of users.

4 Establish Maternal and Child Health Care Knowledge Base

The knowledge base model in the field of maternal and child health care is constructed. The knowledge base expresses the maternal and child health care knowledge in a standardized structural form, provides data model support for the entire upper application, assists the entire treatment process, and enables the maternal and child population and users to independently and quickly obtain relevant knowledge in the professional field. The number of language concept knowledge in language concept lattice is much larger than that in classical concept lattice, and the partial order relationship and data analysis work are also more complex. Therefore, in this section, the Boolean factor analysis method is used to simplify the language concept lattice. The field of maternal and child health care is further combined with the existing high-tech mobile Internet technology, big data technology, artificial intelligence technology and other computer technologies to realize the digitalization, standardization and informatization of maternal and child health care services. Combining the formal background of Boolean matrix and language concept, a knowledge reduction algorithm based on Boolean matrix for language concept lattice is proposed. By calculating the similarity of language concept knowledge in mandatory language concept knowledge, the core language concept knowledge in language concept lattice is extracted. From a practical point of view, we can simply regard the knowledge graph as a multi relationship graph. Determine the field and scope of maternal and child health care knowledge, including what knowledge will be covered by maternal and child health care knowledge, and what questions should be answered by the knowledge in the maternal and child health care ontology knowledge base. In the formal context of language concepts, language values are used to describe attributes, so the data dimensions are greatly increased compared with the classical formal context, so the lattice structure of language concept lattice is more complex than that of concept lattice. Reuse the created maternal and child health care ontology knowledge base, search and query the ontology knowledge base related to the field of maternal and child health care, and learn from the relevant concepts and relationships in the ontology or reuse in building a new maternal and child health care ontology knowledge base. This paper studies the problem of language concept reduction in the formal context of language concepts, and extracts the knowledge base of language concepts from the language concept lattice. A language concept knowledge reduction algorithm is proposed, which processes the mandatory language concept knowledge by calculating the similarity of language concept knowledge, so as to extract the core language concept knowledge base and simplify the language concept lattice. Find out all domain related terms in maternal and child health care, list the terms and give the attributes and concepts contained in the ontology at the same time. The more perfect the domain terms are, the more robust the knowledge base is. In the context of incomplete language concepts, define the similarity between fuzzy objects:

$$S = \frac{|e - d| + f\,|Inc(\alpha, \beta)|}{d\,|\alpha, \beta|} \tag{5}$$

In formula (5), e represents the complete lattice of the language concepts, d represents the language concept set, f represents the language order, α, β represents the upper and lower bounds of the language concepts, respectively.

In the formal context of incomplete language concepts, whether language concepts can be used to describe different fuzzy objects has uncertainty. Therefore, it is used to describe the relationship between fuzzy objects and language concepts, which is closer to human understanding. Determine the hierarchical relationship between classes in the maternal and child health knowledge base, and the hierarchical relationship between classes can be determined by bottom-up, top-down or a mixture of two methods. Determine the attributes of the class in the maternal and child health knowledge base, and the internal structure of the class is described by attributes. The formula for calculating the multi granularity similarity relationship of language concepts is:

$$M = \frac{\left\|e^2 - d^2\right\|}{2} \times d\,|\alpha, \beta| \tag{6}$$

In formula (6), e represents the multi-granular language concept coordination set, d represents the similarity threshold.

However, when expressing the same information, compared with the dimension of attributes in the formal context, the dimension of language concepts in the formal context is greatly increased. Given the similarity threshold, the identification function is transformed into the minimum disjunctive normal form by using the absorption law and the distribution law. Determine the constraints between attributes in the maternal and child health knowledge base. Create instances in the maternal and child health knowledge base, build each instance through the created classes in the maternal and child field, and confirm whether the instance has corresponding attribute values. The convolution neural network structure of maternal and child health knowledge base is composed of four layers: input layer, multiple convolution layers, output layer and full connection layer. First, the maternal and child knowledge data is preprocessed, and the text data is converted into multi-dimensional vectors. Each conjunctive term of the minimum disjunctive normal form is a reduction under granularity, and all its conjunctive terms constitute all the reductions of the formal background of incomplete language concepts under granularity. After the input of the input layer, the multidimensional vector is processed by convolution neurons. A single convolution neural network structure can contain multiple convolution layers and multiple output layers.

5 Design Personalized Recommendation Method Based on Association Rule Mining Algorithm

Workflow of association rule recommendation function: when the user requests to browse resources from the server, the server generates session information, and the session information recording module first judges the content information accessed by the user. The essence of data fusion based on association is to establish semantic relationships between a large number of heterogeneous data. RDF data model is mainly used, that is, heterogeneous digital education resources can be transformed into standard format, so that each knowledge unit is related, and the relationship between existing knowledge bases can be established. Semantic analysis is mainly through processing and analyzing digital resources to obtain valuable content. If the access information has been browsed, it will not be written into the session. If the access information is new, it will be written into the session. There are many kinds of teaching resources in the network. Content-based recommendation is difficult to recommend unstructured resources such as audio and video, and it is difficult to recommend across fields. Association rule-based recommendation has a low degree of personalization, and it is difficult to get better personalized recommendation results. Then, the association rule reading and processing program module is used to find the content information accessed by users in the association rule table, read out the recommended content information, and hand it to the foreground display program related to the recommended content to find and display the recommended content [9]. The system structure of personalized recommendation method of teaching resources is shown in Fig. 2:

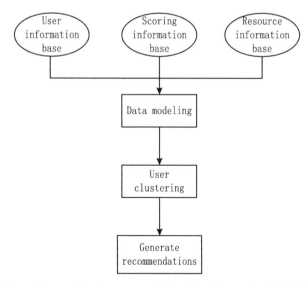

Fig. 2. Architecture of personalized recommendation of teaching methods for Maternal and Child Health care teaching resources

It can be seen from Fig. 2 that the recommendation method inputs the basic information and scoring data of users and resources, and outputs the recommendation results. Return the page data containing the recommended content to the client. When the user leaves the system, the storage access log module stores the contents accessed by the user into the access log table of the database. Workflow of association rule mining function: teachers or administrators log in to the background of the system, select association rule mining algorithm, set basic parameter values such as minimum support and minimum confidence, realize association rule mining, and store the mining results of association rules in the association rule table. Personalized recommendation can be divided into three steps: data processing, recommendation calculation and prediction recommendation. The first unit is to preprocess the data in the user information base, resource information base and scoring information base, and build a data model, that is, get the user feature vector, resource attribute vector, resource attribute preference vector, etc., so as to calculate the user similarity later. In the personalized recommendation method of maternal and child health care teaching resources designed this time, the concept of parameter estimation is introduced. If the difficulty coefficient, guess coefficient and discrimination coefficient of the current project are known, then the answer result data in the score matrix and the known difficulty coefficient, guess coefficient and discrimination coefficient are substituted into the IRT model to establish the maximum likelihood function of capability parameters, as shown in formula (7):

$$N = \prod_{j=1}^{\sigma} (z - \sigma)^{1-j} \tag{7}$$

In formula (7), z represents the positive answer probability obtained by the IRT model function, σ represents the true answer situation of the tested user in the score matrix, j represents the difficulty coefficient of the knowledge point.

Apriori algorithm module realizes content recommendation, that is, when users access the content in the theoretical learning video module, it realizes the function of recommending other learning content to users according to association rules. Besides content recommendation, ml-sh module can also realize the function of recommending access to the user. The second unit is to calculate the similarity of users and find the nearest neighbors according to the recommended method on the basis of the first unit, in which new users are based on user characteristics and information entropy model, and other users are based on scoring and resource attribute preference model. Take logarithm on both sides of formula (7) to get:

$$\ln(N) = \sum_{j=1} \ln(\lambda_j) + \ln(1 - \lambda_j) \tag{8}$$

In formula (8), λ represents the maximum likelihood estimator.

Using association rules to realize content recommendation is the key content of this paper. This paper describes the mining of association rules and the method of using association rules to realize content recommendation. The method is mainly composed of content recommendation and association rule mining module. The third unit is responsible for users' prediction scores and the final top-N recommended resources. There are both registered users and unregistered users in the personalized recommendation method of teaching resources. Unregistered users can retrieve and browse resources and non personalized recommendation services. The content recommendation module of association rules mainly realizes the recommendation function of other content according to the page content accessed by the user and the association rules. The association rules mining module mainly realizes the function that the background administrator uses the association rules mining algorithm to mine the association rules according to the user's access log, and stores the mining results in the database. In addition, for registered users, they can evaluate resources and manage personal information in addition to the rights of unlisted users. At the same time, the recommendation strategies for new registered users and rated users are different.

6 Simulation Experiments

6.1 Build up the Experimental Environment

The verification of the recommended scheme in this paper is realized through the system, using the classic windows + mysql + apache + PHP environment. The personalized recommendation method proposed in this paper is implemented in the development environment equipped with 3.1 GHz Intel Core i5 processor and 8 GB 2133 MHz LPDDR 3. The package management software anaconda and sublime 3 editor are used as development tools, and the programming language is python. The software and hardware environments are as follows: client: IE 4G memory, operating system: Windows, Web server: Apache/2.4.23(Win32), database product: MySQL, server script: PHP, development tool: MyEclipse2020, JDK support: JDK. External network bandwidth 8mbps, memory: DDR4 16 GB, CPU: AMD Ryzen 71700 Eight Core Processor 8-core 16 threads.

6.2 Experimental Results

Select reference [1] method, reference [2] method, reference [3] method as a contrast method, and compare it with the personalized recommendation method of maternal and child health education resources designed this time. Test the response time of Resource Recommendation of the three personalized recommendation methods of maternal and child health education resources under different user numbers, The shorter the time, the better the concurrency performance of the method is proved. The experimental results are shown in Table 1, 2, 3 and 4:

It can be seen from Table 1 that the response time of the personalized recommendation method of maternal and child health teaching resources in this paper and the other two personalized recommendation methods of maternal and child health teaching resources are 1.051 s, 1.540 s and 1.814 s respectively; It can be seen from Table 2 that the response time of the personalized recommendation method of maternal and child health teaching resources in this paper and the other two personalized recommendation methods of maternal and child health teaching resources are 2.851 s, 4.596 s and 4.855 s respectively; It can be seen from Table 3 that the response time of the personalized recommendation

Table 1. Number of users 200 resource recommended response time (s)

The number of experiments	Reference [1] method	Reference [2] method	Reference [3] method	The personalized recommendation method of maternal and child health care teaching resources in the article
1	1.332	1.779	1.515	1.006
2	1.659	1.802	1.822	1.114
3	1.483	1.714	1.977	0.978
4	1.326	1.936	1.549	0.845
5	1.515	1.825	1.866	0.994
6	1.584	1.774	1.917	1.312
7	1.316	1.830	1.833	1.125
8	1.847	1.944	1.892	0.977
9	1.315	1.855	1.847	1.331
10	1.549	1.731	1.779	1.025
11	1.447	1.822	1.685	1.009
12	1.631	1.915	1.793	1.014
13	1.585	1.993	1.689	0.847
14	1.713	1.548	1.943	1.113
15	1.805	1.745	1.982	1.074

Table 2. Number of users 400 resource recommended response time (s)

The number of experiments	Reference [1] method	Reference [2] method	Reference [3] method	The personalized recommendation method of maternal and child health care teaching resources in the article
1	5.616	4.878	4.784	3.415
2	4.878	4.966	5.386	2.748
3	4.316	5.132	4.895	2.495
4	3.997	5.031	5.012	3.006
5	4.022	4.667	4.877	2.142
6	4.116	4.515	4.941	3.475

(*continued*)

Table 2. (*continued*)

The number of experiments	Reference [1] method	Reference [2] method	Reference [3] method	The personalized recommendation method of maternal and child health care teaching resources in the article
7	4.198	5.121	4.978	2.199
8	5.121	4.948	4.976	3.114
9	4.774	4.677	4.997	2.087
10	5.336	4.531	4.822	2.746
11	4.815	5.016	5.748	3.143
12	4.012	4.751	5.495	3.255
13	4.377	5.220	5.006	3.149
14	4.241	4.866	5.142	2.914
15	5.122	4.513	5.475	2.878

Table 3. Number of users 600 resource recommended response time (s)

The number of experiments	Reference [1] method	Reference [2] method	Reference [3] method	The personalized recommendation method of maternal and child health care teaching resources in the article
1	9.487	7.548	9.512	6.544
2	8.645	8.316	9.147	6.483
3	8.991	8.487	9.351	6.102
4	9.612	8.615	8.948	5.947
5	8.147	7.948	9.275	6.314
6	8.351	9.364	8.771	5.349
7	7.948	9.788	9.123	5.717
8	9.215	9.487	8.802	5.612
9	9.336	8.115	8.665	5.318
10	9.148	8.212	8.319	6.771

(*continued*)

Table 3. (*continued*)

The number of experiments	Reference [1] method	Reference [2] method	Reference [3] method	The personalized recommendation method of maternal and child health care teaching resources in the article
11	8.999	8.366	8.771	6.123
12	9.103	9.154	8.544	5.802
13	9.215	9.477	9.483	5.665
14	8.144	9.202	9.102	6.319
15	7.946	8.746	8.947	6.411

Table 4. Number of users 800 resource recommended response time (s)

The number of experiments	Reference [1] method	Reference [2] method	Reference [3] method	The personalized recommendation method of maternal and child health care teaching resources in the article
1	12.301	13.457	13.616	9.154
2	13.548	12.748	13.878	10.031
3	14.917	14.159	13.316	11.120
4	13.645	13.747	13.997	9.748
5	13.747	15.166	15.022	9.789
6	12.871	14.199	15.116	10.551
7	14.522	16.742	14.198	10.374
8	15.334	15.213	15.121	11.885
9	12.008	14.779	14.515	9.677
10	13.494	13.552	15.121	9.644
11	12.548	16.415	14.948	11.122

(*continued*)

Table 4. (*continued*)

The number of experiments	Reference [1] method	Reference [2] method	Reference [3] method	The personalized recommendation method of maternal and child health care teaching resources in the article
12	14.183	15.412	14.677	9.748
13	13.455	14.733	14.531	9.647
14	12.748	15.120	14.585	10.488
15	13.489	14.144	15.191	11.316

method of maternal and child health teaching resources in this paper and the other two personalized recommendation methods of maternal and child health teaching resources are 6.032 s, 8.819 s and 8.721 s respectively; It can be seen from Table 4 that the response time of the personalized recommendation method of maternal and child health teaching resources in the text and the other two personalized recommendation methods of maternal and child health teaching resources are 10.286 s, 13.521 s and 14.639 s respectively. According to the experimental results, it can be analyzed that the less the number of users, the faster the response of the resource recommendation of the three personalized recommendation methods of maternal and child health care teaching resources. In the four experimental scenarios, compared to the other three methods, the performance of the personalized recommendation method of maternal and child health teaching resources in this paper is better.

7 Conclusion

The personalized recommendation method of maternal and child health care teaching resources in this paper provides users with personalized language association rules, and constructs different fuzzy object language formal backgrounds for different users. In the whole learning process, the error prone knowledge points of middle school students' users have been consolidated, and the difficulties have been broken through, so as to improve the learning level of students, promote the personalized development of users of maternal and child health education resources, and further improve the development and utilization of high-quality teaching resources. On this basis, from the perspective of connotation and extension, a cognitive system of fuzzy object language concept lattice is established to better reflect users' cognitive process and provide exploratory suggestions for users. In the subsequent improvement process, the dependence on user participation will be minimized.

References

1. Qin, Z., Zhang, M.: Research on learning resource recommendation model based on collaborative filtering algorithm. Comput. Technol. Dev. **31**(9), 31–35 (2021)
2. He, Y., Xu, W.: Research and application of personalized education resource recommendation algorithm based on high-dimensional tensor decomposition. Wirel. Internet Technol. **18**(10), 114–115 (2021)
3. Wu, H., Xu, X., Meng, F.: Knowledge graph-assisted multi-task feature-based course recommendation algorithm. Comput. Eng. Appl. **57**(21), 132–139 (2021)
4. Chen, L., Lu, S., Zeng, F., et al.: Application of multi-base joint distance learning in practice teaching of nursing specialty based on the internet. Nurs. J. Chin. People's Liber. Army **37**(9), 86–89 (2020)
5. Chen, X.: The application of participatory teaching in the practice teaching of maternal and child health. J. Qiqihar Univ. Med. **41**(5), 611–613 (2020)
6. Xu, Y., Guo, J.: Recommendation of personalized learning resources on K12 learning platform. Comput. Syst. Appl. **29**(7), 217–221 (2020)
7. Zhang, Z., Guo, Y., Yang, H., et al.: Exploration and practice on individualized intelligent teaching based on learning behavior analysis —a case study of "principles of communications" course. J. Beijing Univ. Posts Telecommun. (Soc. Sci. Ed.) **22**(6), 101–107, 118 (2020)
8. Wu, C., Liu, M.: Teaching resource recommendation algorithm based on kernel canonical correlation analysis. J. Univ. Sci. Technol. Liaoning **44**(1), 62–66 (2021)
9. Wang, X.: Interval value attribute data set association rule mining algorithm simulation. Comput. Simul. **37**(1), 234–238 (2020)

Methods of Integrating Ideological and Political Education into Health Management in Colleges and Universities Based on Internet of Things Technology

Wenjuan Xie[1]($\boxtimes$) and Jin Zhou[2]

[1] Shaoyang University, Shaoyang 422000, China
juhfd584@163.com
[2] English Department, Sanya Aviation and Tourism Vocational College, Sanya 572000, China

Abstract. In order to better promote the physical and mental health development of college students, this paper puts forward the method of Integrating Ideological and political education into health management based on Internet of things technology, optimizes the integration mode of Integrating Ideological and political education into health management in Colleges and universities in combination with Internet of things technology, constructs an evaluation system of Integrating Ideological and political education into health management in Colleges and universities, and simplifies the steps of Integrating Ideological and political education into health management in Colleges and universities, which is confirmed by experiments. The method of Integrating Ideological and political education into health management in Colleges and Universities Based on Internet of things technology has high practicability and fully meets the research requirements.

Keywords: Internet of things technology · Ideological and political education · Health management

1 Introduction

The Ministry of education proposed to vigorously promote the classroom teaching reform with the goal of curriculum ideological and political education, improve the teaching design, sort out the ideological and political education elements contained in various professional courses and the ideological and political education functions carried by them, and integrate them into all links of classroom teaching. "Introduction to health service and management" is a compulsory professional Enlightenment Course for freshmen majoring in health management in Colleges and universities. It integrates ideological and political elements into the whole teaching process of the course, and realizes the equal emphasis on knowledge transfer and value guidance, which is conducive to exploring the deeper synergistic educational effect of ideological and political education. The research on the construction of healthy China has achieved rich research results [2].

S. Wang (Ed.): IoTCare 2022, LNICST 501, pp. 159–177, 2023.
https://doi.org/10.1007/978-3-031-33545-7_12

There are still many areas to be studied and explored. For example, how to promote the construction of a healthy China in practice, how to improve the health literacy of the whole nation, and how to implement health education, health promotion and other education. Research on the role of diversified health education models, such as general health education, knowledge and behavior model health education, WeChat health education and sports curriculum, in the prevention and treatment of specific diseases. The third is the current situation of college students' health literacy, health education needs analysis and research on the path to improve college students' health literacy.These studies have fully recognized the importance of College Students' health education, and are actively looking for relevant problems and countermeasures. The diversified education model research also provides valuable experience for this study. These studies are based on the traditional concept of health, and only pay attention to the role of health education in the treatment and prevention of diseases. Under the background of "healthy China", the concept of health in health education has been promoted from "treatment of diseases" and "prevention of diseases" to "health promotion". Under this background, health education focuses on establishing a four-dimensional health concept of disease-free, physical and mental integrity, social adaptation and environmental harmony, It is a "great health concept", which involves ideological education. Y Zhang[3] deeply analyzes the influence of mobile internet on the timeliness of college students' ideological and political education, and on this basis, establishes a new application strategy to ensure the full integration of mobile internet and college students' ideological and political education.Bamakan discuss how blockchain technology meets the requirements of HWM. Therefore, we conducted a comprehensive systematic literature review to determine and critically evaluate the application of blockchain in the research field. These applications are divided into waste generation, waste separation and packaging, waste storage containers, waste collection, temporary waste storage areas, waste treatment, waste off-site and on-site transportation, waste disposal, hospital staff training, waste management regulations, hospital sewage systems, energy, and waste recycling and reuse.Jenkins to study the role of wearable medical sensor devices, machines, deep learning algorithms and medical systems based on the Internet of Things in screening, diagnosis, monitoring and treatment of patients with COVID-19.Under the background of "healthy China", how to carry out health education with the core of "great health concept" is an important joint of College Students' health education and ideological and political education. Based on this, combined with Internet technology, this paper studies the method of Integrating Ideological and political education into health management in Colleges and universities.

2 Integrate Ideological and Political Education into Health Management in Colleges and Universities

2.1 Integration Method of Ideological and Political Education into Health Management in Colleges and Universities

Both college students' health education and ideological and political education take college students as the main educational objects. College teachers and other staff are both educators and educatees. Both college students' health education and ideological and political education require the two-way interaction between college teachers and other staff and college students to be effectively completed. Colleges and universities have conducted in-depth analysis and understanding of college students as an educational object in the process of carrying out health education and ideological and political education, and formulated targeted education plans, The health needs and ideological and political literacy of contemporary college students show distinctive personalized and hierarchical characteristics. The whole process of contemporary college students from entering colleges and universities to graduation is the common research object and educational process of the two major education. The essence of College Students' health education and ideological and political education is "education", so there are many similarities in the way of education. The educational means of both can be divided into two levels, namely, theoretical education and practical education. Theoretical education mainly includes classroom theoretical teaching, theoretical lectures and knowledge publicity. It pays attention to the education and guidance at Ideological and theoretical level, and mainly aims at the transformation of ideas; practical education mainly includes extracurricular practical activities, experiencing real life, educational practice, etc., and mainly aims at the presentation of behavior. The combination of theoretical education and practical education is an effective method commonly used in college students' health education and ideological and political education, and it is also an important methodology to do a good job in college education. The research on the theory of student work mode is the objective basis for its practical transformation. To build a theoretical system of developing student work mode, we must also take "development" as the main line, take promoting the all-round development of students as the starting point and destination of theoretical research, and put the basic concepts, basic principles, basic objectives, basic contents and other structural elements of developing student work mode through the theoretical system. These elements are not only different, but also related to each other. They contain each other and restrict each other. They occupy different positions and have different functions. Together, they constitute a complete theoretical system of development oriented student work mode. As shown in Fig. 1:

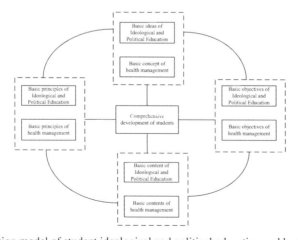

Fig. 1. Integration model of student ideological and political education and health management

The training goal of health service and management specialty is to cultivate compound medical talents with both political integrity and ability, solid medical knowledge and management ability, so as to meet the professional needs of changing from modern medical model to prevention. Due to the particularity of medical services and medical management, medical talents must have good professional ethics and medical ethics. "Introduction to health service and management" is a professional Enlightenment Course for freshmen for the first time. The course covers the basic knowledge of medicine, management and other disciplines, so that students have a deep and comprehensive understanding of the professional knowledge architecture system, stimulate Freshmen's motivation to learn professional knowledge, enabling them to establish correct values, world outlook, cultivate a good style of study, and play a connecting role [6]. In the teaching process of "Introduction to health service and management", relevant ideological and political elements are sorted out from the development process of health service management, health promotion of major infectious diseases, health services of traditional Chinese medicine, grass-roots health service management, health care and elderly care services, relevant laws and regulations of health service industry, health risk assessment and management, and health management ethics, and organically integrated into the teaching practice of curriculum knowledge. As an institutional innovation in the field of higher education in recent years. The ideological and political education curriculum emphasizes that improving the ideological and political quality is the primary requirement of talent training. Cultivate useful talents who are determined to fight for socialism with Chinese characteristics for life, "be both professional and professional, have both ability and moral integrity, and develop in an all-round way". Compared with western developed countries such as Britain and America, China's health service industry started late. However, the implementation of a series of security systems and policies has pointed out the direction for the development of health care and health service industry, which has achieved rapid and orderly development and a series of new historical achievements. It fully demonstrates the advantages of the socialist system with Chinese characteristics and guides college students to support the leadership of the CPC. The belief in the socialist system with Chinese characteristics should cultivate college students to establish values and enhance their confidence in the socialist system with Chinese characteristics [7]. J2EE is a de facto industrial standard that uses Java technology to develop campus level applications. It is the product of the continuous adaptation and promotion of Java technology to campus level applications. It has incomparable advantages over the traditional Internet application model. J2EE provides an independent, portable, multi-user, secure and standard based campus level platform for developing server-side applications using Java technology, so as to simplify the development, management and deployment of campus applications. J2EE platform uses a multilayer distributed application model. The logic of the application program is encapsulated in components according to the different functions it realizes, and a large number of application program components that make up J2EE applications are installed in different machines according to their layers. This model has the ability to reuse components, the security mode of data exchange based on Extended Markup Language, and flexible transaction control. The b/s structure of health management is shown in Fig. 2.

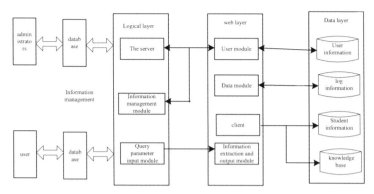

Fig. 2. Health management B/S structure

Manage the activities related to student information consultation. It mainly includes: online counseling, setting up an online psychological counseling room to provide students with online psychological counseling services. The specific functions are as follows: student psychological counseling subject management. Register and manage various psychological counseling services that can be provided, and record the service contents, consultants and service methods, etc.; Consulting service resource management. Electronic management of various resources (including various materials) required in various consulting services, and matching with consulting service projects; Online consultation plan arrangement. Manage the project, personnel and time plan of online consultation; Statistical analysis of consulting services. Carry out statistical analysis on the actual operation of each consulting service project; Consultation case records [8].

The ideological and political team, including counselors, head teachers and other student staff, is the main body and front-line staff for student management. It is of great significance for the arrangement, development and planning of the Student Affairs Office of the college to master the information of the ideological and political team in time and obtain the relevant statistical classification data. The information statistics of Ideological and political team is to collect the basic information of Ideological and political personnel such as name, gender, date of birth, nationality, educational background, and special work-related information such as professional title, position, Department, professional research direction, and make statistics according to department, role, etc. for the use of student work office. There are many league members and Party members among the students, who are advanced elements in the student group and good helpers in carrying out student management. Statistics on the information of these students can increase the understanding of the basic situation of the student group, and have more significance for the ideological and political education of students [9]. Every time, student party and League organizations at all levels will collect and summarize the information of Party and League members to the superior departments. The information statistics of Party and League members is to collect, summarize and count these information, including the student number, name, gender, Department, major, class and political appearance of Party and League members, and can be counted according to the multiple stages of application for League membership, League membership, application for Party membership, promotion of excellence, activists for Party membership, development objects, probationary party members and formal party members, so as to grasp the status of student groups more accurately.

Manage the information of student counselors and head teachers, record their daily work, and complete the evaluation of counselors and head teachers. Mainly includes: counselor information management. Establish the basic information database of counselors (including photos and profiles), maintain and query them; Counselor evaluation. Publish the selection methods of excellent counselors, and each college reports the evaluation materials and publishes the evaluation results of counselors; Counselor evaluation. Design the counselor evaluation questionnaire, conduct a sampling survey on students, enter the survey data, and conduct a preliminary evaluation on the basis of the Counselor's self-evaluation. The student work department (Department) will evaluate according to the self-evaluation, and the preliminary evaluation will be combined with the specific situation of the Counselor's work, record the evaluation results for the record, and notify the College of the evaluation results. Instructor training. Announce the training arrangements for counselors. Regular meetings of counselors and head teachers (tutors). The college uploads regular meetings and training records; Counselors teach. Announce the teaching decision of the new counselor, and report the teaching record and teaching summary. Work exchange. Upload and exchange Counselor's work experience articles; Records of students with learning difficulties; Students with self-discipline difficulties focus on the situation record.

2.2   Evaluation Algorithm of Integrating Ideological and Political Education into Health Management in Colleges and Universities

The college students' health management service system takes the school as the general department, effectively combines the Ministry of sports, the school hospital and the mental health consulting center, fully mobilizes the advantages of all parties, breaks the traditional single department operation mode, and strengthens the linkage between departments, departments and students. At the same time, in order to better ensure the operation of the service system and improve the service quality, it is necessary for schools to set up corresponding supervision systems and incentive mechanisms. Infectious diseases are the common enemies of all mankind. In particular, the prevention and control of severe infectious diseases and health promotion need the joint efforts of the international community. As a large developing country, China pays great attention to and actively participates in the emergency response and health promotion activities of the global epidemic of infectious diseases [10]. Health is the basic need of people for a better life, the capital that the patients yearn for, and the wealth that the patients do not have. The survey found that most people who are not ill are in a sub-health state, they lack active health awareness, and their health behavior choices tend to be passive, and college students are this kind of group. Research shows that the concept of active health has a positive effect on promoting people's health behavior, improving the health literacy of teachers, creating an active and healthy social atmosphere, and promoting national health. Giving full play to the synergistic educational function of College Students' health education and ideological and political education, and cultivating the educatees' active health concept is an important measure to change the passive treatment state of college students. The synergy of the two should not only promote the educatees' practice of diet, rest, exercise and other living habits, but also encourage the teachers to practice active disease prevention, active health management and active enrichment of the spiritual world. The incentive mechanism is mainly to set different material and spiritual rewards for departments and individual students. Its composition mainly includes: additional score reward, certificate trophy and banner reward, material and economic reward. Model management theory provides a solid theoretical basis for the idea. The basic characteristics of model theory are integrity, relevance, hierarchical structure and so on. Nowadays, we integrate model management theory with emerging disciplines such as information theory, computer and modern communication technology in college students' health management services, making health management services more modeled, standardized, quantified and personalized, collecting and evaluating each student's information, and conducting individual health intervention, which makes health management services even more powerful. The organizational structure of the college students' health management service system studied is shown in Fig. 3.

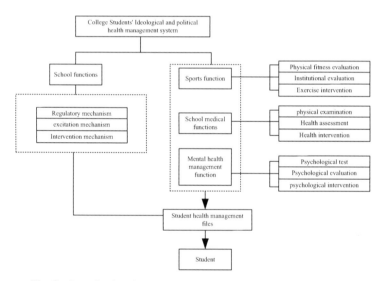

Fig. 3. Organizational structure of health management service system

The communication between managers and students should have the skills of transmitting information, controlling managers, motivating managers and expressing emotions. First of all, communication is the most intuitive goal of communication, and other goals can only be achieved on this basis. This method is mainly divided into online anomaly detection, diagnosis, prediction and evaluation. Fuzzy comprehensive evaluation method is used to evaluate the health status of the model.

$$M = \{m_1, m_2, ..., m_n\} \tag{1}$$

Here, m_n represents N fuzzy factors for the evaluation work Because the influence of these factors may be different, the corresponding weight must be determined according to the influence of each factor in practice.

$$A = \{a_1, a_2, ..., a_n\} \tag{2}$$

In the formula, a_n is the weight corresponding to the n factor m_n. From the perspective of fuzzy comprehensive evaluation, several types can be selected, such as triangle type, normal type, Cauchy type, middle type, degradation, etc. Among them, fuzzy comprehensive evaluation is also called fuzzy comprehensive evaluation problem. When conducting comprehensive evaluation, it is necessary to have the element set recorded as:

$$U = \{\mu_1, \mu_2, ..., \mu_n\} \tag{3}$$

The evaluation set V and the single factor v_m decision are further defined. If the evaluation results are divided into m levels, the group composed of the above results is called the evaluation set.

$$V = \{v_1, v_2, \cdots, v_m\} \tag{4}$$

Here, γ represents the evaluation conclusion of the n layer, and the evaluation of any data is a subset of R.

$$R = \sum U + V/2\gamma n(M - A)^n \tag{5}$$

The generated health management data are fuzzed and the triangular membership function is selected.First, fuzzify the measurement data according to the following formula for unified management.

$$\mu(x) = \begin{cases} 1 - \frac{|\gamma - 1|}{R}, \\ 0 \end{cases} \tag{6}$$

Managers can not implement unified command and coordination to students without communication skills. Secondly, motivation is an important skill to achieve communication. In the process of student management, timely and effective work guidance, affirmation of work performance evaluation, timely reward of some excellent behaviors, etc., these communication methods can achieve the purpose of motivating students, while timely and timely incentives can further achieve comprehensive and in-depth communication; Finally, emotional communication is the most important part of communication. Through some ideological exchanges between each other, exchanging views on a series of problems such as learning and life can help to improve students' satisfaction and self-confidence. Based on the above characteristics of student management, referring to the people-oriented student management mode, this paper puts forward the student management mode in the service-oriented middle school. It is a new way of student management based on the service theory in the new public management theory. It adheres to the purpose of running a service-oriented middle school and absorbs western management concepts. It has new management concepts, behavior and habits management,

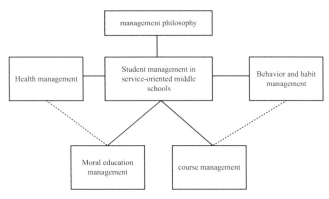

Fig. 4. Ideological and political health management of service-oriented students

accommodation management, learning and curriculum management mode, moral education and health management mode. The ideological and political health management structure of service-oriented students is shown in the following figure (Fig. 4):

In order to ensure that this model adapts to the development of medicine, the expansion of functional application and the needs of environmental changes, the health evaluation model configuration function module is designed. Through this function, users with the role of doctor or administrator can change the scoring rules of physiological detection items, the weight of examination items and the evaluation weight of physiological models, so as to achieve the application purpose of improving the evaluation model with the times and focusing on the evaluation of various aspects of human health. After the doctor or administrator user changes the health evaluation model, the model saves the change record to the corresponding background operation log, and displays the change reminder for the administrator in the foreground interface of the administrator.

2.3 The Realization of Integrating Ideological and Political Education into Health Management

Health management is a medical behavior and process that emphasizes human health as the center and health or disease risk management as the focus, and comprehensively detects, evaluates, effectively intervenes and tracks the health status of individuals or groups and the risk factors affecting health. Health management doctors are required to respect human life, personality, rights and other medical ethics and morality, adhere to the supremacy of life, and serve the physical and mental health of the people wholeheartedly, This is also an important part of medical ethics and moral education. The university health management information model is mainly based on the basic idea of object-oriented. It is designed and developed by combining the structured life cycle method and prototype method in the software development methodology. Users of all roles of the model are invited to intervene in the model planning, requirements analysis and detailed design stages. The rapid construction of the prototype is used for users to compare the application requirements. While following the phased and modular analysis and design ideas of the information model life cycle, give full play to the characteristics of prototype cycle and iteration, and make the model application well match the expectations of users. In addition, as health management is a comprehensive discipline of life science, management science and information science, its modeling environment (University) and users (teachers and students) have distinctive characteristics and commonalities. While constantly improving and providing requirements and model examples, it will focus on the design and implementation of key modules and core algorithms in the model Experts in the medical field are invited to review and discuss with health care workers in Colleges and universities at multiple levels to ensure that the model is scientific, universal and of higher practical value.The key problem of information extraction lies in the classification of information, selecting the maximum information gain $H(a_{max})$, the minimum information gain $H(a_{min})$, and constructing the minimum Greer evaluation index of health management.

$$g(A) = \mu(x)/H(a_{max}) - H(a_{min}) \tag{7}$$

If $F(n)$ is the direct of data set n, $S(x)$ is the conditional direct of data set S to feature x, and φ is the sample subset. Then the gain ratio of Ideological and political management information is:

$$g_R(D) = \frac{F(n)}{S(x)} - g(A) * \varphi \tag{8}$$

Then the Gini index of the ideological and political health management sample set is:

$$\text{Gini}(D) = 1 - \sum_{k=1}^{K} \left(\frac{|g(A) - \varphi|}{|g_R(D)|} \right)^2 \tag{9}$$

On this basis, to establish a network data extraction system with good quality, we need to meet the requirements of versatility, openness, repeatability, flexibility and scalability, so as to better adapt to the application of the model. When evaluating the extraction mode of network data, two commonly used evaluation methods are often used: accuracy rate P and recovery rate κ. Accuracy refers to the ratio of selected information to all selected data; The memory ratio is the proportion of selected information in the selected information. In the performance comparison of two different information extraction modes, F (the sum of accuracy and recovery ratio) is adopted, that is:

$$F = \text{Gini}(D) \frac{(\kappa^2 + 1) \times \text{PR}}{(\kappa^2 \times \text{RP}) - 1} \tag{10}$$

For large-scale medical and health process extraction, first collect the medical record files in EMR, then use the method of ICTCLAS to classify the medical records and tag parts of speech, then extract the samples in batches through syntax tags, vocabulary collection, jape rule writing, batch learning PR and other methods, and finally generate XML files with semantic tags (Fig. 5).

By extracting the medical information of patients, the necessary medical information can be obtained from the patient's medical records. This requires a certain understanding

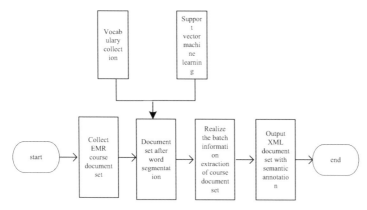

Fig. 5. Technical process of batch extraction of health information

of the knowledge and background knowledge in the field of clinical medicine and the needs of doctors. The pretreatment of medical and health information is the statistical analysis of patients' condition. In order to reduce the interference of noise on the training data, a method based on the course blank is adopted. Then convert the semi-structured data into pure text and load it into gate. There is a large amount of data in EMR data, so only a small amount of data is extracted for training and verification, which not only saves a lot of computing resources, but also improves the efficiency of the test. Since the medical record content of medical and health information is a very complex and changing process, it is difficult to extract relevant data. When the disease occurs, the patient's subjective abnormal feelings or some objective pathological changes are caused by some abnormal changes in body function, metabolism, morphology, etc. The name of the disease causing CD is expressed by the test items in the hospital information model database, and the diagnostic category of the disease is expressed in Roman alphabet or digital table. Through the treatment mode vocabulary, treatment effect improvement vocabulary, efficacy deterioration vocabulary, effect neutral vocabulary and treatment effect vocabulary and other different correlation extraction methods. Because of the complexity and individualization of medical language, the extraction of support vector machine has a better application prospect. In the case of definition and association, a variety of NLP and feature expression methods are used. For entity recognition, it is more effective and efficient to use the lexical language features of the entity itself and its surroundings. Relationship extraction involves the NLP features of two entities and the combined features of these two entities. The combination of vocabulary and part of speech is the basic combination mode of relationship information extraction. The linguistic symbol features, contextual features, semantic types (attributes, predicates, adverbials) and semantic relationships of words are summarized into feature vectors. Finally, the self training method is used to expand the training corpus to form a feature-based support vector machine extraction model architecture. As shown in the Fig. 6.

Using language features to locate the beginning and end positions of entities, this recognition method often has better results than learning each character of entities. In addition, the entity itself and the surrounding characters are also quite effective. Based

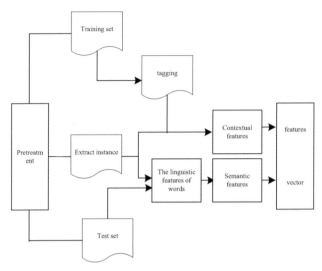

Fig. 6. Feature based health management information feature extraction model architecture

on this, it can effectively extract and manage the health management of a large number of employees in a complex environment, so as to ensure the effect of medical record information management. According to the current form and content of student work management in a certain university, combined with the current situation, institutional setting and staffing, a lot of information has been collected through the investigation of college leaders, leaders of learning and work departments, counselors, class teachers, students and other aspects. Combined with the expected effect of the future student work management model, the functions of the model and the relationship between the modules in the model are determined. Under the leadership of the college Party committee, the student management work is mainly in the charge of the student work department. The student work department is subordinate to the Department at the Department Level - the student work office, and the specific work is directly carried out by the student work office. In order to facilitate work, the Student Affairs Office also has five department level departments: student management department, ideological and Political Education Department, college student assistance center, student apartment management department, and mental health education guidance center. These departments respectively implement various work of student management. The training goal of health service and management specialty is to cultivate compound medical talents with both political integrity and ability, solid medical knowledge and management ability, so as to meet the professional needs of changing from modern medical model to prevention. Due to the particularity of medical services and medical management, medical talents must have good professional ethics and medical ethics. "Introduction to health service and management" is a professional Enlightenment Course for freshmen for the first time. The course covers the basic knowledge of medicine, management and other disciplines, so that students have a deep and comprehensive understanding of the professional knowledge structure system, stimulate the motivation of freshmen to learn professional knowledge, enable them to establish correct values and world outlook, cultivate a good style of study, and serve as a bridge between the preceding and the following. In the teaching process of "Introduction to health service and management", relevant ideological and political elements are sorted out from the development process of health service management, health promotion of major infectious diseases, health services of traditional Chinese medicine, grass-roots health service management, health care and elderly care services, relevant laws and regulations of health service industry, health risk assessment and management, and health management ethics, and organically integrated into the teaching practice of curriculum knowledge.

3   Analysis of Experimental Results

The purpose of testing is to prove that there are faults in the program, and to find out and solve as many faults as possible. The test tries to design the test cases that can expose the problems most. The student office's maintenance of special students is mainly the recording and maintenance of special student information, including the query, addition, modification, deletion, import and export of student data, so as to realize the query of special student maintenance information. The basic information of 420 students is shown in Table 1.

Table 1. Basic information of students' health status and ideological and political concept survey

Features	Category	Number of people
Gender	Male	200
	Female	220
Professional category	Science and Engineering	139
	Literature and history	148
	Arts	153
grade	1	100
	2	97
	3	105
	4	118
Health evaluation	Very good	101
	good	102
	commonly	111
	Poor	96

This result shows that, on the one hand, college students have great health needs, on the other hand, they have the problem of weak awareness of their own health care. In the long run, the health status of college students will be more worrying, and the lack of active health concept at the ideological level is the fundamental reason for this phenomenon. Ideological education is the advantage of Ideological and political education in Colleges and universities. It is the responsibility of health education and ideological and political education in Colleges and universities to carry out correct health concept education. Collaborative education between the two is an important way to solve this practical problem. Based on this, students' suggestions on the content and method of the integration of health education and ideological and political education in Colleges and universities are collected and integrated into the management method of this paper, Based on the positive attitude of college students towards the collaborative education of college health education and ideological and political education, college students gave a positive response to the specific content and mode of integration of the two, and formed effective suggestions. Through statistical analysis, college students' suggestions on the content and mode of integration of the two are shown in Table 2:

Table 2. Students' suggestions on the contents and methods of the integration of health education and ideological and political education in Colleges and Universities

Features	Category	Number of people
Fusion content	Physiological health knowledge	332
	Mental health knowledge	349
	Behavioral health knowledge	400
	Sexual health knowledge	397
	Moral health knowledge	332
Fusion mode	Integration of health concepts in course content	331
	Cultivation of healthy behavior in extracurricular practical activities	401
	Carry out special lectures on health education	359
	Strengthen the correct guidance of college counselors and class teachers on College Students' health concept	360
	Help modern communication media to carry out information fusion publicity and education	333
	other	123

The results show that college students hope to acquire healthy knowledge about physiology, psychological behavior, sex, morality and other aspects in the course of the integration of the two, showing the healthy needs for all-round development, which is of great significance to the all-round development of college students themselves: the suggestions on the integration of the two mainly show diversified and modern characteristics, On the basis of traditional health education and ideological and political education courses and lecture forms, we pay more attention to the integration of ideas and the guidance of ideas. At the same time, we emphasize the use of extracurricular practical activities to strengthen health behavior, and are good at using modern information dissemination carriers for collaborative education. It is highly innovative and feasible. It is of constructive significance for this study to explore the specific ways of educating people. Based on this, the college can manage the information of mental health educators. Establish the information base of mental health education counselors and mental health observers. Add the records of college mental health education activities. In order to test the effectiveness of health evaluation management methods in practice, this paper proposes a web server program background management program and database running under the network environment based on tcp/ip. The server and background administrators of the website should run on Windows NT/Windows 2000/wixp. Based on vision2 of Keil company, with i553b as the core and i553b as the core, this paper uses external devices for simulation. According to the above information, the operation effects of the two modes are compared, and the calculation accuracy and time of the two modes are compared, and they are tested in detail (Table 3).

Table 3. Comparison of performance test results of two methods

Data volume (GB)	Traditional method		Literature [3] Method		Method of this paper	
	Data processing time/S	Accuracy of data processing %	Data processing time/S	Accuracy of data processing %	Data processing time/S	Accuracy of data processing%
500	250	45	230	55	100	85
1000	400	50	300	60	130	88
1500	550	60	350	70	130	91
2000	650	75	450	75	140	95
2500	750	77	550	87	160	92

Based on the information in the above table, it is not difficult to find that the data processing accuracy of traditional health management methods is up to 77%, the data processing accuracy of the method in literature [3] is the highest 87% and that of this method is up to 92%. Compared with the traditional health management methods, this method can process a large number of health management data faster and more effectively in the actual application process, and the processing effect is significantly better than the traditional methods. The test results of students' mental health modules are further compared and analyzed. The specific test results are as follows (Table 4):

According to the data tested in the above table, it is found that under the same circumstances, the overall effect of students' Ideological and political mental health under the guidance of this method is significantly better than the traditional method. Further, the accuracy of the two models in practical operation is compared and compared in a complex environment, and the following data are obtained (Fig. 7):

It can be seen from the above test data that, compared with traditional methods and literature [3] methods, the integration method of ideological and political education in colleges and universities based on the Internet of Things in health management is more accurate and stable, and the time required under the same conditions of use is also greatly shortened.

Table 4. Test results of students' mental health module

Project	Method in this paper	Traditional method
Test title	Mental health test	Mental health test
Importance level	high	–
Preset conditions	Users enter the ideological and political team module	User enters personal module
Operation steps	Users click to view the assessment results	Output results
Expected output	Return to the summary of appraisal results	Return to the summary of appraisal results
Test result	Fully passed	Partially passed

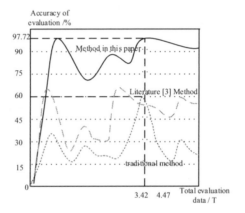

Fig. 7. Comparison test results

4   Suggestions on Integrating Ideological and Political Education into Health Management in Colleges and Universities

In the final analysis, the construction of the great ideological and political pattern is to use all possible forces in society and colleges and universities to do a good job on the ideological and political work of college students. It is an educational model that covers the "whole staff, whole process and all-round" of the educatees. The "great health" education required by the construction of a healthy China is precisely aimed at the education of the educatees in the whole life cycle. The coordination of the two major education is an effective way to establish morality and cultivate people in an all-round way. "Building Morality and cultivating people" is the fundamental task of higher education, and it is also an important part of the comprehensive and healthy development of the educated. The construction of the great ideological and political pattern should not only take the all-round and healthy development of the educated as the premise, but also create a good environment for the all-round and healthy development of the educated. With virtue and talent cultivation as the center, we should start the whole process education mode, and cultivate health education while building a great ideological and political pattern. First of all, the perspective of collaborative education of health education and ideological and political education should cover the education in Colleges and universities, do not ignore the collaborative education function of the two major education due to the nature of specialty and employment direction, and pay attention to and implement the integration practice of the two major education. Secondly, the perspective of collaborative education of College Students' health education and ideological and political education should cover the whole process of educational from enrollment to graduation, and the collaborative education of the two should not be interrupted due to internship and employment. Finally, the perspective of collaborative education of College Students' health education and ideological and political education should cover the study, life and employment of educatees in an all-round way, combined with a variety of counseling and education methods, Guide them to correctly view the pressure in all aspects, correctly deal with and resolve the difficulties of life, and form an environment conducive to the educated to master their own destiny.

Colleges and universities are the main fronts to carry out health education and ideological and political education. The coordinated development of the two must also take colleges and universities as the main battlefield. First of all, colleges and universities should have the enthusiasm and initiative to carry out the collaborative education of health education and ideological and political education in Colleges and universities. The key to the collaborative education is to integrate the two into one, put forward the concept of collaborative education from the leadership area pole, and call for collaborative education action; From the perspective of financial investment, increase the hardware configuration and software application of collaborative development; From the aspect of teachers, we should strengthen the introduction of comprehensive talents and the training of existing teachers; from the aspect of management, we should carry out the integrated management mode of health education and ideological and political education. In addition, colleges and universities also need to actively take the lead in organizing large-scale theme activities, such as visits, seminars, etc., integrate other government agencies, healthy campuses and social forces into the collaborative education action, establish a platform for multi-party participation, and play a leading role in gathering multi-party forces and resources.

Comprehensive healthy talents are the pillar of collaborative education of College Students' health education and ideological and political education, and the capital to realize the collaborative education of the two major education. The absorption of healthy talents by United hospital and other departments is an important way to obtain collaborative education resources. The first is to vertically combine public hospitals of grade II and above, absorb clinical medical staff and party and government managers, and clinical medical staff can obtain first-hand clinical information and authoritative health knowledge: Party and government managers not only have high ideological and political literacy, are familiar with the relevant policies of the party and the state, but also have rich experience in hospital management, and can carry out relevant research in the field of health; the second is that ordinary colleges and universities can horizontally combine medical colleges and universities, Absorb double qualified talents with both clinical experience and teaching experience. The integration of these healthy talents, as well as the integration of resources, can strongly promote the coordinated development of College Students' health education and ideological and political education.

The timeliness, universality and interactivity of network information communication make it an important propaganda position for the collaborative education of great health education and great ideological and political education. According to the behavior change theory of Fromm, a famous psychologist, using the method of enhancing the transformation force in the behavior correction strategy to guide college students to establish correct social values under the conditions of modern network communication, the government and colleges and universities should make full use of and grasp the initiative of modern network environment to carry out integrated education, and use modern network communication carriers such as wechat, microblog, and micro video to promote social positive energy and promote the idea of comprehensive and healthy development, Give publicity and praise to the practice of positive social behavior, and set an example for college students' comprehensive health behavior.

5   Conclusion

It is a new thing to integrate "ideological and political factors" into the course teaching, and there is no experience to learn from in the practice of "Introduction to Health Service and Management". This study is exploratory and experimental. Put forward the method of integrating ideological and political education into health management in colleges and universities based on Internet of Things technology. However, this method has some limitations, that is, it has not been applied to practice and other fields. In the future development, with the continuous in-depth attempt of the construction of ideological and political courses in colleges and universities, we can further explore the "ideological and political course" education and teaching system suitable for domestic college students, and finally form a teaching standard system and characteristic course standards.

Fund Project. General project of Hunan social science achievement evaluation committee (XSP22YBZ168); Key scientific research projects of Hunan Provincial Department of Education (20A452).

References

1. Huang, J., Wu, X., Huang, W., et al.: Internet of things in health management systems: a review. Int. J. Commun. Syst. **34**(4), e4683 (2021)
2. Lian, J., Fang, S., Zhou, Y.: Model predictive control of the fuel cell cathode system based on state quantity estimation. Comput. Simul. **37**(07), 119–122 (2020)
3. Zhang, Y.: Research on the effectiveness of ideological and political education in colleges and universities based on mobile internet. In: 2021 2nd International Conference on Education, Knowledge and Information Management (ICEKIM), pp. 121–125 (2021)
4. Bamakan, S., Malekinejad, P., Ziaeian, M.: Towards blockchain-based hospital waste management systems: applications and future trends. J. Clean. Prod. **349**, 131440 (2022)
5. Jenkins, T.: Wearable medical sensor devices, machine and deep learning algorithms, and internet of things-based healthcare systems in COVID-19 patient screening, diagnosis, monitoring, and treatment. Am. J. Med. Res. **1**, 9 (2022)

6. Parrilla, M., De Wael, K.: Wearable self-powered electrochemical devices for continuous health management. Adv. Func. Mater. **31**(50), 2107042 (2021)
7. Gruß, I., Bunce, A., Davis, J., et al.: Initiating and implementing social determinants of health data collection in community health centers. Popul. Health Manag. **24**(1), 52–58 (2021)
8. Xia, Y.: Big data based research on the management system framework of ideological and political education in colleges and universities. J. Intell. Fuzzy Syst. **40**(2), 3777–3786 (2021)
9. Zheng, P., Wang, X., Li, J.: Exploration and practice of curriculum ideological and political construction reform——take "'information security'" course as an example. ASP Trans. Comput. **1**(1), 1–5 (2021)
10. Bowles, P.: Internet of things-based health monitoring systems, artificial intelligence-driven diagnostic algorithms, and body area sensor networks in COVID-19 prevention, screening, and treatment. Am. J. Med. Res. **1**, 9 (2022)

Data Mining of Psychological Tendency and Health of Ideological and Political Students in Higher Vocational Tourism English Courses

Jin Zhou[1]([⊠]) and Wenjuan Xie[2]

[1] English Department, Sanya Aviation and Tourism Vocational College, Sanya 572000, Hainan, China
zhoujin55400@163.com
[2] Shaoyang University, Shaoyang 422000, Hunan, China

Abstract. In order to improve the quality of students' psychological tendency health data, this paper puts forward the research of mental tendency health data mining based on SVM. By cleaning the students' mental tendency health data and optimizing the SVM with particle swarm optimization algorithm, the classification of students' mental tendency health data is completed. According to the weighted results of mental propensity health data, the primary classification and feature recognition of large-scale mental propensity health data were carried out. Based on the optimal modeling of students' psychological tendency health data, the objective function of maximum difference of students' psychological tendency health data is defined. Maximum likelihood estimation is used to obtain the frequency distribution of the data in the Tourism English Course of higher vocational colleges. Experimental results show that the proposed method can not only improve the accuracy and efficiency of mental health data classification, but also control the integrity of mental health data over 80%.

Keywords: Support Vector Machine · Higher Vocational Colleges · Tourism English · Course Ideology and Politics · Psychological Tendency · Health Data Mining

1 Introduction

In recent years, the development of education in our country is progressing, and the importance of ideological and political education of tourism English courses in higher vocational colleges is also increasing. According to the development of national economic situation, society needs a large number of high-level skilled talents. Higher vocational education is an important part of higher education in our country, aiming at cultivating a large number of highly skilled talents with reasonable structure and good quality. The proportion of professional talents exported from higher vocational colleges will account for a large proportion under the requirement of economic structure. College students leave their parents and hometown to face the brand-new world as a social person, which is called "the second weaning period of life". At this particular stage, it is very easy to experience a wide range of maladjustment [1].

© ICST Institute for Computer Sciences, Social Informatics and Telecommunications Engineering 2023
Published by Springer Nature Switzerland AG 2023. All Rights Reserved
S. Wang (Ed.): IoTCare 2022, LNICST 501, pp. 178–190, 2023.
https://doi.org/10.1007/978-3-031-33545-7_13

In this period, the immature development of human nature, the ability of self-regulation and self-control, and the burden of employment and interpersonal relationship caused by the fierce competitive environment make most students' psychological pressure gradually increase. At the same time, most of the higher vocational students have poor academic performance and have not formed good study habits. Higher vocational students will face more psychological pressure. College students usually shoulder the family and even the country's hope, generally received a good education, should become the pillars of the country, contribute to the country's construction of their own talents. But the emergence of psychological problems led to a variety of tragic events, how to timely detect and intervene in the mental health problems of college students, is particularly important.

With the development of science and technology, the application of computer has gradually entered the operation and management of all walks of life. Through the psychological assessment system, college psychological counselors can quickly collect students' psychological conditions and make judgments, improve work efficiency and reduce work intensity. To a certain extent, it provides a great help, while the database also accumulated a large number of psychological data. But at present most of the psychological assessment conducted by colleges and universities are based on the basic psychological information of students access, query, statistics and backup operations. A large amount of psychological data is not analyzed in depth and not fully utilized. From it, we can mine some hidden information knowledge and grasp the trend of students' psychological development. Therefore, it can not effectively provide decision-making help for psychological counseling.

Wang Feng et al. [2] Considering that the traditional psychological stress testing method is mainly based on questionnaire survey and evaluation with the aid of professional equipment, which has high cost and great intrusion into the evaluated object, etc. Based on the analysis of perceptual data of smartphones, this paper studies the methods of assessing college students' psychological stress, extracts reasonable features from perceptual data, and puts forward a more efficient method of assessing psychological stress. Secondly, this paper introduces how to transform psychological stress assessment into classification problem and construct classification model by semi-supervised learning. Finally, the model is tested on the open data set StudentLife. The experimental results show that this method is superior to the baseline method in the aspects of psychological stress detection accuracy and recall. Zhou Xianyu et al. [3] Aiming at the problems of the traditional evaluation methods, such as low real-time evaluation, poor evaluation effect of single modal data, and biased social desirability response, an automatic evaluation method of college students' mental health based on multi-modal data fusion is proposed in this paper. The model can accurately assess the mental health status of college students. It has a good application prospect in the intelligent learning environment, and can provide decision-making basis and technical support for improving students' mental files and optimizing mental health services.

Data mining is the mining of information and knowledge from massive data. Data mining technology in the retail industry, financial industry, telecommunications and other industries has been fruitful. If data mining technology is applied to the development of mental health management system, a large number of fuzzy and random data information in students' mental health archives can be processed by relevant algorithms. To a certain extent, it will help counselors to make judge and prevent students' psychology more scientifically and quickly, to guide and intervene psychology in time, to improve work efficiency and to reduce psychological events.

Based on the above research background, this paper uses support vector machine to design a mental health data mining method to ensure the healthy development of students' psychology.

2 The Design of Data Mining Method for Students' Psychological Tendency Health

2.1 Cleaning Student Mental Health Data

The data mining method of students' mental health is to clean up the data by two parts: data processing and output. The above two steps are implemented by concurrent [4, 5]. In the part of data processing, we complete the redundant processing, decontamination and determine the expiration time of the data. Using the timer to collect the data of students' mental tendency health in the buffer queue, complete the detection of students' mental tendency health data, and output the real data. When the existing data has expired, using comparative judge to judge the authenticity of students' mental health data, and transmit the output to the online platform of vocational colleges.

Through reading the cache queue, the conflict detection mechanism, the converter and the calculator, the mental propensity health data are processed.

The mental propensity health data processed by calculator were stored in EPC format. Among them, EPC represents the EPC code value of students' mental health data in Tourism English Course of higher vocational colleges. $RSSI$ represents the signal strength of the mental health data. timestamp represents the time to gather data on students' mental health preferences. What expiretime represents is the expiration time of students' mental health data in the Tourism English course of higher vocational colleges. Z represents the value of mental health data of students' psychological tendency in tourism English curriculum of higher vocational colleges.

The data with the same characteristics were detected by conflict detection mechanism. First, the processor is used to collect a characteristic data C from the mental health data of students. According to whether there is the same data in the reading buffer queue, we can judge whether there is conflict in the thinking and politics of tourism English courses in higher vocational colleges. If there is data conflict, get the students' mental health conflict data T in higher vocational colleges tourism English curriculum ideological and political Z value. When the value of Z is 1, C. The expiretime and Z values of the expiration time of the mental propensity health data in the reading cache were modified, where:

$$T(\text{expiretime}) = C(\text{expiretime}) \tag{1}$$

If the value of Z is greater than 1, modify the value of Z in the read buffer of the student mental health conflict data so that:

$$T'(Z) = T(Z) + 1 \tag{2}$$

If there is no conflict, use the converter to process the students' mental health data q, get the caching requirements of the students' mental health data. Convert it to the appropriate format to insert at the end of the queue.

The function of the converter is to change the format of students' mental health data. Uniform data format for easy handling of data.

Using the signal-distance strength propagation model, the washing process time t and the washing process speed v of students' mental health data are calculated as follows:

The data of mental health tendency of students selected for the first time in two consecutive times were recorded as $RSSI_1$ and $RSSI_2$. Based on the signal-distance strength propagation model. The distance between the computing processor and the mental propensity health data at t_1 and t_2 time D_1, D_2:

$$D_1 = 10^{\frac{RSSI_1}{10-N}} \tag{3}$$

$$D_2 = 10^{\frac{RSSI_2}{10-N}} \tag{4}$$

N stands for empirical value.

The comparator is used to compare the given threshold γ and the mental propensity health data Z. According to the comparison results, the authenticity of label data is judged. When the data of students' mental propensity health is real, the data are exported and transmitted to the online platform of vocational colleges.

2.2 Designing an Algorithm of Students' Psychological Tendency Health Data Classification Based on SVM

Based on the cleaning of students' mental health data, the SVM training set is preprocessed to improve the training speed, and the SVM is trained to obtain the decision function. It can be seen that not all training samples work in the SVM classification process. Instead, only the training samples corresponding to the non-zero solution c_i of the dual problem, that is, the support vector, act on the decision function [6]. In other words, the complexity of the SVM decision for an unknown sample is $G(|l|)$. When $|l|$, the number of support vectors, is large, the estimator is large, resulting in a slow classification speed. Based on this, particle swarm optimization algorithm is used to reduce the support vector. After training SVM, the fuzzy membership vector of the set of support vectors is used as the particle in the particle swarm, and the average classification error of the test set is used as fitness function. The optimal set of support vectors is selected to reduce support vectors, so as to improve the classification speed of students' mental health data.

Particle swarm optimization algorithm searches for the solution by adjusting the position of particles. Assuming that the population $X = \{x_1, x_2, \ldots, x_n\}$ is composed of n particles in the D dimension search space, the current position of the i particle is $X_i = \{x_{i1}, x_{i2}, \ldots, x_{in}\}$. The current velocity of the particle is $V_i = \{v_{i1}, v_{i2}, \ldots, v_{in}\}$. The best position for particle i is $P_i = \{p_{i1}, p_{i2}, \ldots, p_{in}\}$. The best place for all particles to pass is $P_g = \{p_{g1}, p_{g2}, \ldots, p_{gn}\}$. The i-particle at time $t + 1$ is:

$$v_{id}^{t+1} = v_{id}^t + \zeta_1 \psi_1 \left(p_{id}^t + x_{id}^t\right) + \zeta_2 \psi_2 \left(p_{gd}^t - x_{id}^t\right) \tag{5}$$

$$x_{id}^{t+1} = x_{id}^t + v_{id}^{t+1} \tag{6}$$

Among them, $1 \leq d \leq D$; $1 \leq i \leq n$; ψ_1 and ψ_2 are random numbers uniformly distributed on the interval of $(0,1)$. ζ_1 and ζ_2 are called learning factors.

In particle swarm optimization algorithm, each particle represents a solution, and particle swarm optimization algorithm is applied to support vector machine to reduce support vector. The number of support vectors obtained by trained SVM is the dimension of particles. Assume that the range of membership of these samples is $[R_{min}, R_{max}]$. This range is chosen as the position range of the initialized particle, and the weight vector of the sample calculated is regarded as a particle in the initialized particle swarm space. Each particle has its position and velocity. The position indicates the membership degree of the sample. The velocity changes the membership degree and sets a threshold. Particle output, when the sample membership is greater than the threshold value, so that its membership to maintain the original value, that the sample was selected. Otherwise, its membership is assigned a value of 0, indicating that the sample is not selected. Therefore, the problem of selecting support vectors is transformed into the PSO optimization problem of selecting optimal particles.

The training set is divided into two parts: one for the training set and the other for the testing set. The training sample set is processed and the training SVM gets the support vector set. The average classification error of the test set is used as the fitness value of the particles. Define the fitness function as:

$$Fitness = \frac{1}{H} \sum_{i=1}^{H} (y_i - g_i)^2 \tag{7}$$

H is the number of samples in the test set, y_i is the predicted value, and g_i is the actual value. The smaller the fitness of the particles, the better.

According to the above process, the classification algorithm of students' mental health data is designed using SVM.

2.3 Calculate the Correlation Between the Characteristics of Students' Psychological Tendency and Health Data

In the process of mining students' psychological tendency health data in the ideological and political ideological and political courses of tourism English courses in higher vocational colleges, the preliminary classification and feature identification of the psychological tendency health data are carried out. The degree of association between various types of features can be calculated. The specific steps are detailed as follows:

Suppose that F_{ij} represents the frequency of the appearance of i in Tourism English Course Thought and Politics D_j. N_i represents the number of times a mental health data feature appears. F_{ik} is the probability of the appearance of i in Tourism English Course Ideological and Political k. Then use the following formula to express the weighted results of the psychological predisposition health data:

$$\chi_{ij} = \frac{U(w) \times F_{ij}}{N_i \otimes D_j} \otimes F_{ik} \tag{8}$$

In the formula, $U(w)$ represents the constant coefficient.

Suppose, the maximum value of information entropy of each feature class is represented by $\sigma(j)$. W represents the number of characteristics of mental disposition health data. Φ represents the total dimensionality of the candidate feature set for mental dispositional health data. f_e represents the th feature of the e-th type of data. Then use the following formula to combine the weighting method of inter-class and intra-class information entropy distribution of feature items [7] to carry out preliminary classification and feature identification of large-scale psychological tendency health data:

$$\lambda(S_{ac}) = 1 - \frac{\max(S_{ac}) \times l}{\phi \otimes coff} \cdot f_e \frac{\Phi(\wp(I) * W)}{\sigma(j) \otimes W} \tag{9}$$

In the formula, $\max(S_{ac})$ represents the correlation between the psychological disposition health data and the maximum correlation coefficient. l represents the feature selection pros and cons evaluation function. ϕ stands for the feature recognition rate of mental tendency health data. $coff$ represents the weight that balances the maximum recognition rate and feature dimension. $\wp(I)$ represents the number of categories.

Suppose that any two mental disposition health data are represented by a_i and a_j. ς represents the threshold between the given mental disposition health data distances. The distance from a_i to a_j in the mental health data is smaller than that of ς. However, the distance between a_i and the mental health data other than a_j is greater than ς. Then use the following formula to calculate the correlation function between the psychological tendency health data:

$$A = \sum \frac{V \times (a_i, a_j)}{\varsigma \times Q(\varsigma_i)} \tag{10}$$

In the formula, V represents the probability of the same feature appearing in the health data of different psychological tendencies. $Q(\varsigma_i)$ stands for independence of mental predisposition health data.

Suppose, a one-dimensional mental orientation health data sequence is represented by n. N''' represents the number of vector points in the phase space reconstruction of mental orientation health data. The similarity between any two psychological tendency health data is defined as the maximum difference between the two vectors, which is expressed by the following formula:

$$K_m(r) = \frac{(x_i - x_j)}{N''' \otimes n} \otimes X(E) \tag{11}$$

In the formula, $X(E)$ represents the similarity between the health data of various psychological tendencies.

To sum up, it can be shown that in the process of mining students' psychological inclination health data in the ideological and political ideological and political courses of tourism English courses in higher vocational colleges, a preliminary classification and feature identification of the large-scale students' psychological inclination health data is carried out. Calculating the correlation between various types of features lays the foundation for the realization of the data mining of students' psychological tendency health.

2.4 Optimal Modeling of Students' Psychological Tendency Health Data

According to the correlation between the characteristics of students' psychological tendency health data, the optimal modeling is carried out on the students' psychological tendency health data. If the mental time series set of different stages in the student's learning process is defined as $\{X(t), t = 1, 2, \cdots, n\}$. Because the rebellious psychology of college students has obvious differences in the form of expression, it is necessary to reconstruct the phase space of the formation process of students' psychology. So get the matrix:

$$
\begin{bmatrix}
x(1) \; x(1+\tau) \cdots x(1+(m-1)\Omega) \\
x(2) \; x(2+\tau) \cdots x(2+(m-1)\Omega) \\
\cdots \qquad\qquad \cdots \\
x(k) \; x(k+\tau) \cdots x(k+(m-1)\Omega)
\end{bmatrix}
\tag{12}
$$

In the formula, m represents the complexity of students' psychology. Ω represents the duration of the student's mentality, satisfying:

$$
k = n - (m-1)\Omega
\tag{13}
$$

Consider each row in the matrix as a variety of influencing factors of students' psychological changes, the total number is k. According to the degree of conflict, the index of the affected categories of each influencing factor in the students' psychological performance status is obtained, and the psychological performance status of different impact categories is obtained. For m-dimensional students, the total number of different mental performance state sequences corresponding to the degree of psychological complexity is m. Assuming that the probability of occurrence of b kinds of different mental performance state sequences is $p_1, p_2, \cdots, p_k$, then according to the form of Shannon entropy, the probability of students' mental state sequence is sorted, then the permutation entropy is:

$$
H_{PE}(m) = -\sum_{j=1}^{b} p_j \ln p_j
\tag{14}
$$

Integrate the state sequence given by the above formula. The following formula is used to express the emotional characteristics of behavior corresponding to the psychological state of students at this stage:

$$
0 \le H_{PE} = \frac{H_{PE}}{\ln(m)} \le 1
\tag{15}
$$

Suppose $\{x(t), t = 1, 2, \cdots, N\}$ represents a time series set of behavioral emotional characteristics of students' mental states. Due to the complexity of the behavioral tendency of college students dominated by rebellious psychology, it is necessary to establish a relational expression with the duration t_i of rebellious psychology. Select the duration time series $X(t_i + \tau)$ to form a new duration phase point column $Y(t)$. The mental duration t_i is determined by calculating the correlation of $X(\tau)$ and $Y(\tau)$.

According to the behavioral emotional characteristics corresponding to the psychological state of students, the ant theory is used to model the health data of students' psychological tendency. It is assumed that t_{ij} represents the behavioral tendency strength of college students' psychology in the τ period. $\Delta t_{i,k}(\tau)$ represents the pheromone that the psychology of college students searched by ant k has hindered the tendency behavior. χ $(0 \leq \chi \leq 1)$ represents the influence of student psychology on tendentious behavior. Use the following formula to calculate the intensity of behavioral tendency to search for the next period, the formula is:

$$t_{ij}(\tau + 1) = \chi \cdot t_{ij}(\tau) + \sum \Delta t_{i,k}(\tau) \tag{16}$$

Assuming that l_k represents the length of the path that the k th ant traveled in this cycle, there are:

$$\Delta t_{ii,k}(\tau) = \frac{R}{L_k} \tag{17}$$

Among them, R is a constant, assuming that ε_{ij} represents the visibility of the path (i, j), which is usually taken as $\frac{1}{d_{ij}}$. Set d_{ij} to represent the length of path (i, j). The corresponding importance of path visibility is $(\beta \geq 0)$. The relative importance of the path trajectories is $\alpha (\alpha \geq 0)$. U represents the feasible point set. The migration probability of ant k in the τ time domain is $p_{ij,k}(\tau)$. Then use the following formula to define $p_{ij,k}(\tau)$:

$$p_{ij,k}(\tau) = \begin{cases} \frac{[t_{ij}(\tau)]^\alpha [\varepsilon_{ij}]^\beta}{\sum\limits_{l \in U} [t_{ij}(\tau)]^\alpha [\varepsilon_{ij}]^\beta}; & j \in U, \\ 0 & ; j \notin U. \end{cases} \tag{18}$$

Based on the above elaboration, the objective function of the influence of students' psychology on behavior is calculated by the following formula:

$$\min B = g(x) \cdot x \in [a, b] \tag{19}$$

Among them, $g(x)$ is the optimization function.

The optimization model of college students' mental health data is constructed using the following formula, namely:

$$\begin{cases} t_j(\tau + 1) = \varphi \cdot t_j(\tau) + \sum\limits_k \Delta t_j \\ \Delta t_j = R/L_j \end{cases} \tag{20}$$

In the above formula, Δt_j represents the increase in the regional attraction strength of the j th ant in this cycle. L_j represents the amount of change in $g(x)$ in this cycle, which is defined as $g(x + r) - g(x)$. The optimization of the function is carried out with the help of the continuous movement of m ants. When $\varepsilon_{ij} \geq 0$ is satisfied, ant i transfers from its nearest neighbor I to the neighbor of ant j according to probability p_j. When $\varepsilon_{ij} \leq 0$ is satisfied, the ant i searches the nearest neighbor I, and the search radius is r, that is, each ant or the place where the other ants are located. Or perform a near-neighbor search and gradually converge to the global optimal solution of the problem.

By solving the problem of students' psychological predisposition behavior disorder, the optimal modeling of students' psychological predisposition health data was carried out.

2.5 Realization of Students' Psychological Tendency Health Data Mining

Suppose that the frequency of occurrence of the i-th feature is represented by $\lambda_i^{(c)}$. ∂_i represents the frequency vector of the mental orientation health data i. $V_m(r)$ represents the maximum difference between the two psychological orientation health data. Its objective function is defined by the following formula:

$$\arg\min A = \frac{\Omega(y(c) - y(d))}{V_m(r) \otimes \lambda_i^{(c)}} \otimes \partial_i \tag{21}$$

In the formula, $y(c)$ represents the amount of information including c data. $y(d)$ represents the frequency of d features. Ω stands for the best classification scheme.

Suppose that $p(d|\hat{c})$ represents the probability of generating students' psychological tendency health data d in the ideological and political course $\hat{c}$ of tourism English in higher vocational colleges. $p(c|\hat{c})$ represents the probability of generating the health data $\hat{c}$ of all students' psychological inclinations in the students' psychological inclination health database in the ideological and political c of the tourism English course in vocational colleges. The frequency distribution of each data in the ideological and political $\hat{c}$ of the tourism English course in higher vocational colleges is obtained by using maximum likelihood estimation, which is expressed as:

$$\hat{c}(q) = \frac{p(d|\hat{c}) \otimes p(c|\hat{c})}{LLR \otimes \ell_{(W)} * t_m^{(d)}} \times \frac{\mu(S)}{\sigma(A)} \tag{22}$$

In the formula, *LLR* represents the log-likelihood ratio obtained by taking the logarithm. $\ell_{(W)}$ represents the current feature correction set. $t_m^{(d)}$ represents the distribution of the $i + 1$-th important feature symbol after searching for d second-important feature symbols. $\mu(S)$ stands for calculating the objective function value from the classification result and the dimension of the feature subset. $\sigma(A)$ represents the minimum feature dimension.

Assuming that $\arg\max D_E$ represents the optimization objective function under a certain number of categories, it can be expressed by the following formula:

$$\arg\max D_E = \Omega(d) * X(Z) \frac{\delta(u)}{\beta(q)} * K(N) \tag{23}$$

In the formula, $\Omega(d)$ represents the similarity data execution value between the cluster centers. $X(Z)$ represents the similarity between two close cluster centers. $\delta(u)$ represents the probability of symbolic distribution constructed from the feature space u of students' psychological tendency health data. $\beta(q)$ represents the relationship between students' psychological predisposition health data. $K(N)$ represents the optimized feature subset from the original student mental orientation health data features.

According to the above elaboration, the following formula is used to complete the mining of students' psychological tendency health data:

$$\partial(\hat{c}) \frac{\arg\max D_E * \hat{c}}{\delta(u)} \tag{24}$$

To sum up, by defining the objective function of the maximum difference of students' psychological tendency health data. The frequency distribution of each data in the ideological and political courses of tourism English courses in higher vocational colleges is obtained by using maximum likelihood estimation, and the data mining of students' psychological tendency and health is realized.

3 Experimental Comparative Analysis

3.1 Experimental Data Source

The data used in this paper come from 941 records in a university student psychological survey database. The SCL-90 scale is used to measure the mental health of college students.

The mental health indicators recorded in the database included somatization, interpersonal sensitivity, obsessive-compulsive symptoms, anxiety, depression, hostility, paranoia, phobia, psychosis and positive average scores.

The psychological data used in this paper have the following characteristics:

1. Being scientific: The SCL-90 Psychological Measurement Scale used in this school is widely used in the professional field of psychology and has high popularity. Moreover, it can quantify the students' behavior and psychological symptoms, and the data obtained is very professional and scientific.
2. High reliability: The measurement data of this part are stored in the database of relevant parts of the school. Data collected under the unified leadership of the school student department, distributed through questionnaires, or scattered online are more reliable.
3. Data imbalance: 941 student records used in this article measured the results of "abnormal" data only 76, measuring the results of "normal" data only 865. That is, the original data results are "abnormal" and results are "normal" data serious imbalance. This will affect the feasibility of data mining and the accuracy of test results.

3.2 Data Purification

Data cleansing is to delete the untrue and incomplete data from the original data, which can not meet the quality requirements of decision tree algorithm. Thus, the quality of data analysis can be ensured and more accurate data mining results can be obtained.

1. Purge False Records: Because the SCL-90 test has 90 multiple choice questions. After statistics that the test time is less than 4 min of the record is not earnest answer left unreal data. This part of the record is therefore culled.
2. Purifying unrelated attribute factors: Because the scope of the census was all college students, the data of students' name, sex, age, specialty, grade and time consumption had no effect on the model. It will increase the time and cost of data analysis and reduce the efficiency of data. Therefore, these factors are not considered in constructing the decision. After data purification, 886 relatively reliable records were obtained. After the adjustment of the database, the score table of each factor in the sample set

of decision tree training is obtained. The scores of each field in the sample set of decision tree training correspond to the scores measured by SCL-90, that is, the score of attribute factor of mental health index.

3. Purify the status of students: Because the SCL-90 is not always accurate, it can not be directly used as a basis for the diagnosis of psychological crisis, only as a reference. Therefore, a status attribute is attached to mark whether the students have psychological crisis. State refers to the mental health education center after the relevant workers screened to confirm the existence of psychological crisis.

After data purification, 886 relatively reliable records were obtained. Among them, 100 were selected as test samples and 786 as training samples.

3.3 Result Analysis

Data mining method based on smartphone perception, Ecological Instantaneous Assessment Theory and this paper's method are used to carry out the mental health data mining experiment. The results of the accuracy and efficiency tests for classifying student mental health data are shown in Figs. 1 and 2.

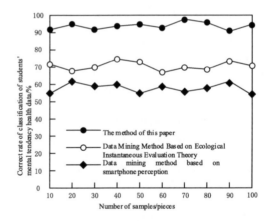

Fig. 1. Correct rate of classification of students' mental tendency health data

It can be concluded from Fig. 1 and Fig. 2 that the accuracy and efficiency of this method are higher than those of traditional data mining methods based on smartphone perception and ecological instantaneous assessment. The main reason is that SVM is used to classify and recognize the data features of mental health of students, and to calculate the degree of association among the features. Thus greatly improved the accuracy and efficiency of this method in the classification of mental health data.

On the basis of ensuring the accuracy and efficiency of the classification of students' psychological inclination health data. When mining students' mental health data, it is also necessary to ensure the integrity of the data, as shown in Fig. 3.

According to the results of Fig. 3, the data integrity of mental health data mined by this method is over 80%, and the data integrity of mental health data mined by smartphone is

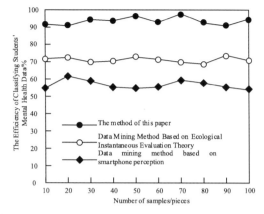

Fig. 2. The Efficiency of Classifying Students' Mental Health Data

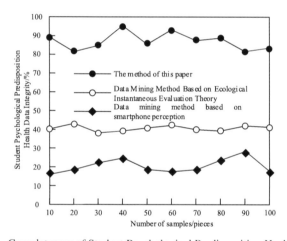

Fig. 3. Completeness of Student Psychological Predisposition Health Data

under 30%. When the data mining method based on ecological instantaneous assessment theory is used to mine students' mental health data, the data integrity fluctuates at 40%. Compared with the test results of three different methods, this method can be used to mine students' mental health data with higher integrity.

4   Conclusion

This paper puts forward a data mining research on mental health of students in Tourism English Course based on SVM. Experimental results prove that this method can improve the classification efficiency of mental health data. It can guarantee the integrity of mental health data to more than 80%. But there are still many deficiencies in this study. In the future research, we hope to introduce principal component analysis to extract the characteristics of students' mental health data and ensure the quality of data mining.

Fund Project. 2022 Hainan Higher Education and teaching reform research project: Research on the generation path of integrating curriculum ideology and politics into tourism professional English Curriculum -- a case study of Higher Vocational Colleges in Hainan Province (Project No.: Hnjgzc2022–111).

References

1. Wei, Z., Yong, W., Ning, Z.: Improved student psychology based optimization algorithm using hybrid strategy. Appl. Res. Comput. **39**(6), 1718–1724 (2022)
2. Rahman, M.M., Singh, M.K.M.: English Medium university STEM teachers' and students' ideologies in constructing content knowledge through translanguaging. Int. J. Biling. Educ. Biling. **25**(7), 2435–2453 (2022)
3. Shi, Q., Cai, N., Jiao, W.: Monitoring and evaluating college students' mental health based on big data analysis. Am. J. Health Behav. **46**(2), 164–176 (2022)
4. Zhou, X., Liu, L., Chen, Y., et al.: Research on design and application of an automatic assessment model for college students' mental health based on multimodal data fusion. E-educ. Res. **42**(8), 72–78 (2021)
5. Mou, K., Xu, B.: Research on emotional analysis platform of college students' public opinion information based on big data. In: 2022 IEEE 6th Information Technology and Mechatronics Engineering Conference (ITOEC), vol. 6, pp. 2105–2110. IEEE (2022)
6. Yu, Y., He, A., Zheng, S., et al.: Association between school bullying and mental health of adolescent students in low-income and middle-income countries. Chin. J. School Health **06**, 842–875 (2021)
7. Liu, Y., Chen, Q.: Personalized information mining of mobile terminal users based on tag mapping. Comput. Simul. **39**(1), 177–180, 208 (2022)

Intelligent Imaging Method of Nuclear Magnetic Resonance Medical Devices Based on Compression Sensing

Xuchu Deng[1]([⊠]), Zongying Lai[1], and Lizhi Chen[2]

[1] School of Ocean Information Engineering, Jimei University, Xiamen 361012, China
dd612p@163.com
[2] Chengdu Neusoft University, Chengdu 611844, China

Abstract. Aiming at the problems of low peak signal-to-noise ratio and slow imaging speed in the imaging method of nuclear magnetic resonance medical devices, an intelligent imaging method of nuclear magnetic resonance medical devices based on compression sensing is designed. The imaging space of nuclear magnetic resonance medical devices is limited to two dimensions, and the nuclear magnetic resonance pulse sequence is designed to determine the current proton state by receiving the energy attenuation signal. The imaging data is compressed and sampled, and the original signal is reconstructed according to the collected data and the measurement matrix to ensure the image quality. Finally, the intelligent imaging mode based on compressed sensing optimization is realized. The experimental results show that the peak signal-to-noise ratio of the intelligent imaging method of NMR medical devices in this paper is higher than that of the other two intelligent imaging methods of NMR medical devices, which proves that the performance of the intelligent imaging method of NMR medical devices can be improved after combining the compression sensing technology.

Keywords: Compression sensing · Nuclear magnetic resonance · medical apparatus and instruments · Intelligent imaging · Gradient magnetic field · Natural signal

1 Introduction

The intelligent imaging method of nuclear magnetic resonance medical devices based on compression sensing can present various dynamic processes, including the physiological movements of tissues and organs (such as heart, bone and joint, swallowing, etc.), as well as the changes of contrast agents and surgical intervention, which has broad application prospects. Compression sensing collects and compresses signals during signal acquisition, combining sampling and compression, greatly reducing the number of samples and data storage. However, the problem of long imaging time has been restricting the further development of MRI. On the one hand, the long imaging time greatly increases

S. Wang (Ed.): IoTCare 2022, LNICST 501, pp. 191–205, 2023.
https://doi.org/10.1007/978-3-031-33545-7_14

the possibility of patient movement during the imaging process, causing artifacts, blurring and other problems in the image, and even having to sacrifice image quality to shorten the imaging time, but it causes the lack of diagnostic information. Applying compressed sensing to image and video fields can effectively reduce data acquisition costs and data storage costs. Compression sensing can sample data at a frequency much lower than Nyquist's, and is widely used in image compression, medical imaging, atomic force microscope imaging, radar imaging, pattern recognition, channel coding and many other fields. It is considered to be an important key technology to promote the development of social informatization. On the other hand, the long imaging time limits the time resolution of imaging, resulting in the inability to fully present the real dynamic process, which directly hinders the trend of real-time dynamic imaging to clinical application [1, 2]. Therefore, accelerating the speed of magnetic resonance imaging has important theoretical significance and practical value for improving image quality, improving time resolution, and expanding the application field of magnetic resonance medical device imaging.

The imaging time of magnetic resonance medical devices is mainly composed of scanning time and image reconstruction time. In the theory of compressed sensing, the measured signal is required to be sparse or compressible. In practice, most signals are not strictly sparse, but studies have shown that most natural signals are compressible. That is, although it is a non sparse signal in the time domain, the signal can be sparse after a series of domain transformations, such as discrete cosine transform, discrete wavelet transform and curvelet discrete transform. In principle, dynamic imaging is the repeated application of conventional static imaging methods, that is, a frame of data is completely scanned, and then the image is directly reconstructed by inverse Fourier transform. Due to the application of fast Fourier transform, the imaging time mainly depends on the scanning time. That is to say, most natural signals are sparse in Fourier domain, discrete cosine domain, discrete wavelet domain and curvelet basis. Another representation of signal sparsity, redundant dictionary representation, is also a commonly used signal sparse transformation method. In order to meet the real-time requirements, the scanning speed is required to be higher than the physiological movement speed. However, hardware (gradient magnetic field intensity and its switching rate) and physiological (such as nerve stimulation) factors limit the application of fast scanning. No matter two-dimensional image or three-dimensional image, as long as the conditions of compressed sensing are met, the measurement of data can be greatly reduced, so as to shorten the reconstruction time. Therefore, how to shorten the scanning time and image reconstruction time and improve the imaging speed has become the main research problem of magnetic resonance medical device imaging. In this paper, an intelligent imaging method of nuclear magnetic resonance medical devices based on compression sensing is proposed. The imaging space of nuclear magnetic resonance medical devices is limited to two dimensions, and the nuclear magnetic resonance pulse sequence is designed to determine the current proton state by receiving the energy attenuation signal. The imaging data is compressed and sampled, and the original signal is reconstructed according to the acquired data and measurement matrix to ensure the image quality. The results show that the mean value of the peak signal-to-noise ratio of the method studied is high, which proves that the performance of the intelligent imaging method of nuclear magnetic resonance medical devices is improved after the combination of compression sensing technology. Fast imaging speed and high quality of reconstructed images are of great significance both from the perspective of patients and doctors.

2 Collect Magnetic Field Imaging Signal

Imaging with magnetic resonance technology actually reflects the distribution of hydrogen atoms in the body. Usually, at a certain resonance frequency, RF excitation often excites the whole solid, so we can use the gradient transformation to selectively excite a part of the solid when we locate the hydrogen atom in space. If the sampling is dense enough, a continuous signal can be represented by its sampling values at equal time intervals, and all the signals can be recovered through these sample values, which is the content of the sampling theorem. Therefore, in magnetic resonance imaging, three gradient magnetic fields are used for imaging operation. One gradient magnetic field is used to determine the plane. After determining the plane through the gradient magnetic field, the imaging space is limited to two dimensions. Then the corresponding signals are spatially encoded in this two-dimensional plane, and this process realizes the collection of data at a specific level. The importance of sampling theorem is that it acts as a bridge between continuous time signals and discrete-time signals [3–5]. Under certain conditions, a continuous time signal can be completely recovered from its samples, which provides a theoretical basis for discrete signals to represent continuous signals, because in many aspects, the processing of discrete signals is more flexible and convenient than that of continuous signals. The static magnetic field is the external magnetic field, pointing in the longitudinal direction, and its magnetic field strength determines the net magnetic moment and resonance frequency of the atomic nucleus. The uniformity of magnetic field is particularly important for imaging. If the magnetic field is uneven, the imaging image will often produce deformation or artifacts. In the process of magnetic resonance imaging, due to external factors, the external magnetic field strength is often difficult to achieve complete uniformity. According to the multiplication property of Fourier transform, the spectrum calculation formula of finite frequency band is obtained:

$$L(\delta) = \frac{1}{2\pi} \left[D(\delta) \times \sqrt{G(\delta - 1)^2} \right]$$ (1)

In Eq. (1), D represents continuous time signal, G represents sampling frequency, and δ represents periodic function. The concept of sampling makes people think of using discrete-time system technology to realize continuous time and indirectly process continuous time signals: first, convert continuous time signals into discrete-time signals through sampling, then use discrete-time system to process the discrete-time signals, and finally convert discrete-time signals into continuous time. Therefore, in order to ensure a good MRI effect, the uniformity of the external magnetic field must be guaranteed within a specific range. Gradient magnetic field is generated by several groups of coils located in the magnet cavity through current. Attached to the main magnetic field, it can increase or decrease the strength of the main magnetic field, so that the spin protons along the gradient direction have different magnetic field strengths, so there are different types of resonance frequencies. The structure of human eyes leads people to understand that images are not as sensitive to uniform or linear changes in the image field as data stored on binary media. For example, it is insensitive to some distortions and cannot detect some subtle changes in the image. Even if these subtle changes are directly lost, the human eye cannot feel them. Through the purposeful change of the static magnetic field, we can change the uniformity of the magnetic field, and then interpret the spatial information of the signal through the transformation law of the static magnetic field strength, so as to obtain the spatial code of the signal. RF coil can also be used as receiving coil (induction coil) under normal circumstances. For one-dimensional signals, the characteristic information is represented by the sensing matrix, and the expression formula of linear measurement sparsity is:

$$Y = \varepsilon \times \frac{H}{2} \tag{2}$$

In Eq. (2), ε represents the orthogonal basis composed of column vectors, and H represents the original signal. Therefore, within a certain range, the image changes caused by quantization errors cannot be detected by human eyes. The usual way of recording raw data is based on the assumption that the human visual system is uniform and linear, which leads to the equal treatment of the visually insensitive part and the visually sensitive part, resulting in more data than the ideal coding. This redundancy is called visual redundancy. According to Ferrari's law of electromagnetic induction, the change of magnetic flux in a closed circuit will produce induced electromotive force. Therefore, place a coil in a suitable position within the range swept by the transverse magnetization component. Make the coil cut the magnetic induction line, and the induced electromotive force will be generated in the coil, so that the magnetic resonance signal can be detected. In the process of free precession, the decrease of transverse magnetization vector makes the electromotive force received by its coil also decrease. This signal is called free induction attenuation signal. In order to reconstruct the original signal, it is necessary to calculate all the projection data, then select several data with large amplitude, and encode their positions, while all the remaining projection data with small amplitude are discarded. Then through the ring coil to collect the free attenuation signal, the changing magnetic field intensity signal will be obtained, and then the magnetic field intensity signal will be converted into the corresponding electrical signal to complete the signal acquisition. The received signal is the superposition of the overall magnetization vector. Therefore, the entire detection system can detect spatial information only when each magnetic field is a gradient magnetic field.

3   Extracting NMR Pulse Sequence

Nuclear magnetic resonance refers to the phenomenon of resonance absorption transition between Zeeman levels under certain conditions. RF pulse, coding gradient field, parameter setting during signal acquisition and their sequence are called pulse sequence of nuclear magnetic resonance. In magnetic resonance imaging, in order to observe the current state of protons, RF pulses are usually used as excitation elements. When the frequency of RF pulses is the same as the precession frequency of protons, resonance will occur [6]. The space allowed to receive digitized original data is k space, and its unit is spatial frequency (hz/cm). The pulse sequence includes 90° pulse and 180° pulse. After 90° pulse excitation, the elapsed time: apply another 180° RF pulse, the proton will flip 180° in the transverse plane, and then after time, the spin echo signal will be generated. The generation of resonance will transfer the energy of the RF pulse to the proton. After removing the RF pulse, this part of energy will decay slowly. Therefore, by receiving the decay signal of this part of energy, the current proton state can be determined. Assuming that the external magnetic field intensity is Z_0, the proton precesses at the angular velocity of η_0. Using a magnetic field with a magnetic field strength of Z_1, an RF pulse is generated, and the pulse angular velocity is η_1. By using the pulse sequence, changing the interval between the two pulses, the peak signal of the spin echo at each time interval is obtained, and the echo signal is obtained by connecting each peak point. Human body imaging needs to determine the spin density, not the size of the magnetization vector. To obtain proton density weighted images, pulse sequences with long repetition time and short echo time should be used. The magnetic field Z_1 is much smaller than the field strength of the external magnetic field. To generate resonance, the frequency of the RF pulse must be the same as the precession frequency, that is, the angular velocity must be the same. When the two frequencies are the same, the proton precession direction will deflect towards the Z_1 magnetic field. That is, when $\eta_0 = \eta_1$. Resonance will occur, and the proton precession direction will deflect. Since the external magnetic field is a stable magnetic field, and the magnetic field strength Z_1 is much smaller than the external magnetic field strength Z_0, the influence of precession reversal on the external magnetic field strength can be ignored. With the increase of the action time of the magnetic field Z_1, the deviation of the proton precession direction is also increasing, and the magnetization vector in the corresponding action direction is also gradually increasing. Finally, the proton precession direction is overturned into the same plane. According to the RF pulse intensity and action time, the turning angle γ can be determined, and the formula is as follows:

$$\gamma = \frac{\phi \times h \times l}{2} \tag{3}$$

In Eq. (3), ϕ represents the gyromagnetic ratio, h represents the intensity of RF pulse, and l represents the action time of RF pulse. In the relaxation process, we call the phenomenon that the vertical component of the magnetization vector gradually increases and returns to the level before excitation as longitudinal relaxation. The phenomenon that the horizontal component of the magnetization vector gradually decreases until it disappears is called transverse relaxation. Nowadays, the pulse sequences that can obtain proton density weighted imaging are mainly spin echo pulse sequence and gradient echo pulse sequence. The basic idea of gradient echo pulse sequence is to form echo through the reverse of frequency coding gradient. When the magnetization vector returns to the original state in the vertical direction, its vector just disappears in the horizontal direction, so the time required for the longitudinal relaxation process is the same as that for the transverse relaxation process [7, 8]. When the RF pulse acts, the corresponding magnetization vector will deflect. The gradient echo sequence of 90° pulse is a simple pulse sequence. RF pulse is a sinc function in time domain, corresponding to square pulse in frequency domain. The phase coding gradient is represented by a series of horizontal lines, indicating that it steps in incremental rules in different repetition periods. Through the phase coding and frequency coding, the specific spatial coding at the specific level is formed. Spatial frequency is a vector, which refers to the phase change per unit length in a certain direction. When generating NMR images, two gradient fields of frequency and phase are used. The original data are collected in the frequency domain and can be directly stored in k space. The reconstructed images can be obtained by Fourier transform of these data. The data with positive phase of spatial coding will be filled to the top of the specific space, and the data with negative phase will be filled to the bottom of the specific space. In this particular space, the signal of the middle row is the strongest. In most cases, the main data are concentrated in the center of the specific space. The NMR signals encoded by three gradients carry the information of layer, frequency and phase respectively. The image can be obtained by Fourier transform of the data stored in k space. Fourier transform can be used between the reconstructed image and its corresponding k space, which is the remarkable feature of k space.

4   Recognizing Dynamic Features of Medical Device Images

According to the time relationship between signal acquisition and imaging, the imaging methods of magnetic resonance medical devices can be roughly divided into two categories: offline and online. In the process of horizontal and vertical relaxation, the atomic nucleus releases energy and transitions from the high-energy state to the original equilibrium state. The process of medical image reconstruction is to complete intelligent imaging by analyzing the voltage signal released in this process. Online imaging method is to reconstruct the image separately for the single frame data at the current time, that is, the form of reconstruction while sampling. When the reconstruction speed of online imaging is fast enough to be faster than the data acquisition speed, this method can be called real-time imaging. The NMR signal is jointly contributed by the spin in the excited volume of the sample. The relationship between the signal and the spin density is as follows:

$$W = \int \frac{\phi \times h \times l}{2} - |\vec{\mu}| \times \varpi^3 \qquad (4)$$

In Eq. (4), μ represents time-frequency domain signal and ϖ represents time-domain signal. There is no phase shift in spatial coding, and the data obtained after frequency coding will usually be filled into the middle of a specific space. By applying a certain frequency of RF signal, the plane geometric distribution of the whole human body structure can be obtained. However, it is impossible to image the designated part to be detected, so the received signal must be spatially located. Real time magnetic resonance imaging of medical devices has a wide range of applications, such as dynamic imaging of human joint function, quantitative analysis of cardiovascular blood flow, magnetic resonance guided cardiac surgery and so on. At present, the magnetic resonance imaging system in medicine completes the positioning and coding of spatial information by applying three gradient magnetic fields that are perpendicular to each other and change linearly. Generally, for an image signal, the energy is mainly concentrated in the low-frequency band, that is, the central area of k space. The high-frequency part of the image contains less energy distribution, that is, the surrounding part of k space. This paper first reconstructs the frame difference image, and then obtains the current frame image by adding the reconstructed frame difference image to the previous frame image. Therefore, the previous images are the basis of the whole movie reconstruction, and their reconstruction quality will affect the reconstruction quality of the next frame image of the movie. Therefore, the traditional equal interval uniform density scanning sampling method often leads to the generation of image aliasing artifacts. Therefore, this paper considers using a variable density sampling method to collect more low-frequency bands with high information and less high-frequency bands with low information, which may obtain a more accurate reconstruction effect and reduce the generation of image aliasing artifacts. Therefore, this paper constructs an imaging mode in which the sampling rate gradually decreases to a stable level. Use 2 × down imaging for the first image, 4x down imaging for the second image, and 8 × down imaging for each subsequent image. Generally, the ability of the transform sparse basis to transform the signal sparsely is expressed by the decay rate of the transform coefficient:

$$v = \left| \frac{r}{d} \right| - \beta \times \left(|\vec{\mu}| \times \varpi^3 \right) \tag{5}$$

In Eq. (5), r refers to the orthogonal transformation set, d refers to the transformation coefficients, and β refers to the coefficient index representation after the coefficients are arranged in power exponential descending order. According to the calculation results of formula (5), the most critical step for unequal interval variable density imaging is the selection and definition of sampling density. In this paper, we choose to conduct under sampling in the direction of x axis, that is, the size of sampling interval in the direction of x axis affects the sampling density. Compared with the film as a whole, the high sampling rate of the first two images will not significantly increase the film sampling rate, so it will not have a significant impact on the average sampling time. Nuclear magnetic resonance imaging of medical devices uses the resonance effect of atomic nuclei to image the human body by collecting the electromagnetic signals released after nuclear resonance. Theoretical analysis shows that the total variation regularization constraint can not only reduce the noise in the reconstructed image, but also smooth the edge of the image. However, due to the piecewise smoothness of the image, the piecewise constraint sometimes directly leads to the excessive blur of the fine texture structure of the image. The number of hydrogen atoms in the human body is the largest and the most widely distributed. When imaging the human body with nuclear magnetic resonance medical devices, the resonance effect of hydrogen atoms is generally used to detect its resonance signal. However, wavelet basis function has the characteristics of good time-domain locality and moment cancellation, and can well represent the mutation characteristics of image signals, such as jumping singularity, and well represent the local smooth part. Due to the different content of hydrogen atoms in different parts and tissues of the human body, the detected signal intensity is also different when imaging different parts with NMR medical devices. Therefore, the resonance effect of hydrogen atoms can be used to image human tissues and distinguish pathological tissues.

5 Optimization of Intelligent Imaging Mode Based on Compressed Sensing

Compressed sensing is mainly composed of three parts: signal sparse representation, random signal acquisition, i.e. linear measurement process, and sparse reconstruction. Compared with the traditional data compression method, the most distinctive feature of compressed sensing is that it bypasses the inefficient link of sampling and then compression, and uses the sensing matrix to directly obtain the characteristic information of sparse signals or compressible signals. The premise of using compressed sensing is that the signal is sufficiently sparse. Because the actual measured signal is usually not sufficiently sparse, a suitable transform basis is selected to make the signal more sparse in the transform domain, so as to obtain better reconstruction results. If the original signal with sparse representation is sampled randomly, the original signal can be recovered under the condition of breaking through Nyquist. The compressed sensing algorithm breaks through the limitation of Nyquist Shannon sampling theorem, and can greatly reduce the sampling rate of the signal, and accurately reconstruct the original signal with only a small amount of sampling data [9, 10]. In the theory of compression sensing, the linear measurement process is often represented by a stable set of linear equations. The main process of compression sensing is shown in Fig. 1:

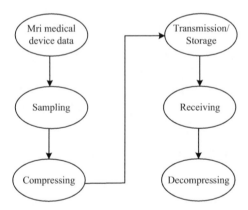

Fig. 1. Main process of compression sensing

It can be seen from Fig. 1 that in the imaging process, the signal can be compressed while sampling, reducing the compression cost of the signal. Applying compressed sensing technology to the measurement process of atomic force microscope can reduce the sampling rate of atomic force microscope and shorten the originally long imaging time. The process of intelligent imaging is to use reconstruction algorithm to reconstruct the original signal according to the collected data and measurement matrix. Before explaining the structure of the discriminator, first of all, it briefly introduces the content of the loss function related to the training of the discriminator [11]. In the previous research, the loss function used by the traditional generation countermeasure network in training the generator has two types, one is saturated and the other is unsaturated.

Conduct continuous magnetic resonance imaging operations for many times in a certain time period to capture the operation of human organs and tissues in that time period. Unlike static magnetic resonance imaging, intelligent imaging requires faster imaging speed. And due to the reduction of sampling rate, the interaction force between the probe tip of the atomic force microscope and the sample surface is reduced, so as to reduce the wear of the probe and the damage of the sample surface, and further improve the imaging accuracy of the atomic force microscope. Because the time-varying of human organs and tissues, such as the heart, is moving all the time, and the corresponding space will also change with it [12, 13]. To capture the spatial data at the current time point, we need a very fast data acquisition speed to ensure that the data acquisition is completed before the heart shape changes, otherwise it will inevitably cause data distortion. Under some conditions, when the real data is completely distinguished from the generated data, the saturation loss tends to have a gradient of zero, while the unsaturated loss, although the gradient is not zero, has the problem of instability. This will eventually lead to the discriminator often unable to train to the optimal or the learning rate is too high, otherwise it may make the gradient disappear and the training stop. Therefore, it is necessary to minimize the time of data acquisition without sacrificing spatial resolution.

6 Simulation Experiment Analysis

6.1 Experimental Preparation

It is composed of NMR spectrometer, RF power amplifier, gradient power amplifier, preamplifier, unilateral NMR equipment, duplexer and computer. CUDA architecture is composed of CPU and GPU. CPU plays the role of host and GPU plays the role of device. Among them, GPU mainly completes threaded parallel processing, while CPU is mainly responsible for serial computing and logical transaction processing. Use coaxial cable to connect the unilateral NMR equipment with the spectrometer. They all have relatively independent memory address space. CPU corresponds to host side memory and GPU corresponds to device side memory. CUDA calls the memory management function in CUDA API to realize the operation of memory and video memory. First, the two-phase coded pulse sequence is written in the tnmr sequence editing software of tecmag NMR spectrometer, and the imaging parameters are set. The NMR signal generated by the sample is directly output to the NMR spectrometer after being amplified by the preamplifier after passing through the duplexer, and then transmitted to the computer, which displays the signal. During the whole experiment, the RF coil has two functions: transmitting and receiving. The operation of memory is basically the same as that of general C programs. The operation of memory mainly includes opening up space, initializing space, releasing space, and completing data transmission at the device end and the host end.

6.2 Experimental Result

In order to get intuitive experimental results, the intelligent imaging method of MRI medical devices based on deep learning and the intelligent imaging method of MRI medical devices based on generation countermeasure network are selected to compare with the intelligent imaging method of MRI medical devices in this paper. Test the peak signal-to-noise ratio of the three MRI medical device intelligent imaging methods under different signal-to-noise ratio conditions. The larger the value, the higher the accuracy. The experimental results are shown in Tables 1, 2, 3 and 4:

Table 1. Signal to noise ratio 10 dB peak signal to noise ratio

Number of experiments	Intelligent imaging method of magnetic resonance medical devices based on deep learning	Intelligent imaging method of magnetic resonance medical devices based on generated countermeasure network	The intelligent imaging method of NMR medical devices in this paper
1	21.203	23.655	29.363
2	22.166	22.421	28.345
3	21.245	21.944	31.266
4	23.123	22.106	30.151
5	22.331	21.303	29.009
6	21.228	23.005	31.154
7	22.545	22.146	29.136
8	21.612	20.616	28.483
9	22.144	21.074	27.212
10	21.714	23.099	31.514
11	23.162	24.548	29.217
12	22.495	23.316	28.649
13	21.317	22.157	27.157
14	22.445	21.159	29.166
15	21.147	23.301	30.337

It can be seen from Table 1 that when the signal-to-noise ratio is 10 dB, the peak signal-to-noise ratio of the intelligent imaging method of nuclear magnetic resonance medical devices in this paper and the other two intelligent imaging methods of nuclear magnetic resonance medical devices are 29.0344, 21.992 and 22.390 respectively.

It can be seen from Table 2 that when the signal-to-noise ratio is 30 dB, the average peak signal-to-noise ratio of the NMR medical device intelligent imaging method in this paper and the other two NMR medical device intelligent imaging methods are 45.395, 34.656 and 33.494 respectively.

It can be seen from Table 3 that when the signal-to-noise ratio is 50 dB, the average peak signal-to-noise ratio of the NMR medical device intelligent imaging method in this

Table 2. Signal to noise ratio 30 dB peak signal to noise ratio

Number of experiments	Intelligent imaging method of magnetic resonance medical devices based on deep learning	Intelligent imaging method of magnetic resonance medical devices based on generated countermeasure network	The intelligent imaging method of NMR medical devices in this paper
1	32.154	36.474	42.944
2	35.811	32.151	43.847
3	34.326	32.215	45.554
4	32.177	31.933	46.564
5	31.494	34.467	44.518
6	33.547	32.485	43.334
7	36.315	31.120	45.102
8	34.194	34.648	43.174
9	35.477	32.971	46.946
10	36.515	31.479	45.994
11	36.152	34.944	46.741
12	34.483	33.154	48.166
13	35.788	35.747	46.331
14	34.455	33.316	46.559
15	36.949	35.299	45.144

Table 3. Signal to noise ratio 50 dB peak signal to noise ratio

Number of experiments	Intelligent imaging method of magnetic resonance medical devices based on deep learning	Intelligent imaging method of magnetic resonance medical devices based on generated countermeasure network	The intelligent imaging method of NMR medical devices in this paper
1	42.313	43.347	48.202
2	43.255	41.152	46.147
3	41.649	42.474	52.105
4	42.636	44.518	49.947
5	41.552	43.166	48.466

(*continued*)

Table 3. (*continued*)

Number of experiments	Intelligent imaging method of magnetic resonance medical devices based on deep learning	Intelligent imaging method of magnetic resonance medical devices based on generated countermeasure network	The intelligent imaging method of NMR medical devices in this paper
6	43.255	41.481	49.747
7	42.144	42.121	51.946
8	41.263	43.333	52.441
9	42.102	42. 154	52.646
10	43.447	41.744	51.488
11	44.894	42.849	52.117
12	43.548	44.556	52.599
13	42.474	42.314	53.415
14	41.165	43.415	55.116
15	42.415	41.112	49.212

paper and the other two NMR medical device intelligent imaging methods are 51.040, 42.541 and 42.684 respectively.

Table 4. Signal to noise ratio 70 dB peak signal to noise ratio

Number of experiments	Intelligent imaging method of magnetic resonance medical devices based on deep learning	Intelligent imaging method of magnetic resonance medical devices based on generated countermeasure network	The intelligent imaging method of NMR medical devices in this paper
1	52.447	49.994	55.748
2	49.752	48.516	56.851
3	46.188	51.054	58.263
4	48.146	50.477	57.499
5	49.258	52.366	56.205
6	51.481	53.845	57.211
7	49.515	49.211	55.171
8	49.499	48.314	56.447
9	51.515	46.151	57.211

(*continued*)

Table 4. (*continued*)

Number of experiments	Intelligent imaging method of magnetic resonance medical devices based on deep learning	Intelligent imaging method of magnetic resonance medical devices based on generated countermeasure network	The intelligent imaging method of NMR medical devices in this paper
10	50.162	47.207	58.319
11	48.147	46.499	56.408
12	49.311	48.515	58.523
13	48.487	50.212	56.545
14	51.941	49.324	57.641
15	52.157	48.544	55.109

It can be seen from Table 4 that when the signal-to-noise ratio is 70 dB, the peak signal-to-noise ratio of the intelligent imaging method of nuclear magnetic resonance medical devices in this paper and the other two intelligent imaging methods of nuclear magnetic resonance medical devices are 56.877, 49.867 and 49.349 respectively.

Table 5. Signal to noise ratio 90 dB peak signal to noise ratio

Number of experiments	Intelligent imaging method of magnetic resonance medical devices based on deep learning	Intelligent imaging method of magnetic resonance medical devices based on generated countermeasure network	The intelligent imaging method of NMR medical devices in this paper
1	53.991	55.488	62.164
2	52.415	57.415	63.314
3	51.547	56.549	62.331
4	53.316	54.211	61.158
5	54.448	55.099	63.207
6	52.220	56.147	62.849
7	53.147	55.305	63.541
8	54.466	55.488	62.662
9	52.848	56.501	63.315
10	53.502	54.215	64.548
11	54.433	53.490	63.547
12	55.548	54.155	62.644
13	54.699	55.649	63.102
14	53.147	56.007	62.106
15	52.331	54.413	63.113

It can be seen from Table 5 that when the signal-to-noise ratio is 90 dB, the average peak signal-to-noise ratio of the NMR medical device intelligent imaging method in this paper and the other two NMR medical device intelligent imaging methods are 62.907, 53.471 and 55.342 respectively. It can be seen from the experimental results in Tables 1, 2, 3, 4, and 5 that the intelligent imaging method of NMR medical devices in this paper can maintain good performance under different signal-to-noise ratio experimental scenarios.

7 Conclusion

(1) This paper discusses the sparse representation of MRI images in different transform domain spaces, and designs and implements the spatial sparse sampling track with random variable density. At the same time, it studies the peak signal to noise ratio of the intelligent imaging method of MRI medical devices.
(2) The variance of image pixels is used to adaptively estimate the weighting matrix, which is solved under the framework of compressed sensing. A random variable density sampling method is designed to collect low-frequency regions with high information content.
(3) The intelligent imaging method of MRI medical devices studied in this paper can maintain good performance in different SNR experimental scenarios.

In the future, it is necessary to continue in-depth research to find an efficient reconstruction algorithm suitable for MRI application scenarios and parallelize it.

Fund Project. Project supported by the Scientific Research Foundation of Jimei University, China, ZQ2019034, and Fujian Province Young and Middle-aged Teachers Education Research Project, JAT190303.

References

1. Wang, M., Wang, Y., Yu, M., et al.: Preliminary application of artificial intelligence-based image optimization in coronary CT angiography. Chin. J. Radiol. **54**(5), 460–466 (2020)
2. Phasinam, K., Kassanuk, T.: Machine learning and internet of things (IoT) for real-time image classification in smart agriculture. ECS Trans. **107**(1), 3305–3311 (2022)
3. Li, S., Zhang, X., Gao, X., Sun, H.: Research on black-and-white image processing method of smart car camera. J. Meas. Sci. Inst. (2), 23–26 (2022)
4. Chierchie, F., Moroni, G.F., Stefanazzi, L., et al.: Smart readout of nondestructive image sensors with single photon-electron sensitivity. Phys. Rev. Lett. **127**(24), 1–6 (2021)
5. Li, Y., Chen, Y., Yang, X.: Edge segmentation of brain tumor based on MRI image. Comput. Simul. **37**(10), 369–373 (2020)
6. Cai, W., Wang Y.: Advances in construction of human brain atlases from magnetic resonance images. Chin. J. Magn. Reson. **37**(2), 241–253 (2020)
7. Li, Q., Zhu, H., Huang, G., et al.: Low-power in-pixel buffer circuit for smart image sensor. Sens. Rev. **40**(5), 585–590 (2020)
8. Fan, J., Ma M., Zhao, S.: Research on high reflective imaging technology based on compressed sensing. J. Electron. Inf. Technol. **42**(4), 1013–1020 (2020)

9. Xia, K., Yin, H., Jin, Y., et al.: Cross-domain brain CT image smart segmentation via shared hidden space transfer FCM clustering. ACM Trans. Multimedia Comput. Commun. Appl. (TOMM) **16**(2), 1–21 (2020)
10. Bao, Y., Cai, M., Zhao, M., et al.: A comparative research on the efficiency and image quality between manual and artificial intelligence post-processing of coronary CT angiography. J. Pract. Radiol. **36**(8), 1322–1325 (2020)
11. Wang, W., Zhang, X., Wang, S.-H., Zhang, Y.-D.: Covid-19 diagnosis by WE-SAJ, systems science & control. Engineering **10**(1), 325–335 (2022). https://doi.org/10.1080/21642583.2022.2045645
12. Huang, C., Wang, W., Zhang, X., Wang, S.-H., Zhang, Y.-D.: Tuberculosis diagnosis using deep transferred EfficientNet. In:IEEE/ACM Transactions on Computational Biology and Bioinformatics (2022). https://doi.org/10.1109/TCBB.2022.3199572
13. Hida, Y., Makariou, S., Kobayashi, S.: Smart image inspection using defect-removing autoencoder - ScienceDirect. Procedia CIRP **104**(1), 559–564 (2021)

Evaluation of Post Fitness of Employees in Health Care Enterprises Based on Big Data

Lizhi Chen[1](✉) and Xuchu Deng[2]

[1] Chengdu Neusoft University, Chengdu 611844, China
clz200111162022@163.com

[2] School of Ocean Information Engineering, Jimei University, Xiamen 361012, China

Abstract. Under the background of big data, the structure of health care enterprises is constantly upgrading, and there is a misplaced matching relationship between employees and posts. In order to promote the development of health care enterprises and optimize the allocation of talents, this paper studies the post fitness evaluation of health care enterprises based on big data. Put forward the selection principles and ideas of fitness evaluation indexes, and provide the basis for index selection; Establish an evaluation index system of fitness, screen high-frequency factors and select sequencing parameters; Through index identification and quantification, this paper analyzes the coordination and adaptation relationship between employees and post structure in medical and health care enterprises. Calculate the fitness, divide the fitness grade type according to the fitness evaluation grade type standard, and complete the evaluation. Through empirical analysis, the post coordination fitness of employees in 10 medical and health care enterprises showed a tortuous upward trend from 2016 to 2021, with 5 enterprises suffering from weak degree imbalance and 5 enterprises suffering from weak degree coordination. Among them, the average fitness of enterprise 7 is the highest, which is 0.59, but the overall level still has much room for improvement, and it is necessary to adjust and supplement the appropriate talents in time.

Keywords: Big Data · Enterprise Health Care · Algorithm Fusion · Employee Position · Fitness Evaluation · Evaluation Index Selection

1 Introduction

The 19th National Congress of the Communist Party of China clearly pointed out the transformation of the main social contradictions in our country in the new era-"The main social contradictions in our country have been transformed into the contradiction between the people's growing need for a better life and the unbalanced development". With the development of China's economy and society, people's living standards are constantly improving, and the demand for health is increasing day by day. The quantity and quality of social medical resources have great influence on national physical and mental health, but the quantity and quality of existing medical resources can hardly meet people's growing health needs [1]. Under the situation that supply is less than

S. Wang (Ed.): IoTCare 2022, LNICST 501, pp. 206–220, 2023.
https://doi.org/10.1007/978-3-031-33545-7_15

demand, a new wave of developing medical technology and resources with the help of information technology industry has arisen, and the development of medical industry has also ushered in the spring. Although the concepts of mobile medical care, artificial intelligence medical care and internet hospital have been put forward until now, a large number of internet medical care trendsetters have emerged. Internet giants such as Ali, Tencent, JD.COM and Baidu have also laid out the internet medical care industry, which has the potential to be shared by the whole world. Various medical and health care enterprises have sprung up. Medical care refers to people who maintain or improve their health through prevention, diagnosis, treatment, improvement or cure of diseases, diseases, injuries and other physical and mental disorders. Health care is provided by health professionals and related health fields. Medicine, dentistry, pharmacy, midwifery, nursing, optometry, audiology, psychology, occupational therapy, physical therapy, sports training and other health professions are all part of medical care. Including its work in providing primary health care, secondary health care, tertiary health care and public health. Under the background of big data, the state has issued a series of policies and measures to promote the healthy development of Internet medical industry, and comprehensively standardized and guided the healthy development of "Internet + medical care" enterprises [2]. Domestic "Internet + Medical" enterprises have successively appeared different modes, such as non-interactive medical health information service, online consultation, medical e-commerce, health monitoring and management, and medical service process optimization. Integrate several departments dedicated to providing health care services and products in the medical industry. As the basic framework for defining this sector, the International Standard Industrial Classification of the United Nations classifies medical care as generally including hospital activities, medical and dental practice activities and "other human health activities". The last category involves the activities of nurses, midwives, physiotherapists, scientific or diagnostic laboratories, pathological clinics, residential health facilities, patient advocates or other related health professionals or activities under their supervision. In addition, according to industry and market classifications, such as global industry classification standard and industry classification benchmark, medical care includes many categories of medical equipment, instruments and services, including biotechnology, diagnostic laboratories and substances, drug manufacturing and delivery. However, by analyzing the current medical environment, the shortage of medical resources is not only insufficient in quality, but also unevenly distributed in time and space, which is mainly manifested in: asymmetric information among patients, hospitals and doctors, which leads to a large number of patients "voting with their feet" and blindly pouring into second and third-class hospitals, but few grassroots community health institutions are interested in it; Second, the doctors in the third-class hospitals are burdened with heavy tasks and exhausted, and the medical resources are stretched, while the medical resources in the grassroots community hospitals cannot be effectively utilized. Therefore, higher requirements are put forward for the employees of various medical and health care enterprises, and the matching degree between the positions and employees of enterprises has become a hot issue in current research. Under the background of big data era, with the adjustment and change of enterprise structure, the type and level of talent demand should also be continuously optimized in factor allocation to ensure the matching and adaptation between employees and enterprise positions, thus promoting the sustainable development of the whole industry economy. Therefore, it is an important practical task for the whole industry to guide the fitness between employees and posts in health care industry. Based on big data, this paper studies the evaluation of the fitness of employees in health care enterprises, first, establish the fitness evaluation index system, screen high-frequency factors, and select the order parameters; Then, through the identification and quantification of indicators, it analyzes the coordination and adaptation relationship between the employees and the post structure of the health care enterprise; Finally, the fitness is calculated, and the fitness grade types are divided according to the fitness evaluation grade type standards to complete the evaluation. The conclusions drawn from the empirical analysis provide a basis for promoting the development of health care enterprises and are of practical significance for improving the fitness of the health care industry under big data.

2   Health Care Enterprise Staff Post Fitness Evaluation

2.1   Selection Principles and Ideas of Fitness Evaluation Indicators

In medical and health care enterprises, there are many factors that affect the fitness between employees and posts. To evaluate the fitness of employees in medical and health care enterprises under big data, it is necessary to follow certain scientific criteria and objectively and truly reflect the current status of employees in medical and health care enterprises. The research on the fitness between employees' structure and the structure of health care enterprises is an all-round and multi-dimensional research process, ranging from the top-level design of the industry to the individual's employment choice, which involves many social fields. Therefore, the selection of evaluation indicators should be both systematic and comprehensive, and have certain internal logic [3]. It is easy to quantify, and the selected indicators should have reliable data sources, that is, the selected indicators must be mentioned in the official documents of our country or have corresponding statistical caliber. The selected indicators should not only meet the requirements that different regions in the same period are comparable, but also meet the requirements that the same region is comparable in different periods. The selected indicators should be able to truly reflect the current situation of regional development, or adapt to the actual economic development. Follow the principles of systematicness, scientificity, operability, comparability and timeliness. In order to realize the unity of structure and function between employee structure and health care enterprise structure, the optimization of employee structure is divided into four sequential links: input-generation-allocation-application. Two dimensions including rationalization and upgrading of industrial structure are respectively connected, and the sequence parameters are extracted as evaluation index system. The specific selection process is shown in Fig. 1.

As can be seen from Fig. 1, according to synergetics theory, the necessary condition for the long-term stable existence of a new system is the "orderliness" among the subsystems that make up the system, which is mainly manifested in the regularity of "the combination of elements and functions, the combination of space-time structure and the order of evolution process" in the material system. Only when employees and enterprise structure subsystems are coordinated, that is, orderly, can their parent system,

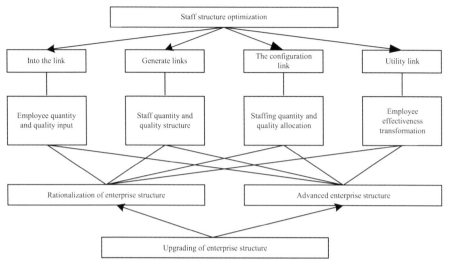

Fig. 1. Schematic diagram of docking extraction sequence parameters of employee structure optimization and enterprise structure upgrading

the economic system, develop sustainably for a long time. Therefore, the research on the theme of this paper can be transformed into a measure of the orderliness of the composite system formed by employees and enterprise structure subsystems. In the synergetic thought, only when the employee structure and the enterprise structure are realized from disorder to order can the coordination between the two systems be ensured, thus making the economic parent system develop sustainably. The measurement mark of two systems from disorder to order is "order parameter", which can quantify the degree of order. Order is derived from the cooperation between subsystems and plays an important role. Therefore, in order to quantify the degree of coordination between employees and enterprise structure, it is necessary to extract the order parameters that meet the requirements [4, 5]. The order degree of the composite system formed by the two subsystems can be divided into three levels from low to high, and the highest level is the unity of the structure and function of the subsystems, which means that the two systems are highly ordered. Based on this, when quantitatively studying the coordination and adaptation relationship between employees and enterprise structure, it is necessary to unify their functions and structures, and on this basis, complete the extraction of order parameters.

2.2 Establish a Fitness Evaluation Index System

According to the above principles and ideas of index selection, this paper divides the employee structure into four links: input-generation-allocation-utility, and divides the enterprise structure into two levels: structure scale and structure quality, which are coupled and docked to extract sequence parameters. The evaluation system is established from four levels: system level-target level-criterion level-index level, and the quantitative formula of each index is calculated to form the evaluation index system, as shown in Table 1.

Table 1. Framework of evaluation index system

System level	Target layer	The standard layer	Index layer
Adaptability of employees to enterprise positions	Input link	Number of employees and quality input of enterprises	The proportion of education investment in GDP a1
			Growth rate of education expenditure per student in higher education a2
			Location entropy of educational expenditure per student in higher education a3
			Share of R & D input in GDP a4
			Location entropy of R & D input in GDP a5
			The R & D input growth rate a6
	Generation link	Number and quality structure of employees	The density of talent b1
			The ratio of talent to employees b2
			Location entropy of talent ratio to employees b3
			Under the big data, the number of talents in healthcare enterprises has increased highly b4
			In terms of big data, the proportion of talents in healthcare enterprises is highly proportional b5
	Configuration link	Productivity of post employees in enterprises	Static coordination degree of traditional healthcare enterprises c1

(continued)

Table 1. (*continued*)

System level	Target layer	The standard layer	Index layer
			Static coordination degree of healthcare enterprises under big data c2
			The whole enterprise static coordination degree c3
	Utility link	Employee's utility play	Number of patent applications d1
			Location entropy of patent application quantity d2
			Patent authorization d3
			Location entropy of patent authorization quantity d4
			The increase rate of the number of patent invention applications granted d5
			Number of contracts traded in the technology market d6
			The number of contracts traded in the technology market is in the national proportion d7
			Technical market transaction contract amount d8
			The contract amount of transactions in the technology market is represented in the whole country d9
			Enterprise employee productivity d10

By sorting out the evaluation indexes in the collaborative system of employee structure and enterprise post structure, the high-frequency factors are screened out, and a reasonable weight is determined for each attribute. To study the coordination and adaptation of the two subsystems of enterprise post and employee structure, according to the above evaluation index system, it is necessary to select the order parameters for quantitative calculation [6].

2.3   Index Identification and Quantification

In order to objectively study the coordination status of talents in enterprises, the index of "static coordination degree" is introduced. Taking the index of "static coordination degree of healthcare enterprises under big data" as an example, its formula can be set as follows:

$$Q_I = \frac{w_i}{W} - \frac{s_i}{S} \tag{1}$$

where, W is the labor productivity of each department of health care enterprise, S is the proportion of post talents, and w_i and s_i are the labor productivity and the proportion of post talents of i departments respectively [7]. If $Q_i = 0$, it means that the coordination and adaptation degree of this department is consistent with that of the enterprise; if $Q_i > 0$, it means that the proportion of talented employees in this department is relatively high but the output is relatively low, indicating that the employees in this department are not fully functioning; if $Q_i < 0$, it means that the proportion of talented employees in this department is relatively low but the output is relatively high; when there are more talented employees, structural transfer to this enterprise can help the growth of the enterprise. The quantitative calculation formulas of each index are shown in Table 2.

The quantification of each evaluation index is realized by the quantification method in Table 2. In order to more accurately analyze the coordination and adaptation relationship between employees and post structures in medical and health care enterprises, this paper quantitatively analyzes the indicators extracted by coupling and docking of the two systems [8]. Each index in the system has a development target value. Compared with the actual development value of the index, the ratio obtained is the efficacy coefficient. The mathematical expression of the efficacy function of index e_i is:

$$F_i = f(e_i) \tag{2}$$

where, F_i is the efficacy coefficient, and when the value ranges from $0 \leq F_i < 1$, $i = 1, 2, ..., n$, when $F_i = 1$, the target value is the best, which means the target value is the worst. According to the synergetic theory, if the synergetic system is stable and orderly, the efficiency function presents a linear relationship, and the maximum or minimum value of the efficiency function is the critical point of the system without qualitative change. Based on this, the following efficacy function is established:

$$\begin{cases} F(e_i) = (x_i - \alpha_i)/(y_i - \alpha_i), \alpha_i \leq x_i \leq y_i, \text{When } F(e_i) \text{ is positive} \\ F(e_i) = (\alpha_i - x_i)/(y_i - \alpha_i), y_i \leq x_i \leq \alpha_i, \text{When } F(e_i) \text{ is negative} \end{cases} \tag{3}$$

Table 2. Quantitative calculation method of evaluation index

Index layer	Quantitative calculation formula
a1	= Education investment funds/ GDP
a2	= Higher education students average education expenditure in that year/Higher education students are all spent on education in the previous year-1
a3	= Higher education per student education expenditure/Enterprise education expenditure per student in higher education
a4	= R&D Investment funds/GDP
a5	= The proportion of departmental R & D investment in GDP /The proportion of enterprise R & D investment in GDP
a6	= R & D is spent on the current year/ R & D invested for the previous year-1
b1	= The number of talent/Number of employees
b2	= The ratio of talent to the department's employees/The ratio of enterprise talent to employees
b3	= The ratio of department talent to employees/The ratio of enterprise employees to employees
b4	= The number of talents in healthcare enterprises has increased under departmental big data/The number of traditional healthcare professionals in the sector has increased
b5	= The number of talents in health care enterprises under departmental big data/The number of the traditional health care personnel in the enterprise
c1	= Department of the traditional industry talent ratio/Department talent ratio-Labor productivity ratio of sector traditional industries / sector labor productivity
c2	= Department of high-tech industry talent ratio/Department talent ratio-Labor productivity ratio of regional high-tech industries/Department of labor productivity
c3	= 1/2(Static coordination degree of traditional healthcare enterprises + Static coordination degree of healthcare enterprises under big data)
d1	straight forward calculation
d2	= The number of departmental patent applications/Number of enterprise patent applications
d3	straight forward calculation
d4	= Amount of departmental patents granted/Enterprise patent authorization amount
d5	= The department of invention application for the current year of authorization quantity/Department invention application for the last year of authorization amount-1
d6	straight forward calculation

(*continued*)

Table 2. (*continued*)

Index layer	Quantitative calculation formula
d7	= Number of contracts traded in the enterprise technology market/Number of contracts traded in the national technology market
d8	straight forward calculation
d9	= Enterprise technology market contract amount/Contract amount traded in the national technology market
d10	= enterprise GDP/The number of enterprise employees

In the formula, x_i is the actual value of e_i, and α_i and y_i are the extreme values of e_i when the system is stable. The function value reflects the measurement of the degree of coordination and adaptation of a single index to the whole system. According to the above various calculations, the efficacy function value can be obtained.

2.4 Calculate Fitness

In order to comprehensively describe the efficacy and benefits of system indicators and comprehensively reflect the fitness of the whole system, a single efficacy function value cannot be used, so it is necessary to establish a functional relationship that takes efficacy coefficient as an independent variable and can reflect the coordination and fitness between the two subsystems. In this paper, the fitness function is used to judge the employee's post fitness, and the range of fitness function value is $0 \leq HD \leq 1$. The larger the fitness function value is, the higher the fitness of employees in medical care enterprises is, and vice versa [9].The efficacy of each index on the coordination and fitness evaluation system is regarded as the goal of the system's own development. It is assumed that there are N goals, of which N_0 are negative indicators and N_1 are positive indicators. The larger the index value, the better. The other $N - N_0 - N_1$ goals are close to a certain value. Then, a total efficacy function is established with a certain efficacy coefficient. The total efficacy function value is that the coordination and fitness of this complex system is easy to get results and ensure accuracy.

$$HD= \sum_{i=1}^{n} w_{ij} * Fe(v_{ij}) \tag{4}$$

where, $\sum_{i=1}^{n} w_{ij} = 1$, w_{ij} is the weight coefficient of $Fe(v_{ij})$, the coordination fitness is the calculated weighted sum. Next, determine the weight of each evaluation index. Subjective weighting method and objective weighting method are the main two ways to establish the weight evaluation index. Ring comparison analysis, analytic hierarchy process, Delphi and fuzzy comprehensive evaluation are the main calculation methods of subjective weighting method; Factor analysis, correlation coefficient, variation coefficient, principal component analysis and entropy are the main calculation methods of objective weighting method. Through comprehensive analysis, this paper selects the entropy method in the objective weighting method to establish the weight of each index [10]. A method to measure uncertainty is called entropy. The smaller the amount of information, the greater the uncertainty and entropy; The greater the amount of information, the smaller the uncertainty and the smaller the entropy. Entropy can not only judge the randomness and disorder degree of an event, but also can be used to judge the dispersion degree of an index. If the index with greater dispersion degree is selected, it will have a greater impact on the comprehensive evaluation [11]. The steps of calculating entropy and establishing weight are as follows: Set n observation values and k indicators, then x_{ij} is the j th indicator of the i th observation value. The greater the difference between x_{ij}, the more information this indicator contains and transmits, and the greater the comparative effect of this indicator on complex systems. Entropy can be used to measure the amount of information [12], that is, the increase of information represents the decrease of entropy.Calculate the specific gravity value of the characteristic index, and set x_{ij} as the initial value and x_{ij} as k_{ij}, then the calculation formula of the specific gravity value of the i th observation value under the j th index is:

$$k_{ij} = x_{ij} / \sum_{i=1}^{n} x_{ij} \tag{5}$$

If the information entropy of the j st index is d_j, the calculation formula of information entropy is:

$$d_j = -\gamma \sum_{i=1}^{n} k_{ij} * \ln k_{ij} \tag{6}$$

Among them, $\gamma > 0$, if x_{ij} are all equal to the given j, there are $k_{ij} = 1/n, d_j = \gamma \ln n$. For a given j, x_{ij}, the smaller the difference is, the greater is d_j. When x_{ij} are all equal, $d_j = d_{max} = 1(\gamma = 1/\ln n)$. At this time, as the comparison between observed values, index x_{ij} has no effect, and it is necessary to calculate the difference coefficient. The greater the difference between x_{ij} and d_j, the greater the comparison effect of index on observed values. Therefore, the difference coefficient is defined as:

$$l_i = 1 - d_i \tag{7}$$

l_i the larger, the more attention should be paid to the role of this indicator, and finally determine the weight, whose formula is:

$$w_j = l_i / \sum_{j=1}^{k} l_i, j = 1, 2, ..., k \tag{8}$$

After the above calculations, the weight of each index is calculated. Finally, for the classification standard of fitness grade, 0.00–1.00 is divided into 10 continuous grade intervals [13]. It can be seen that the coordination adaptation grade is a continuous ladder, then a coordination grade represents an interval, and each grade is a kind of coordination state. Among them, the fitness value greater than 0.50 is the coordination interval, and

Table 3. Standard table for evaluation grade type of coordination fitness

Coordination level	Coordinate the adaptation value	Coordination degree
1	0.00—0.10	extreme disorder
2	0.11—0.20	High disorder
3	0.21—0.30	Moderate disorder
4	0.31—0.40	low disorder
5	0.41—0.50	weak disorder
6	0.51—0.60	weak coordination
7	0.61—0.70	low coordination
8	0.71—0.80	Moderate coordinatio
9	0.81—0.90	High coordinatio
10	0.91—1.00	extreme coordinatio

the fitness value less than or equal to 0.50 is the imbalance interval. The specific division of the standard is shown in Table 3.

According to Table 3, the post suitability of employees in healthcare enterprises based on big data in this paper is evaluated.

3　Empirical Analysis

3.1　Experimental Preparation

In order to analyze the fitness of employees' positions in healthcare enterprises under big data in more detail, this paper selects 10 healthcare enterprises as parameter objects, and selects the relevant index data from 2016 to 2021 to evaluate the fitness of employees' positions in healthcare enterprises. The weight calculation results of each index calculated above are shown in Table 4.

After obtaining the index values and their weights from Table 4, the post fitness and average value of employees in 10 medical and health care enterprises are calculated, and the coordination fitness curve is drawn in turn. According to the standard table of fitness evaluation grade type, the grade of post fitness of employees in each enterprise is judged, the evaluation of post fitness of employees in medical and health care enterprises is completed, and the evaluation results are counted.

3.2　Overall Analysis of Fitness

According to the calculation results of job fitness and average value of employees in 10 health care enterprises, the coordination fitness curve is drawn, and the change trend of fitness of different enterprises in 2016–2021 is analyzed, as shown in Fig. 2.

According to the results of Fig. 2, the time series comparison and analysis of the position coordination and adaptability of employees in 10 medical and health care enterprises shows that the adaptability of each enterprise shows a tortuous upward trend. It

Table 4. Weight value of each index

Metric	Weight	Metric	Weight
a1	0.0156	c2	0.0601
a2	0.0432	c3	0.0610
a3	0.0141	d1	0.0523
a4	0.0285	d2	0.0603
a5	0.0416	d3	0.0421
a6	0.0187	d4	0.0612
b1	0.0453	d5	0.0401
b2	0.0385	d6	0.0254
b3	0.0299	d7	0.0264
b4	0.0164	d8	0.0293
b5	0.0180	d9	0.0415
c1	0.0159	d10	0.0288

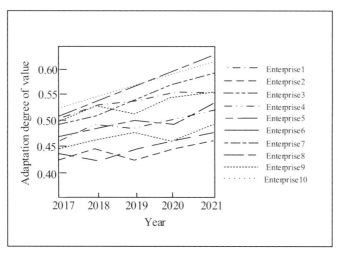

Fig. 2. Change trend of job fitness of employees in 10 health care enterprises from 2017 to 2021

can be seen that from 2017 to 2021, the position structure and employee talents of each enterprise are constantly optimized, so that the adaptability is improved. The position order of the fitness degree of each enterprise changes little, showing a trend of alternating fluctuations. According to the trend chart of fitness change, the change range of enterprise 7 is small and shows a slow growth trend, but the annual level has always been the highest among the 10 healthcare enterprises.

According to the average value of the fitness degree of each enterprise, the grade type of the post coordination fitness degree of employees in 10 medical and health care enterprises is determined, as shown in Table 5.

Table 5. Grade types of post coordination adaptability of employees in 10 medical and health care enterprises

Enterprise	Grade	Level	Average fit
1	6	weak coordination	0.52
2	5	weak disorder	0.44
3	6	weak coordination	0.51
4	5	weak disorder	0.48
5	5	weak disorder	0.46
6	6	weak coordination	0.51
7	6	weak coordination	0.59
8	5	weak disorder	0.45
9	5	weak disorder	0.43
10	6	weak coordination	0.56

Table 5 clearly shows the grade types of the job fitness of employees in various medical and health care enterprises. It can be seen that the job fitness grades of employees in these 10 enterprises are not high. Five enterprises are weak degree maladjustment and five enterprises are weak degree coordination. Among them, the average value of the fitness of enterprise 7 and enterprise 10 is high, ranging from 0.51 to 0.60. Although the coordination level is the same, and it is also in the weak degree imbalance level, the average fitness of enterprise 4 is the highest, and the average fitness of enterprise 9 is the lowest, indicating that enterprise 9 has obvious disadvantages in fitness, and the overall level still needs to be improved. The range of fitness level needs to be substantially changed, which proves that there is a large room to improve the fitness of employees in health care enterprises, and it needs to adjust and supplement appropriate talents in time.

4   Concluding Remarks

In this paper, by proposing the principles and ideas for the selection of fitness evaluation indicators, establishing the fitness evaluation indicator system, identifying and quantifying indicators, and calculating fitness, we have completed the research on the evaluation of job fitness of employees in healthcare enterprises under big data, and achieved certain research results. The details are as follows:

(1) This paper uses the basic theory of collaboration to bring the post structure of employees and enterprises into the scope of enterprise economic system, and uses the principle of synergy correlation as a support to build a connection channel - order

parameter, which describes the interaction between the post structure of employees and enterprises.

(2) The position order of the fitness of each enterprise does not change much, showing a trend of alternating fluctuations.

(3) There is much room for improvement in the fitness of employees in medical and health care enterprises, and it is necessary to timely adjust and supplement the appropriate talents.

At present, there is still a misplaced supporting relationship between posts and employees in healthcare enterprises under big data. In the future, we should also change our development ideas, increase talent input, give full play to employee communication, and promote the transformation of achievements. In the future research, evaluation indicators can also be continuously optimized to provide a more scientific and effective basis for the development of health care enterprises. The healthcare industry under big data will certainly become a very vibrant industry, promote the medical and health level to a new level with healthy and stable development, and share the achievements of social development.

References

1. Zhu, X., Z., Sen, W., He, Qin.: Impact of Skill Requirements on Employees' Thriving at Work: From the Perspective of Artificial Intelligence Embedding[J]. Foreign Economies & Management 43(11), 15–25 (2021)
2. Jin, Y., Yang, T., Tang, C.: High-skilled talent team construction policy supply and demand adaptation deviation and correction: Taking Sichuan Province as an Example[J]. Human Resour. Develop. China 37(01), 127–142 (2020)
3. Chun-tao, L., Xiang-rong, S., Ai-yin, W.: Impact of household disposable income on education, culture and entertainment expenditure based on quantile regression. Math. Practice Theory 50(20), 162–168 (2020)
4. Qifeng, C.: The promotion of basic medical insurance to the health of the elderly: a dual path analysis of medical treatment and health care. Social Secur. Stud. 5, 63–69 (2020)
5. Yong, X.: The differential implications of technological upgrading on skill levels of workers: evidence from manufacturing enterprises in Guangdong province. Human Resource Develop. China 37(10), 64–74 (2020)
6. Yue, Q.: Allocation efficiency of human capital considering educational heterogeneity——based on the calculation of enterprise-employee matching survey data. China Indust. Econ. 8, 24–41 (2020)
7. Ke, J., Qun, D.: The effects of entrepreneurial leadership on employees' work attitudes and innovation performance in start-ups——the mediated role of workplace spirituality and the moderating effect of LMX. Res. Econ. Manage. 41(1), 91–103 (2020)
8. Abe, S.: Shigeyuki Abe comment on how did Japan cope with COVID-19? big data and purchasing behavior. Asian Econ. Papers 20(1), 170–174 (2021)
9. Ran, L., He, Y.: Simulation of Big Data Cross-Access Authorization Technology Based on Gradient Sampling. Computer Simulation, 37(2), 188–191,420 (2022)
10. Audenaert, M., Decramer, A., George, B.: How to foster employee quality of life: the role of employee performance management and authentic leadership. Eval. Program Plann. 85(1), 101–110 (2021)

11. Huang, Y., Sheng, K., Sun, W.: Influencing factors of manufacturing agglomeration in the Beijing-Tianjin-Hebei region based on enterprise big data. Acta Geogr. Sin. **32**(10), 2105–2128 (2022)
12. Stergiou, C.L., Psannis, K.E.: Digital twin intelligent system for industrial internet of things-based big data management and analysis in cloud environments. Virtual Real. Intell. Hardw. **4**(4), 279–291 (2022)
13. Ali, H.B., Helgesen, F.H., Falk, K.: Unlocking the power of big data within the early design phase of the new product development process. INCOSE Int. Symp. **31**(1), 434–452 (2021)

Design of Telemedicine and Health Care System Based on Embedded Technology

Shufeng Zhuo[1], Yi Hu[2], Xinyao Liu[3], and Zixiu Zou[4,5($\boxtimes$)]

[1] The Internet of Things and Artificial Intelligence College, Fujian Polytechnic of Information Technology, Fuzhou 350003, China
[2] Henan Information Engineering School, Zhengzhou 450000, China
[3] Imperial Vision Technology Company Limited, Fuzhou 350001, China
[4] Fuzhou Institute of Technology, Fuzhou 350506, China
55607@qq.com
[5] SEGI University, 47810 Petaling Jaya, Selangor, Malaysia

Abstract. In order to improve the monitoring accuracy of physiological parameters and the effect of telemedicine, a new telemedicine and health care system based on embedded technology was designed. Use the embedded server to realize the information interaction between the client and the Web server. Send data to the server through the monitoring network terminal, and use the data acquisition module to obtain two parts of the data of the blood pressure module and the blood oxygen module. Monitor physiological signals with embedded monitors. Use embedded technology to search for telemedicine information, and combine encryption algorithms to encrypt the information. Calculate the distance between the monitoring signal to be authenticated sent by the embedded server and the storage database to ensure the safe transmission of the signal and avoid external interference, thus completing the design of the remote medical care system. It can be seen from the experimental results that the blood pressure fluctuation range monitored by the system is 100mmHg-160mmHg, the maximum error between the blood oxygen measurement value and the actual data is only 1%, and the pulse rate data is consistent with the actual data, indicating that the monitoring results using this system are accurate, the practical application effect is good.

Keywords: Embedded Technology · Telemedicine · Health Care System · Monitoring Network End · Server · Encryption Algorithm

1 Introduction

With the improvement of people's living standards, people pay more and more attention to the health of themselves and their families. Coupled with the popularity of PC and the improvement of Internet speed and bandwidth, people are more longing for and need a practical home telemedicine and health care system to facilitate access to doctor diagnosis services. In China, the development of telemedicine is still in its infancy. It

S. Wang (Ed.): IoTCare 2022, LNICST 501, pp. 221–238, 2023.
https://doi.org/10.1007/978-3-031-33545-7_16

mainly targets a small number of patients with difficult diseases. Due to the high medical price and less civil use, the popularity of telemedicine system is low and the market promotion is difficult, which limits the rapid development of telemedicine technology and its industry to a certain extent. Telemedicine mainly provides people with medical information and services through the use of telecommunication, computer, multimedia and other technologies, that is, the basic physiological data information of human body needed for medical treatment is transmitted in different places [1]. The transmission of this medical and physiological information can be realized by using various existing communication technologies such as telephone line, ISDN, frame relay, ATM and satellite. Current telemedicine systems mainly use two types of technologies, one is to store data and then transmit it to transmit physiological data from one end to the other, which are non-real-time applications, such as electrocardiograms, CT scans and Transmission of images such as X-rays. Another more and more widely used is the two-way interactive, face-to-face visualization technology, that is, real-time mutual communication, consultation and consultation through PCs, cameras, and audio equipment terminals.

According to the logical relationship between the constructed telemedicine and healthcare system and various architecture levels of different platforms, combined with the Internet of Things technology to analyze the "sensing and knowing" characteristics of the telemedicine and healthcare system, so as to realize the real-time monitoring of the telemedicine and healthcare system; The proposed method based on SpringMvc the telemedicine health care system of the architecture model uses the SpringMvc architecture model to build software programs, combines user needs with qualitative problems in the medical system, and establishes a complete telemedicine health care system. Traditional medical technology is easily limited by time and space, often has very large limitations, and cannot provide guaranteed medical services for a wide range of people. Generally speaking, to realize a stable and reliable telemedicine system, we must solve two important problems: one is to have a stable, reliable and flexible front-end data acquisition equipment; The second is how to realize the interaction between server and client. In view of the above problems, the design of telemedicine and health care system based on embedded technology is proposed. Through the integration of user-side detection instruments, the signals of different detection instruments are coordinated and processed, and the detection data is transmitted through the computer serial interface. At the same time, it is displayed in the user terminal and saved in the network system database. Through programming, the examination data stored in the database of patients can be compared and classified, so as to form a permanent electronic medical record, which can more clearly analyze the pathological conditions of patients and determine the treatment plan. The system also provides emergency treatment, information center and real-time communication system to meet the needs of patients' health care information and real-time dialogue with doctors.

Based on the above analysis, this paper designs a telemedicine system based on embedded technology. The main structure of this paper is as follows:

(1) Analyze the embedded application of telemedicine system, and determine the overall structure of the medical care system.
(2) The hardware structure of the healthcare system is designed, mainly including embedded server, monitoring network, data acquisition, and embedded monitor.

It mainly uses embedded server to realize information interaction between client and Web server. The monitoring network terminal sends data to the server, and the data acquisition module is used to obtain the data of blood pressure module and blood oxygen module.

(3) Embedded technology is used to search telemedicine information, and encryption algorithm is used to encrypt the information. The distance between the monitoring signal to be authenticated sent by the embedded server and the storage database is calculated to ensure the safe transmission of the signal and avoid external interference, thus completing the design of the telemedicine system.

(4) The fluctuation range of blood pressure monitored by the system in this paper is to verify the error between the blood oxygen measurement value and the actual data, and the gap between the pulse rate data and the actual data, so as to verify the accuracy of the system monitoring results designed in this paper.

(5) Summarize the full text and draw a conclusion.

2   Embedded Applications of Telehealth Care Systems

Telemedicine is a medical model that uses modern telecommunication and multimedia technology to realize a variety of medical functions such as disease diagnosis, treatment and health care in different places. Telemedicine system is usually composed of three-level structure, namely client, application server and database server [2]. As a kind of telemedicine system, home health care system will collect the physiological parameters and video, audio, video and other data of the monitored person, and then transmit them to the server monitoring center in real time through the network for dynamic tracking of pathological development, so as to ensure timely diagnosis and treatment.

In recent years, with the rapid development of computer network communication technology and the continuous increase of wired network bandwidth, the content of telemedicine has been further enriched, and its connotation and practical significance have been increased. In the application of remote consultation, from the original transmission of pictures and words in advance before consultation, it can now transmit patient information in real time and realize "face-to-face" HD video dialogue [3]. In order to strengthen the modern information management of hospitals and improve work efficiency, a family medical care system based on embedded technology and a three-tier architecture of "family service network doctor" with family as the core is studied and implemented. The terminal is connected to the Internet through Ethernet, and uses TCP/IP protocol for data transmission to realize the collection, transmission and telemedicine of physiological parameter signals. The server side provides corresponding health data and services for different end users [4]. The working process collects various physiological parameters of the elderly through digital instruments such as blood pressure meter, heart rate meter, blood glucose meter, etc., and sends it to the embedded medical care terminal system through the RS232 serial port or USB port, and then the terminal system packages the data and transmits it through the network. It is transmitted to the server side, and the server side will get in touch with the hospital and the attending physician in time after processing the data [5]. The client and the server can be connected to a camera and a microphone, and both sides can conduct video telemedicine.

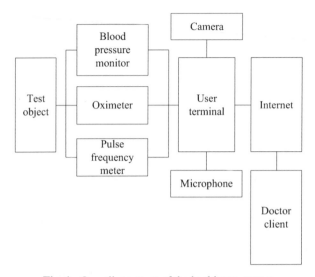

Fig. 1. Overall structure of the healthcare system

Figure 1 is a general structural diagram of the health care system.

The significance of embedded health care system is to break through regional boundaries, so that the elderly can enjoy high-level medical services at home, so as to allocate medical resources more reasonably. The system introduces high-definition image monitoring technology. While providing remote medical health detection data services (realizing the function of doctors' remote "cutting"), it adds technical support for front-end patient audio and video monitoring, which makes the basis of doctors' diagnosis more sufficient, the interaction between doctors and patients more direct and convenient, closer to the medical environment of local diagnosis, and realizes the function of doctors' remote "looking, smelling and asking". Secondly, in the past, telemedicine systems generally used PC as the front-end acquisition device, and used C/S service architecture to realize the doctor client. The data processed by the client software needs the help of the intermediate transfer server [6]. This not only makes the front-end system less mobile, but also the back-end doctor terminal relies too much on the service mode and performance of the intermediate server, resulting in poor system compatibility. The system adopts an embedded Web server as the transmission core of telemedicine data, and the front-end hardware adopts a multimedia SoC solution. Thirdly, the disadvantage of the software terminal is that if the doctor wants to browse the real-time medical information of the patient, he must install the software separately. For different telemedicine front-end acquisition systems, the data protocol is not standardized, so that the compatibility of the software cannot be guaranteed, which will bring a lot of inconvenience to the end user. With the support of embedded web server, this system uses web browsers as client terminals to improve the compatibility and adaptability of clients, so that doctors can diagnose patients in real time on PCs, mobile phones and even TVs.

3 System Hardware Structure Design

The system design adopts the client/server/application software/database structure, and the Internet connects the client and server. The client is mainly composed of audio and video system, physiological sensor, signal conditioning circuit, data acquisition card, virtual instrument application software and self diagnosis information database. The signal conditioning circuit is to amplify and filter the physiological electrical signal obtained by the sensor to achieve the appropriate electrical signal.

3.1 Embedded Server Side

The server is mainly composed of the website of online hospital, online doctor and user/doctor information database. Among them, online doctors need to be equipped with application software and audio and video system. The main function of the server website is to provide Internet access services, user authentication management, open interactive health care and medical environment, and the generation of dynamic web pages; Firstly, the information database is mainly used for the code authentication management of users and network doctors, the generation of dynamic web pages, and other services provided in the website; Another main function is to store, open and process the data files of doctors' acceptance and diagnosis; The application software used by online doctors is the same as that used by customers [7, 8]. Users and network doctors in health care and medical centers have their own fixed codes and passwords. After logging in to the website server, the user can actively choose a doctor to consult and see a doctor by checking the resume of the doctor on duty [9].

The embedded server module is an ARM embedded structure running in the SoC. It is based on the Linux real-time operating system and a web server. The web browser function is implemented at the front end. The client can realize the connection with the web server as long as the browser downloads and browses the web page [10]. In addition, the embedded web server is also responsible for the IP protocol transmission of medical health and physiological data, audio, and video monitoring data. At the same time, the server can also respond to the setting instructions of the web client terminal and transfer them into corresponding serial port or FPGA instructions. Set data acquisition module, audio and video encoding hardware equipment.

3.2 Monitoring Network Terminal

Telemedicine monitoring network can monitor patients remotely through different communication media, which is generally composed of front-end monitor, communication media and monitoring center station. Front end monitors are usually placed in family or community clinics. The monitoring center station can be located in community clinics or large hospitals, while telephone lines, power lines, ISDN (Integrated Services Digital Network), satellites, Internet and some private networks can be used as the communication media of the network. A telemedicine monitoring system composed of multiple medical monitors based on the embedded microprocessor module RCM3000 and the monitoring center station through the Internet [11].

In the network design, a client/server structure is adopted. The embedded monitor used by each family is the client, and the monitoring center station with three slave servers is the server. The embedded monitor can measure and display Sao2 (blood oxygen saturation), HR (heart rate), ECG (electrocardiographic waveform), T (body temperature) and NIBP (non-invasive blood pressure) and other physiological parameters, and when the client and the server require connection after the application is allowed, it can continuously send data to the server through the Internet. At the same time, the emergency call signal of the patient being monitored can also be sent to the server. According to the different identifiers of the data received by the server, the data is processed by the Sao2 slave server, the NIBP slave server and the ECG slave server, and the server can also send relevant commands to the client. The server will receive the monitoring data of multiple clients at the same time and save the data records. Doctors can select certain patients on the screen for real-time observation or view historical records for analysis and diagnosis.

3.3 Data Acquisition Terminal

The data acquisition module includes a blood pressure module and a blood oxygen module. Both modules have corresponding measurement circuits, and the measurement circuit includes a power supply circuit, a signal processing circuit, an analog-to-digital conversion circuit, an ARM control circuit, and a protection circuit. Each data acquisition module only needs to connect the corresponding external electrodes and sensors to complete the acquisition of physiological parameters under the control command of the ARMS processor.

Blood Pressure Collection Module
Blood pressure is a very important physiological parameter of the human body. The prevalence of hypertension is high in our population, especially in the elderly. Generally, what we are familiar with is the high and low pressure value, which refers to the systolic and diastolic blood pressure in medicine. The systole and diastole of the heart in a cycle will form two beats in blood pressure, so we can test these two values. The normal range of blood pressure values is: high pressure 90-130mmHg, low pressure 60-90mmHg. Blood pressure measurement adopts non-invasive vibration measurement method, which can measure systolic blood pressure, diastolic blood pressure and mean blood pressure. The noninvasive vibration measurement method is similar to the Coriolis sound method. During the measurement, the arterial blood flow is blocked through the cuff, and the pressure sensor is used to detect the shock wave of the gas in the cuff during the gradual deflation of the cuff. The slow deflation of the cuff causes the gradual change of the cuff volume, and then changes the air pressure inside the cuff. Through the pressure sensor, the signal quantity with the air pressure value of an approximate slope can be obtained. The real-time cuff pressure can be obtained after filtering, amplification, analog-to-digital conversion and other processing.

Blood Oxygen Collection Module
Blood oxygen refers to blood oxygen saturation, which is the ratio of hemoglobin that has

been combined with oxygen in the blood to the total hemoglobin, and the unit is percentage. The premise of blood oxygen measurement is that hemoglobin and oxyhemoglobin in human blood have different absorption coefficients for light of different wavelengths. Blood oxygen represents the oxygen content in human blood, and is defined as the concentration of oxyhemoglobin in tissues to total hemoglobin (including hemoglobin and oxyhemoglobin). At present, there are few measurement methods of blood oxygen saturation, which mainly distinguish the different component concentrations and blood oxygen saturation in the blood pressure in the finger by the conduction strength of the blood in the finger to the light. Therefore, the measurement method is the fingertip photoelectric sensor measurement method. The sensor is made into a fingertip and put on the finger. 660nm red light and 940nm near-infrared light are injected into the finger blood container. The transmitted light has different intensity due to different refractive index, so as to measure the amount of hemoglobin in blood and blood oxygen saturation, which provides a non-invasive blood oxygen measurement method for clinic. During blood oxygen measurement, two different photodiodes on the blood oxygen probe emit two kinds of light with different wavelengths at the same time, and the light passes through human fingers and is detected by the photoelectric detector. When the artery beats, the light intensity measured by the photoelectric detector is small, while during the interval between two pulses of the artery, the light intensity measured by the photoelectric detector is large. The difference between the two light intensity measurements is the value of the light intensity absorbed by the pulsatile arterial blood. It can be seen that the signal of blood oxygen measurement also contains pulse information, and the pulse parameters of human body can be obtained by blood oxygen measurement.

3.4 Embedded Monitor

CThe embedded monitor is composed of the Ethernet microprocessor module of Z-WORLD Company in the United States and three physiological parameter detection modules, keyboard and its trigger circuit, liquid crystal display and module switch, etc., as shown in Fig. 2.

The RCM3000 module includes the microprocessor Rabbit3000, 512K Flash for storing programs, 512K SRAM for storing data, 54 parallel input and output ports and 6 serial ports. In addition, it has a Base-T LAN or internet interface, and provides the source code of TCP/IP protocol stack without edition fee.

The ECG module can detect parameters such as full-lead ECG signal, respiration wave, heart rate, respiration rate and body temperature; It has four-level ECG signal gain, four-level respiratory wave program-controlled gain, and three-level filtering; PC2 and PC3) are connected to it. The NIBP module can measure the blood pressure of adults or children; it has manual or automatic measurement function; it is connected to it through the serial port D (PC0 and PC1) of the RCM3000. Sao2 module can measure blood oxygen saturation, plethysmogram, intensity, pulse rate and other parameters; can change patient mode and sensitivity level, can perform low perfusion measurement, and can resist motion interference; through serial port B (PC4 and PC5) of RCM3000 connected to it. The three switches connected to PD0-PD2 determine whether the above three modules work.

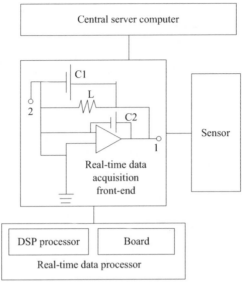

Fig. 2. Schematic diagram of the structure of the embedded monito

4 Software Part Design

The hardware platform constitutes the overall framework and trunk of the telemedicine system. On the basis of the hardware platform, we also need to develop the application software through the software platform, so that the hardware platform can run. Hardware platform and software platform work together to form a complete telemedicine system. The monitoring terminal is an important part of the telemedicine system, which realizes the physiological data acquisition function of terminal patients. At the same time, it can realize the data communication with the upper computer monitoring terminal through the data transmission module, and transmit the measured physiological parameters to the doctors or experts in the monitoring center for diagnosis. The main function of embedded operating system is to be responsible for the allocation of software and hardware resources, task scheduling and the control and coordination of various concurrent activities of the whole system. The main components are composed of underlying driver software, system kernel, driver interface, communication protocol and image interface. The application software is at the top of the embedded system, and it is oriented to users to complete specific functions and requirements.

4.1 Telemedicine Information Search Based on Embedded Technology

The telemedicine information search engine based on embedded technology mainly connects various systems in a point-to-point way. The purpose of embedded technology search is to prevent developers from using HTTP, HTML and JavaScriPt, but it can be used if necessary. Users can customize web applications through HTML, style sheets, and templates. Using the embedded technology search structure to achieve a variety of data integration, the key is to integrate the middleware application interface, and use point-to-point interaction and information-based middleware interaction to ensure the consistency of data sources, and thus perform data encryption search.

The symmetric encryption algorithm is used to encrypt the data, and the data attribute is AND type access structure tree. The structure tree is transformed into the main disjunctive access structure tree through the disjunctive normal form solution method. The symmetric key is encrypted through the access structure tree. Assuming that the sub access structure belongs to different attribute institutions, the ciphertext corresponding to the sub search structure can be expressed as:

$$k_x = \left(D_x, c_0, \{c_i'\}_{i=1,2,\dots,i} \right) \tag{1}$$

In formula (1), x represents the data collected by the sensor; D_x represents the access structure; c_0 represents the ciphertext component; c_i' represents the main disjunctive access structure tree ciphertext component. With the support of this ciphertext, the data encryption access process is designed as follows: For each attribute except the last attribute in the sub-search structure tree, a random number is selected for each attribute, and the value corresponding to the attribute is obtained. The formula is:

$$\varsigma_n = m - \sum_{n=1}^{i} \varsigma_i \tag{2}$$

In formula (2), m represents the total number; ς_i stands for random number. Upload the ciphertext corresponding to all sub search structure trees to the cloud storage server. To judge whether the initial uploaded data meets the optimal upload value, based on the distance between each cluster center, the formula is:

$$d(l_1, l_2) = \sqrt{\sum_{m=1}^{n} (l_{1,m} - l_{2,m})^2} \tag{3}$$

In formula (3), l_1 and l_2 are the inter-class distances of the actual clustering centers; n is the clustering item. A threshold β is set. When $d \leq \beta$, the initial upload data meets the optimal upload value, otherwise, it does not. The clustering effect is adjusted in real time to improve the rationality of classification and provide data support for data encryption processing, thus completing data encryption search.

4.2 Physiological Signal Monitoring

The Web application established by the embedded technology search component is registered on the server. Through the registration of the embedded technology search component, the whole medical service for patients, including flow, flow direction and processing process, can be completed. Using this engine, physiological signals can be searched.

Blood Pressure Monitoring
Blood pressure monitoring is to monitor the blood flow of a certain cross-section in the

blood vessel, that is, to monitor the volume velocity, that is, the ratio of the pressure at both ends of the blood vessel to the friction resistance between the blood flow and the blood vessel wall [12]. Friction resistance depends on blood viscosity and vessel radius, which can be described as:

$$\alpha = \frac{\rho \cdot d}{\pi r^2} \tag{4}$$

In formula (4), r is the radius of the blood vessel; ρ is the viscosity of the blood; d is the length of the blood vessel. The monitoring of blood pressure is the monitoring of human vascular function. In clinical practice, the blood pressure of patients can be known by monitoring frictional resistance.

Pulse Oximetry Monitoring

Oxyhemoglobin is formed by the combination of hemoglobin and oxygen, and these proteins flow through the blood throughout the body and release oxygen throughout the body to maintain normal cellular metabolism. Pulse oximetry monitoring is based on the principle of different light absorption rates of proteins in blood vessels to monitor, which is determined by the ratio of transmitted light to incident light. Based on this, the absorbance of a substance can be expressed as:

$$\delta = \ln \frac{1}{\lambda \rho' H} \tag{5}$$

In formula (5), λ represents the absorption coefficient; ρ' refers to the concentration of light absorbing substance; H is the thickness of the substance. In the infrared region, there is little difference between the absorbance coefficients of hemoglobin and oxygen; In the red light area, the absorption coefficient of hemoglobin is larger, and the absorption coefficient of oxygen is basically not [13].

4.3 Monitoring Signal Transmission Based on Multi-threading

In the process of physiological monitoring signal transmission, initiating the conversion and reading the converted result is an asynchronous process. After the program starts the conversion of the physiological monitoring signal, it has been querying the status of the converted flag bit. Once the conversion is completed, it will read the result, otherwise it will be in a waiting state. This processing method is obviously problematic, because when an error occurs in the conversion process of the physiological monitoring signal and the process cannot be carried out smoothly, the system will be deadlocked by waiting. This situation in the physiological monitoring signal test system will cause the system to respond slowly and reduce its efficiency. In order to solve the above problems, a multi-threading mechanism can be introduced into the program. Physiological monitoring signals are centrally monitored through multi-threading to create interrupts and handle two sub-threads, as shown in Fig. 3.

Once a thread is created, it will run independently of the thread that created it. All threads in a process share the virtual address space of the process, so that all global

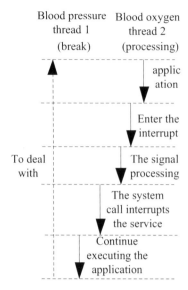

Fig. 3. Physiological monitoring signal centralized monitoring thread

variables of the process can be monitored [14]. The process requires signal encryption, and the formula can be expressed as:

$$c' = E(\psi(a) + \psi(b) - \psi(e)) \tag{6}$$

In formula (6), $\psi(a)$, $\psi(b)$, $\psi(e)$ represents the processing result, encryption result and random information respectively. Calculate the distance between the monitoring signal to be authenticated sent by the embedded server and the storage database, the formula is:

$$H(u, o) = \sum u[B] \oplus o[B] \tag{7}$$

In formula (7), both $u[B]$ and $o[B]$ indicate that the fuzzy monitoring signal to be authenticated corresponds to the symbol of the stored database; B means code; $\oplus$ stands for exclusive or operation. The smaller the Hamming distance is, the stronger the anti-interference ability of the code group is. When the embedded server uses the private key to decrypt, the Hamming distance is compared with the preset threshold. If the Hamming distance is greater than the set threshold, it indicates that the security of the monitoring signal cannot be effectively protected; If the Hamming distance is less than the set threshold, then the safety of the monitoring signal is effectively protected. Based on the strong security of multi-threaded processing technology, all signals can be safely transmitted, avoiding external interference, and providing technical guarantee for multi-party encryption of monitoring signal transmission [15]. Using this mechanism, the main thread can monitor the sub threads through the global flag, which can effectively overcome the stagnation and untimely response in the transmission of physiological monitoring signals, and greatly improve the efficiency of the system.

5 Experiments

5.1 Construction of Virtual Experimental Environment

Constrained by the limited resources of the embedded platform, the first step in the development of embedded software is to establish a cross-compilation environment on the PC host, that is, the code written on the host is generated after cross-compilation and can be applied to the target platform. Binary executable program. The operating system of the PC host is RedHat Linux9.0, and the specific implementation method is to use the virtual machine VMware Workstation software platform to completely install the RedHat Linux9.0 operating system. The ARMS development board of TQ2440 is selected to transplant the Linux2.6 system as the operating system of the embedded software platform. As an open source operating system, Linux is completely free, safe and reliable, supports multi-user multi-tasking and runs independently at the same time, and has sufficient follow-up support. In addition, the Linux system supports a wide range of file systems and drivers, has a good graphical interface, and supports QT testing. To successfully transplant the Linux operating system on the TQ2440 development board, you need to burn the Linux kernel and file system separately. The kernel ensures the realization of functions such as management, communication, and network support for each application on the development board. The file system is the basis of all data in the entire system, and all file information of the system is contained in the file system. In this topic, the supporting resources of the TQ2440 development board include the successfully compiled kernel and file system images, which can be programmed directly on the development board. The process of programming uses the download mode of u-boot, and connects the development board with the HyperTerminal on the PC to realize the mutual data transfer. The specific steps are as follows:

Step 1: Connect the development board to the PC, and turn on the super terminal of the PC, and set the port to 100000 bits/second. 8 data bits, 1 stop bit, no parity and data flow control.

Step 2: Long press the space bar on the keyboard, and power on the development board to enter the USB Download mode.

Step 3: Enter in the super terminal, find the kernel image file zImage.bin in the specified path of the development board resource package and transfer it, and select the default factory-programmed kernel image file. After the transfer is completed, uboot will perform the programming of the kernel file by itself.

Step 4: After the kernel is burnt, enter and choose to burn the Linux file system in the HyperTerminal, and find the corresponding file system root.bin in the specified path for transmission. In this design, the default factory-programmed file system is selected. After the file is transferred, uboot will automatically complete the burning of the file system. It can be seen from the programming information that during the programming process of the file system, there are bad blocks in the NAND Flash, and during the programming process, uboot automatically skips them, and the bad blocks will not cause the normal use of the development board. Unnecessary influence. After completing the programming of the Linux kernel and file system in turn, the QTopia platform with a friendly user interface can be established on the development board to complete the real-time display of physiological parameters such as blood pressure, blood pressure, ECG, body temperature, and respiration.

5.2   Experimental Setup

The medical information search engine based on IntraWeb is used to obtain medical information, and data encryption access is carried out through symmetric encryption algorithm. Therefore, the experimental device selected is the medical information integration device, as shown in Fig. 4.

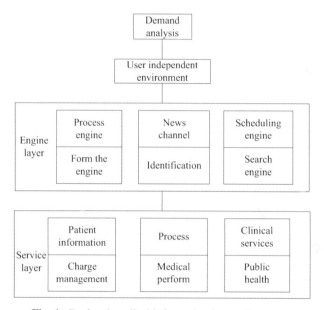

Fig. 4. Regional medical information integration model

According to the selected regional medical information integration device, this process needs the support of information sharing. The simulation analysis method is used to verify the process model, and the rationality analysis and optimization of the medical business process are carried out before the implementation of the project.

5.3   Analysis of Experimental Data

During system debugging, the IP address of the monitoring terminal is uniformly set to 192.168.10.20. After the connection between the monitoring terminal and the upper computer monitoring software is completed, the three physiological parameters of blood pressure, blood oxygen and pulse rate are collected to debug the collection and transmission functions of each module software. The LCD screen of the monitoring terminal and the upper computer software have the function of displaying physiological parameters. The complete overview of the display interface is shown in Fig. 5 respectively.

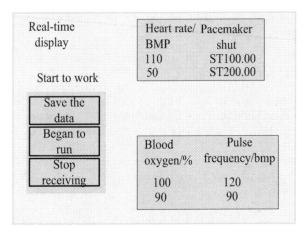

Fig. 5. Monitoring terminal data display interface

The right side of the interface diagram is the value display area of physiological parameters, which can display the real-time display values of physiological parameters; The left side is the waveform display area of physiological parameters, which can display the real-time waveform of measured physiological parameters.

Blood Pressure Data
In the debugging of the blood pressure module, in order to test the accuracy of the blood pressure measurement software, seven different time points were selected at 16:00 and 22:00 on the same day, and the same measurement object was measured seven times. The measurement results are as follows: The fluctuation range of human diastolic blood pressure measured 7 times is 100 mmHg–160 mmHg. During measurement, set the upper and lower limits of diastolic blood pressure to 170 mmHg and 90 mmHg respectively. When the value of diastolic blood pressure is higher than 170 mmHg or lower than 90 mmHg, it means that the measured value is abnormal, and the measurement module will issue an abnormal alarm.

Blood Oxygen Data
The blood oxygen value of human body is calculated according to the different absorption rate of red light under the pulsation of human artery. Therefore, the information collected by the blood oxygen module used in this design also includes the pulse information of human body, that is, the pulse frequency of artery (pulse rate, unit: bpm). In order to accurately reflect the soft measurement performance of blood oxygen measurement, seven different measurement objects are selected to measure blood oxygen at the same time, numbered 1, 2, 3, 4, 5, 6 and 7 respectively, and all seven measurement objects are in a calm state. The measurement results showed that the measured blood oxygen values of the seven subjects were 88%, 91%, 92%, 90%, 89%, 90% and 95% respectively, and the pulse rate values were 60 bpm, 80 bpm, 90 bpm, 70 bpm, 62 bpm, 64 bpm and 70 bpm respectively. Set the normal range of blood oxygen to 90%-100%, and the normal range of pulse rate to 50bpm-120bpm. When the measured value exceeds this range, the system will send an alarm message.

5.4   Experimental Results and Analysis

In order to verify the rationality of the design of the telemedicine health care system based on embedded technology, it is compared with the monitoring data of the system based on the Internet of Things technology and the system based on the SpringMvc architecture pattern.

Blood Pressure Data Analysis
The blood pressure data monitoring results of the three systems are shown in Fig. 6.

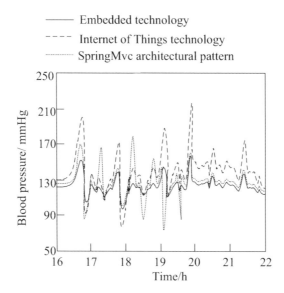

Fig. 6. Monitoring results of blood pressure data from three systems

It can be seen from Fig. 6 that the fluctuation range of human diastolic blood pressure in the system based on IoT technology is 75 mmHg–220 mmHg; The fluctuation range of diastolic blood pressure in the system based on SpringMvc architecture mode is 65 mmHg–190 mmHg; The fluctuation range of diastolic blood pressure in the system based on embedded technology it is 100 mmHg–160 mmHg, and the data obtained by using this system is consistent with the actual data. It can be seen that the blood pressure data monitoring results of the system based on embedded technology are accurate.

Blood Oxygen Data Analysis
The blood oxygen data monitoring results of the three systems are shown in Fig. 7.

It can be seen from Fig. 7 that the blood oxygen measurement values of the system based on the Internet of Things technology are 85%, 83%, 89%, 85%, 87%, 84% and 93%, respectively, and there is a maximum error of 8% with the actual data; The measured values of blood oxygen in the system based on the SpringMvc architecture mode are 86%, 88%, 99%, 95%, 91%, 93% and 95% respectively, and there is a maximum error of

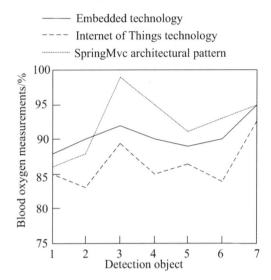

Fig. 7. Monitoring results of blood oxygen data in three systems

7% with the actual data; The system blood oxygen measurement values are 88%, 90%, 92%, 90%, 89%, 90% and 95% respectively, and there is only a maximum error of 1% with the actual data. It can be seen that the monitoring results of blood oxygen data of the system based on embedded technology are accurate.

The pulse rate data monitoring results of the three systems are shown in Fig. 8.

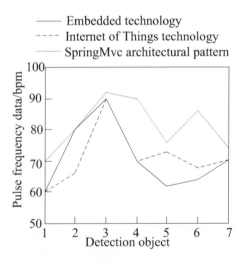

Fig. 8. Monitoring results of pulse rate data for three systems

Figure 8 shows that the system pulse rate data based on IoT technology are 60 bpm, 66 bpm, 90 bpm, 70 bpm, 62 bpm, 64 bpm and 70 bpm respectively, and there is a maximum error of 8% with the actual data; using the system pulse rate data based on the SpringMvc architecture mode 70 bpm, 80 bpm, 92 bpm, 90 bpm, 76 bpm, 96 bpm, and 74 bpm, respectively, with a maximum error of 7% from the actual data; the system pulse rate data based on embedded technology are 60 bpm, 80 bpm, 90 bpm, 70 bpm, 62 bpm, 64 bpm, respectively and 70 bpm, the data obtained by using this system is consistent with the actual data, it can be seen that the monitoring results of pulse rate data based on embedded technology are accurate.

6 Conclusion

(1) The designed telemedicine and health care system based on embedded technology can easily and accurately collect and process the basic physiological information of the human body, provide the online doctors with physiological data information, realize the interaction between users and doctors, make people conveniently and quickly get their own health information, facilitate health care prevention and early treatment, and to a certain extent, realize the self diagnosis information for reference.

(2) The idea of using embedded technology to develop software makes the system easy to maintain and upgrade, reduces the development cycle of products, reduces the development cost of the system, and improves the cost performance of the system, so that the telemedicine service can go to the market, enter the home, serve more people, and provide an effective design scheme for the design of the home telemedicine system.

(3) However, in the process of experimental verification, the response time of the system was not verified, and the response time of the system is closely related to user satisfaction. The verification of the system is not comprehensive, and there are certain limitations. Therefore, the next step needs to verify the response time of the system, to further optimize the comprehensive performance of the system in this respect, and promote the wide application of the system in practice.

References

1. Keke, G., Yang, Z., Xu, D.: Design of remote home medical system based on springmvc architecture mode. Packa. Eng. **41**(04), 160–165+176 (2020)
2. Qu, J., Li, Y.: An authentication protocol for telecare medicine information system. J. Wuhan Univ. Nat. Sci. Ed. **66**(02), 117–125 (2020)
3. García-Villena, J., Torres, J.E., Aguilar, C., et al.: 3D-printed portable robotic mobile microscope for remote diagnosis of global health diseases. Electronics **10**(19), 2408–2420 (2021)
4. Huang, H.W., Hsu, W.Y., Lee, C.H., et al.: Development of a light-weight deep learning model for cloud applications and remote diagnosis of skin cancers. J. Dermatol. **48**(3), 310–316 (2021)
5. Ac, A., Ml, B., Sm, A.: Applying telemedicine for stroke remote diagnosis: the telestroke system. Procedia Comput. Sci. **198**(1), 164–170 (2022)
6. Qin, L., Zhang, R.: Mobile medical system design based on behavior design. Pack. Eng. **42**(22), 191–203 (2021)

7. Tong, W., Hou, Z., Zeng, S., et al.: Design of positioning and remote control system based on NB-IoT. Inst. Techn. Sensor (10), 94–97+119 (2021)

8. Wang, D., Li, C., Sun, J., et al.: Discussion on the clinical value of ultrasonic artificial intelligence diagnosis system combined with telemedicine. Chin. J. Ultrasound Med. **37**(07), 765–766 (2021)

9. Chen, X., Yue, W.: Exploration on mobile terminal guidance service design in smart healthcare system. Pack. Eng. **41**(12), 143–149 (2020)

10. Li, T., Yan, F., Yu, Z., et al.: The design and application of remote monitor data acquisition system based on ARM. Electric Drive **50**(07), 103–107 (2020)

11. Liu, Z., Liu, J.: Accurate test simulation of operation stability and performance of wireless medical monitoring system. Comput. Simul. **36**(4), 375–378 (2019)

12. Wei, W., Xin, Z., Wang, S., Zhang, Y.: Covid-19 diagnosis by WE-SAJ, systems science & control. Engineering **10**(1), 325–335 (2022). https://doi.org/10.1080/21642583.2022.2045645

13. Huang, C., Wang, W., Zhang, X., Wang, S.-H., Zhang, Y.-D.: Tuberculosis diagnosis using deep transferred EfficientNet. IEEE/ACM Trans. Comput. Biol. Bioinf. (2022). https://doi.org/10.1109/TCBB.2022.3199572

14. Lin, H.C., Chou, F.Y., Hong, Y.X., et al.: Fast elevator vibration signal cloud collection system using data compression and encryption algorithms. Sens. Mater. Int. J. Sensor Technol. **34**(Pt.4), 2311–2324 (2022)

15. Li, J.: Research on safe transmission of broadband fm laser signal based on particle swarm optimization algorithm. Laser J. **42**(7), 118–121 (2021)

Anomaly Detection Method of Healthcare Internet of Things Gateway Supporting Edge Computing

Zixiu Zou[1,2], Yi Hu[3], Xinyao Liu[4], and Shufeng Zhuo[5(✉)]

[1] Fuzhou Institute of Technology, Fuzhou 350506, Fujian, China
[2] SEGI University, 47810 Petaling Jaya, Selangor, Malaysia
[3] Henan Information Engineering School, Zhengzhou 450000, China
[4] Imperial Vision Technology Company Limited, Fuzhou 350001, China
[5] The Internet of Things and Artificial Intelligence College, Fujian Polytechnic of Information Technology, Fuzhou 350003, China
55607@qq.com

Abstract. As the link between the perception layer and the network layer, the Internet of Things gateway is of great significance to the safe and stable operation of the healthcare Internet of Things. Once the gateway is abnormal, it will directly affect the information transmission in health care work. Therefore, an anomaly detection method for the gateway of the Internet of Things in health care supporting edge computing is proposed. Several representative gateway status indicators are selected by using the maximum uncorrelation method, and the gateway anomaly detection task is unloaded to the edge server by using edge computing. An anomaly detection model based on SOFM neural network and random forest is constructed to realize the anomaly detection of the Internet of Things gateway in health care. The experimental results show that the determination coefficients of the six types of samples of this method are more than 0.9, which is close to 1, which shows that this method has better anomaly detection performance of the Internet of Things gateway in health care.

Keywords: Edge Calculation · Medical Care · Internet Of Things · Gateway Is Abnormal · Test Method

1 Introduction

What is the Internet of Things? The notes attached to the 2010 Chinese government work report explained: "The Internet of Things refers to the use of information sensing devices (radio frequency identification RFID, infrared sensors, global positioning systems, laser scanners, etc.). According to the agreed protocol, any item is connected to the Internet for information exchange and communication, so as to realize intelligent identification, positioning, tracking, monitoring and management. It is a network that extends and expands on the basis of the Internet." This explanation may appear in the medical and

© ICST Institute for Computer Sciences, Social Informatics and Telecommunications Engineering 2023
Published by Springer Nature Switzerland AG 2023. All Rights Reserved
S. Wang (Ed.): IoTCare 2022, LNICST 501, pp. 239–254, 2023.
https://doi.org/10.1007/978-3-031-33545-7_17

health field in the future: the mobile phone, watch or belt we carry with us suddenly sends out a signal to remind our health problems; this signal can be sent to the hospital, and if the situation is urgent, the ambulance will go directly. to your place; If it is not too serious, community doctors can call and directly view medical files, conduct remote consultations, and make appointments for medical treatment; They can even deliver medicines to homes according to prescriptions through pharmaceutical logistics. The Internet of Things can play an important role in the application of "barcode" patient identity management, mobile medical orders, electronic entry of symptoms and signs, mobile drug management, mobile test specimen management, mobile medical record management, data storage and transfer, infant theft prevention, nursing process, clinical pathway and other management in the medical and health field [1, 2].

With the rapid development of the Internet of Things in the healthcare industry, the gateway of the Internet of Things, which connects the sensing network and the traditional communication network, is playing an important role. As the manager of the Internet of Things, the gateway controls the operation of the whole Internet of Things, and its management authority and reliability requirements are the highest. Because the Internet of Things usually works in a complex environment, and the gateway is the most important field equipment of the Internet of Things, some inevitable important or urgent problems will inevitably appear in its work. Many factors will make it difficult for the gateway to work normally all the time [3]. Once the gateway is abnormal, the whole network will be paralyzed. All sensor nodes managed by the gateway listen to network messages for a long time, resend data repeatedly, channel congestion, data collision and other phenomena, which affect the effectiveness of medical care tasks. In response to the above situation, anomaly detection of healthcare Internet of Things gateways has attracted great attention from both academia and engineering. However, due to the huge amount of gateway status information, and each piece of status information contains a large number of attributes, it is extremely difficult to label each piece of information; with the continuous development of network applications, the amount of data will increase exponentially, and the central the system appears powerless. Faced with the above situation, a method for anomaly detection of healthcare Internet of Things gateways supporting edge computing is studied. The overall structure of the method is as follows:

(1) The maximum uncorrelation method is used to select several representative gateway status indicators, and edge computing is used to unload the gateway anomaly detection task to the edge server. An anomaly detection model based on SOFM neural network and random forest is constructed to realize anomaly detection of healthcare IoT gateway.

(2) During the experiment, the gateway status indicators are set, and the IoT gateway anomaly detection experiment is carried out through sample preparation and task unloading scheme determination. The anomaly detection structure is obtained, and the performance of this method is verified.

(3) Summarize the full text, analyze the limitations of the anomaly detection method of the healthcare IoT gateway that supports edge computing, and further explain the future work.

2 Research on Anomaly Detection of Internet of Things Gateways Based on Edge Computing

The ultimate goal of the Internet of Things is to realize the interconnection of all things in the world and the barrier free information exchange between people, people and things, and things and things. As an Internet interconnection device in the Internet of Things, the gateway of the Internet of Things plays a connecting role, realizing the protocol conversion and data interaction between the sensing network and the communication network. Gateway is also known as inter network connector and protocol converter. The default gateway realizes network interconnection at the network layer. It is the most complex network interconnection device and is only used for the interconnection of two networks with different high-level protocols. The structure of the gateway is similar to that of the router, except for the interconnection layer. Gateway can be used for both wide area network interconnection and LAN interconnection. To go from one room to another, one must pass through a door. Similarly, sending information from one network to another must also pass through a "gateway", which is the gateway. As the name suggests, a gateway is a "gateway" that connects a network to another network, that is, a network gate. Once there is a problem with the gateway, it will directly affect the communication quality of the entire Internet of Things, so it is necessary to perform accurate status detection on the gateway.

2.1 Determination of Gateway Status Indicators

There are many indicators that can reflect the status of the gateway. In the past, one or two indicators were selected for anomaly detection, which has great limitations, making the accuracy of anomaly detection not high. In the face of this situation, the maximum uncorrelation method is used to select several representative gateway status indicators.

If indicator s_1 and other indicators $s_2, s_3, \ldots, s_m$ are independent, it means that s_1 cannot be replaced by other indicators, so the reserved indicators should be as small as possible. Under the guidance of this method, a method of maximum irrelevance is derived. The maximum irrelevance method mainly selects indicators according to the relationship between the complex correlation coefficient and the set critical value, where the complex correlation coefficient refers to the degree of correlation between an indicator and other indicators [4]. The basic principle is as follows: Firstly, the correlation coefficient matrix Y of the sample is obtained, and then according to the correlation coefficient y_{ij}, the complex correlation coefficient z_i^2 is obtained (the complex correlation coefficient refers to the degree of correlation between one indicator and other indicators), and the critical value T is defined. Judging the relationship between the complex correlation coefficient z_i^2 and the critical value T, if $z_i^2 > T$, the index can be removed. The specific calculation process is as follows:

Step 1: Find the correlation coefficient matrix Y of the sample, such as:

$$Y = \{y_{ij}\}_{mm} = \begin{Bmatrix} y_{11} & y_{12} & \cdots & y_{1m} \\ y_{21} & y_{22} & \cdots & y_{2m} \\ \cdots & & & \\ y_{m1} & y_{m2} & \cdots & y_{mm} \end{Bmatrix} \tag{1}$$

$$y_{ij} = \frac{s_{ij}^2}{\sqrt{\frac{s_{ii}^2 s_{jj}^2}{m}}}, i, j = 1, 2, \ldots, m \tag{2}$$

where, y_{ij} reflects the linear correlation between s_i and s_j.

Step 2: Calculate the complex correlation coefficient z_i^2 according to y_{ij}. The value of z_i can be calculated by Y. The specific steps are as follows: Y is divided into blocks in the following way, and Y blocks can be expressed as the following formula:

$$Y = \begin{bmatrix} Y_{-m} & y_m \\ y_m^T & 1 \end{bmatrix} \tag{3}$$

At this time, the main diagonal element of Y is 1, so the complex correlation coefficient of each index can be calculated according to formula $z_i^2 = y_m^T Y_{-m} y_m$, and $z_1^2, z_2^2, \ldots, z_m^2$ can be obtained.

Step 3: Determine the relationship between the critical values T and z_i^2. First determine the critical value T. The critical value T is generally the F test of z_i^2. If $\alpha = 0.1$ is taken, if $F > F_{0.10}$, it means that the multiple correlation is significant. Finally, judge the relationship between T and z_i^2. If $z_i^2 > T$, delete the index.

Finally, due to different dimensions, the indicators cannot be put together for comparison and analysis, so it is necessary to standardize each indicator, and the calculation formula is as follows:

$$\hat{s}_{ij} = \frac{s_{ij} - (\bar{s}_j)}{\sqrt{\text{var}(s_j)}} \tag{4}$$

In the formula, $\hat{s}_{ij}$ represents the standardized index; $\bar{s}_j$ represents the mean of the j index; $\text{var}(s_j)$ represents the mean square error of the j index; s_j represents the j index.

2.2 Anomaly Detection Task Offloading Based on Edge Computing

In the face of a large number of anomaly detection tasks of medical and health Internet of Things gateways with multiple indicators, the traditional central system has been unable to meet the needs of rapid data processing, and edge computing can effectively solve this problem by establishing nodes near the data source to reduce the data transmission delay and divert the tasks of the computing center. Edge computing has the characteristics of real-time, high bandwidth, heterogeneity, etc. by extending the computing power closer to the end user, it makes up for the shortcomings of cloud computing and is the optimization and expansion of cloud computing [5]. With the advent and development of the Internet of Things, edge computing, as a developing computing paradigm, is considered to be one of the key architectures of the next generation communication network. Edge computing architecture is to add edge servers between terminal devices and cloud servers to expand services at the edge of the network. The system architecture of edge computing is generally divided into terminal layer, edge layer and cloud layer.

(1) The terminal device layer, including various mobile terminals connected to the edge network and many Internet of Things devices, such as smartphones, various sensors,

and smart cars. At the terminal layer, the device is not only a data consumer, but also a data provider. In order to reduce the terminal service delay, only the perceptual capabilities of various terminal devices are considered, and the computing capabilities are not considered. Therefore, several devices at the terminal layer collect various raw data and transmit them to the upper-layer architecture, where data tasks are stored and calculated.

(2) The edge layer is the core of the three-tier architecture. It is located at the edge of the network and consists of edge nodes widely distributed between terminal devices and the cloud. It usually includes base stations, access points, routers, switches and edge gateways. The edge layer supports the terminal to access downward, store and calculate the data uploaded by the terminal, connect upward with the cloud, and upload the processed data to the cloud. Because the edge layer is close to users, data transmission to the edge layer is more suitable for real-time data analysis and intelligent processing, which is more efficient and secure than cloud computing. Among the joint services of edge cloud computing, cloud computing server is still a very powerful data processing center.

(3) The cloud layer, composed of multiple high-performance servers and storage devices, has powerful computing and storage capabilities, and can play an important role in areas where there are many data analysis services such as regular maintenance and business decision support. The cloud computing center has the function of storing the data uploaded by the edge computing layer for a long time. In addition, analysis tasks that cannot be processed by the edge layer or other heavy computing tasks can also be implemented in the cloud. The cloud module can also dynamically adjust the edge computing layer according to the control strategy. Deployment strategy.

The edge computing system architecture was proposed in the Edge Computing White Paper 3.0 released in December 2018. The edge computing reference architecture presents the architectural content from different perspectives in a multi-view manner, as shown in Fig. 1, and displays each layer through multiple perspectives function.

The bottom device layer of the framework connects the whole framework, including management services, data lifecycle services and security services. Management services provide unified management and monitoring, and provide information to the management platform. Data lifecycle services provide integrated management for the preprocessing, analysis and execution of machine data. Security services can flexibly deploy and optimize data services to meet the real-time needs of business.

Computing offload is performed by migrating the computing tasks on the terminal device to the extended cloud or edge platform. The computing platform assists the terminal to complete the user's task request, and returns the computing results to the specified device. The task unloading technology mainly includes two problems: unloading decision and resource allocation. The main research points of unloading decision are whether to unload the task, the unloading destination and the unloading amount of the task. The main research points of resource allocation are how much communication and computing resources the server needs to allocate to the task. Generally speaking, there are a series of application tasks with different amounts of data that need to be executed on the terminal device. Firstly, the device needs to detect whether there is a server in

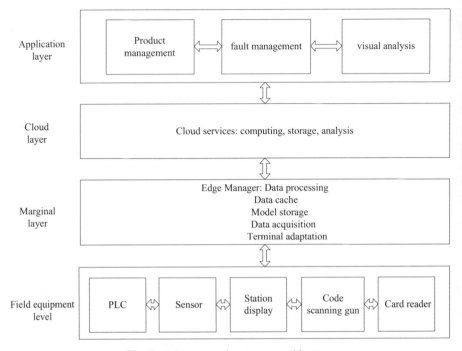

Fig. 1. Edge computing system architecture

the environment that can perform the uninstallation operation. Then, considering the partial uninstallation and binary uninstallation of the task, determine whether the task can be uninstalled, how to uninstall it, and when to uninstall it. The task on the terminal device can be executed locally or on the edge server. If the resources on the edge side are insufficient or cannot meet the demand, the task can be further sent to the cloud server. For local execution, only the computing power of the device itself needs to be considered and the calculation results are output. For remote execution, submit the computing task to the upper-layer server through Wi-Fi and other methods, so that the server will allocate computing resources, communication resources and storage resources for the received task, and execute the computing task. The task result is returned to the user and the occupied resources are released.

After completing task clustering and server resource integration, we need to consider the problem of system resource allocation, that is, which server the task needs to be allocated to perform the most reasonable. Because the communication and computing resources of mobile edge computing server are relatively limited, and the terminal devices are usually heterogeneous, considering the dynamic nature of task unloading and resource load, the optimization goal of most current research work is to comprehensively consider the measurement of delay and load balance when the task does not exceed the bandwidth, storage and computing capacity of the server [6].

Load Balancing

In mobile edge computing, there are many load factors that affect task offloading and resource allocation. We assume that A_i represents the CPU utilization of the i server, B_i represents the memory utilization of the i server, and C_i represents the bandwidth utilization of the i server. Assuming that each server can normally receive requests from resource requesters, the load of each server is defined as follows:

$$D_i = w_1 A_i + w_2 B_i + w_3 C_i \tag{5}$$

Calculate the average load of all servers. The formula is as follows:

$$\overline{G} = \frac{\sum\limits_{i=1}^{N} D_i}{N} \tag{6}$$

Among them, w_1, w_2, w_3 represent the weight coefficient; $\overline{G}$ represents the average load; N represents the number of servers.

Therefore, the load balance degree is expressed as formula (7). The more average the value of the load balance degree is, the more balanced the load distribution of the entire edge computing network system is, and the more average the task distribution is.

$$H = \sqrt{\frac{\sum\limits_{i=1}^{N} \left(D_i - \overline{G} \right)}{N}} \tag{7}$$

In the formula, H represents the load balance degree.

Time Delay

The processing speed of the server for different exception detection tasks is different, and the execution time will affect the user's quality of service. Therefore, the main optimization goal is to effectively reduce the completion time of the task. Assuming that P_j represents the amount of data of exception detection task j, the server's execution time is defined as:

$$Q_{ij} = \frac{P_j}{A_i} \tag{8}$$

In the formula, Q_{ij} represents the time when the i server executes the anomaly detection task j.

Since the resource requester has requested multiple anomaly detection tasks, the calculation time of the task execution required for all mobile devices to complete the task is expressed as follows:

$$U = \sum_{i=1}^{N} \sum_{j=1}^{M} Q_{ij} \tag{9}$$

where, U represents the total execution time of anomaly detection task; M represents the number of tasks.

Based on the above description, the task unloading problem in the mobile edge computing scenario is usually NP problem, which is difficult to solve directly. At present, most of the research to solve this kind of problem is to consider the use of intelligent colony algorithm. The intelligent colony algorithm used here is the fireworks algorithm [7]. Firstly, in the whole feasible solution space, an indefinite number of initial fireworks populations are randomly generated, each fireworks is equivalent to a feasible solution, and then the corresponding fitness function value of each fireworks is determined. By generating different fireworks explosion radius, the fireworks set is updated, and the next generation of explosion sparks and Gaussian mutation sparks are generated. Whether the algorithm meets the cycle end condition is judged, and if so, the search is stopped. Otherwise, select a certain number of individuals in the candidate set as a new fireworks population to enter the iteration of the next process. From the above process, we can see that the fireworks algorithm has an adaptive radius adjustment mechanism, and has certain exploration and mining capabilities. The adaptation of anomaly detection task unloading and fireworks algorithm parameters is shown in Table 1 below.

Table 1. Anomaly detection task offloading problem and parameter adaptation of fireworks algorithm

Fireworks algorithm	Uninstall problems
Individual dimension	Number of user tasks
Individual	Single unloading scheme
Population	Collection of different unloading schemes
Fireworks location	Unloading schemes for different user tasks
Fitness value	Combined value of load balancing and task delay

The specific process is as follows:

Step 1: Initialize. Determine the fireworks individual dimension M (number of anomaly detection tasks) and the value range N (number of servers) of each dimension, as well as the number of fireworks in each generation and other algorithm parameters. Through the reverse learning strategy, a certain number of fireworks are generated as the initial fireworks population.

Step 2: Calculate the fitness value. The location information of fireworks is the unloading decision variable. Under the current unloading decision, the resource allocation variable is solved by convex optimization formula (7), and then the total delay cost value of the task is obtained. As the fitness value of this fireworks individual, the fitness value of all individuals is solved.

Step 3: Solve the explosion radius r and the explosion number k.

Step 4: Generate offspring fireworks. Within the explosion radius r, k-number fireworks are generated by random strategy as offspring fireworks.

Step 5: Generate mutation sparks. Through the mutation operator, the mutant firework individual is generated.

Step 6: Select the next generation of fireworks individuals and update the optimal value of the population. The optimal fireworks are selected among the parent fireworks, offspring fireworks and mutant fireworks to enter the next generation, and other fireworks are selected as the next generation fireworks through the championship strategy, and the optimal value of the population is updated.

Step 7: Judge whether the termination conditions are met. That is, if the maximum number of iterations is reached, the cycle will exit, and the minimum value of the total delay cost of the task and the corresponding unloading decision and resource allocation scheme will be searched. Otherwise, repeat steps 2 to 6 until the termination conditions are met.

Step 8: Output the optimal solution, that is, the anomaly detection task unloading scheme that can meet both the load balancing requirements and the delay requirements.

2.3 Gateway Anomaly Detection Based on Deep Learning

After the above exception detection task is uninstalled, the exception detection task is executed on each edge server. The detection algorithm used here is a combination of SOFM neural network and random forest algorithm. Clustering is carried out through SOFM neural network, and different clusters are divided. The samples in the cluster are sampled for data balancing. Finally, the balanced data set is trained with random forest algorithm to obtain multiple classifiers [8]. Each edge server has a classifier based on random forest for edge operation, and the prediction category corresponding to the maximum value of the calculated comprehensive weight is the final detection result.

SOFM Neural Network

SOFM neural network, the full name of self-organizing feature mapping neural network, is a neural network model proposed by Finnish scholar Kohonen study [9]. The SOFM network has two layers, namely the input layer and the output layer. The output layer is usually composed of a one-dimensional or two-dimensional network matrix. In actual use, the SOFM neural network will learn to map the input data to the corresponding position of the output layer over a period of time. The neuron areas activated by different input data are also different. If the data structure is similar, the adjacent areas will be activated. The difference in the activation area will reasonably distinguish the input data. This process achieves the purpose of learning by changing the connection weights, and these processes are done automatically internally, so this method is called self-organizing feature mapping.

The learning process of SOFM neural network is to input training samples in the input layer. The network can self-organizing adjust the weight vector between neurons, so that the weight vector changes with the change of input mode, and finally make the neurons in the output layer more sensitive to input data. All connection weight vectors are separated from each other to form a set that can represent the input mode, so as to achieve the effect of self-organizing clustering [10].

The gateway status indicator sample has a relatively obvious feature in the data structure, that is, the number of abnormal samples is much smaller than the number of normal samples. Generally speaking, when the ratio of positive and negative samples is greater than 4:1, if these data sets are directly classified and trained, then The prediction results of the trained classification model in actual use will be heavily biased towards the sample category with a high proportion, resulting in poor performance of the algorithm model. In this regard, the state index data of unbalanced gateway is processed based on SOFM neural network.

For an unbalanced data set, find the g nearest neighbors of each minority sample v_i, and select h samples from the g nearest neighbors of the minority sample (ensure that $g > h$). These h samples are assumed to be $v_1, v_2, \ldots, v_h$, and then interpolate through the interpolation formula (see Eq. 10) to get new samples. In this way, it is equivalent to adding h new samples to each minority sample.

$$\hat{v} = v_i + f(0, 1)(u_j - v_i), j = 1, 2, \ldots, h \qquad (10)$$

Among them, $\hat{v}$ represents the new sample; v_i represents the sample point of the minority category, u_j represents the sample point selected from the g nearest neighbors of v; $f(0, 1)$ represents the number between $(0, 1)$ randomly generated.

Random Forest Algorithm
Random forest algorithm is actually an improved version of bagging algorithm, which is equivalent to introducing random attribute selection into bagging algorithm based on decision tree. Random forest algorithm is easy to implement in practical application, with good effect and low time cost, which benefits from the two random measures of random forest, that is, based on the random sample selection of bagging algorithm itself and the random attribute selection, the generalization performance of random forest algorithm is further improved [11].

In the iterative process of the random forest algorithm, the self-service sampling method is used for the selection of samples. By sampling the sample set with replacement, the samples drawn each time are put into the inBag. In addition, according to the content of Chapter 2, there are probably 37% of the samples will not be drawn, put them into the outBag. The data in the inBag is trained by the decision tree algorithm to generate a classification model, and then the model effect is tested through the given test set. The evaluation indicators of the model effect generally use the precision rate η, the recall rate μ, and the F1 value. From the formula (11), the F1 value integrates the precision rate η and the recall rate μ, which can measure and evaluate the performance of the model more objectively. The confusion matrix is shown in Table 2.

$$F1 = \frac{2 \cdot \eta \cdot \mu}{\eta + \mu} \qquad (11)$$

Among them,

$$\eta = \frac{T_1}{T_1 + T_3} \qquad (12)$$

$$\mu = \frac{T_1}{T_1 + T_2} \qquad (13)$$

Table 2. Confusion matrix

Project		Actual results	
		Positive class	Negative class
Prediction results	Positive class	T1	T2
	Negative class	T3	T4

In the formula, F1 represents the harmonic mean between precision η and recall μ.

Assuming that the number of base classifiers in the random forest is β, the F1 value of each decision tree calculated by the given test set is $\psi_1, \psi_2, \ldots, \psi_\beta$, respectively, and the weights of the decision trees in the random forest are as follows:

$$\lambda_i = \frac{\psi_i}{\sum\limits_{i=1}^{\beta} \psi_i} \tag{14}$$

After giving weight to each decision tree, predict and judge the new sample $\hat{v}$ through these decision trees. Assuming that the probability of each decision tree predicting that the new sample $\hat{v}$ belongs to a certain category ε is $\xi_a(\hat{v})$, then in the final voting decision, combined with the weight of the decision tree and the prediction probability, the comprehensive weight of sample $\hat{v}$ belonging to category ε can be obtained as follows [12]:

$$\varpi_\varepsilon(\hat{v}) = \sum_{i=1}^{\beta} \psi_i \times \xi_a(\hat{v}) \tag{15}$$

In the formula, $\varpi_\varepsilon(\hat{v})$ sample $\hat{v}$ belongs to the comprehensive weight of category ε.

Combining the above content, the detailed idea of the classifier can be obtained: in the random forest algorithm [13, 14], multiple sample sets are extracted by the self-help method, and each sample set is trained to obtain a decision tree mode, and then a given test sample set is used to pair the the performance of multiple decision tree models is evaluated, and the evaluation index is the F1 value. According to the principle that the larger the F1 value, the better the model effect, the ratio of the performance index F1 value of each decision tree to the sum of the F1 values of all decision trees is used to determine each decision tree. The weight of the decision tree, then for the prediction of the new sample, first use each decision tree model to judge it, predict the probability that the sample belongs to a certain class, multiply and sum all the decision tree weights and the predicted probability, and get a certain class Finally, the maximum comprehensive weight is calculated by comparison, and the prediction category corresponding to this value is the final result predicted by the random forest algorithm [15].

3   Detection Method Application Test

3.1   Gateway Status Indicators

There are 9 gateway status indicators selected based on the maximum uncorrelation method, as follows:

(1) Throughput: The packet forwarding capability of the device. It usually refers to the ability of the tested equipment to forward data without packet loss, which is generally expressed as a percentage of the line speed (or passing rate) that can be achieved.
(2) Latency: The time interval between receiving packets and forwarding packets within the throughput range of the device.
(3) Packet loss rate: The ratio of the number of discarded packets to the number of received packets under different loads.
(4) Back to back frame: The maximum number of packets that the device can process without packet loss when it receives transmission at the minimum packet interval.
(5) System recovery: The time for the equipment to resume normal operation after overload. If the network equipment has line speed capability, the test is meaningless.
(6) System reset: The time interval from software reset or power off restart to normal operation of the device. Normal operation refers to the ability to forward data with throughput.
(7) Maximum number of concurrent connections: the maximum number of connections that can be established simultaneously between hosts passing through the conversion gateway or between the host and the conversion gateway.
(8) Breakpoint resume transmission capability: In the event of network interruption, the gateway continues to accurately collect data, cache the data in non-volatile devices, and retransmit the cached data to the industrial cloud platform through the forwarding channel when the network returns to normal. Ability.
(9) Local alarm capability: In the case of network failure, equipment failure, etc., the gateway should provide local alarm information based on configuration information and real-time data, and support multiple alarm types such as switch value and analog value. And when sending monitoring data packets to the device, when the return speed reaches a certain threshold, the device will give an early warning to remind the operator to pay attention.

3.2   Sample Preparation

Based on the gateway status index, training samples and test samples are generated with the help of MATLAB, and the results are shown in Fig. 2 below.

It can be seen from Fig. 2 that there are 6 types of samples, and each type of sample includes several small samples.

3.3   Task Offloading Scheme

The sample detection tasks in Fig. 2 are evenly distributed to 15 servers, and the number of tasks allocated to each server is shown in Table 3 below.

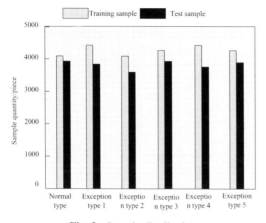

Fig. 2. Sample distribution

Table 3. Gateway anomaly detection task offloading scheme

The server	Training tasks		Test task	
	Normal sample	Abnormal sample	Normal sample	Abnormal sample
1	464	355	125	156
2	315	257	144	124
3	235	220	123	144
4	235	325	125	133
5	185	56	120	125
6	174	87	122	158
7	152	145	322	187
8	263	252	214	183
9	241	145	210	32
10	187	102	54	55
11	166	135	87	289
12	254	66	565	188
13	146	283	222	176
14	225	36	345	133
15	255	255	146	165

3.4 Anomaly Detection Results

Use the training samples in Fig. 2 to train the anomaly detection model based on SOFM neural network and random forest, and then input the test samples into the trained model. Some results are shown in Table 4 below.

Table 4. Example of anomaly detection results

Small sample	Type	Comprehensive weight	Detection category
1	Normal type	6.25	Exception type 5
	Exception type 1	4.12	
	Exception type 2	3.87	
	Exception type 3	5.55	
	Exception type 4	5.47	
	Exception type 5	7.45	
2	Normal type	2.58	Exception type 5
	Exception type 1	2.47	
	Exception type 2	3.68	
	Exception type 3	5.36	
	Exception type 4	5.47	
	Exception type 5	2.58	
3	Normal type	7.45	Normal type
	Exception type 1	5.32	
	Exception type 2	3.65	
	Exception type 3	3.22	
	Exception type 4	3.20	
	Exception type 5	1.77	

3.5 Method Performance Test

All abnormal detection results are counted, and then the coefficient of determination, also known as goodness of fit, is calculated, which can effectively reflect the difference between the detection results and the actual results. The closer the coefficient of determination is to 1, the closer the detection result is to the reality, and the result is shown in Fig. 3 below.

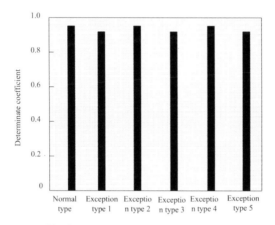

Fig. 3. Method performance test results

It can be seen in Fig. 3 that under the application of the studied method, the determinable coefficients of the six types of samples are more than 0.9, which is close to 1, which illustrates the performance of the studied anomaly detection method.

4 Conclusion

(1) To sum up, once the gateway is abnormal, the entire Internet of Things will be paralyzed. Faced with this situation, this paper proposes an anomaly detection method for healthcare IoT gateway that supports edge computing.
(2) This method assigns the anomaly detection task to the edge server, and implements gateway anomaly detection through the detection model on the server and the classifier. Finally, through testing, the determination coefficients of the test results are all above 0.9, which proves the effectiveness of the method.
(3) However, the SOFM neural network used in this method has some defects, such as slow learning convergence speed, and the network performance is sensitive to initial conditions. However, this paper does not propose a solution to overcome the defects of SOFM neural network, so there are some limitations. In the future, this problem needs to be studied in depth to optimize the comprehensive performance of SOFM neural network, so as to maximize the quality of anomaly detection of healthcare IoT gateway.

References

1. Wang, W., Zhang, X., Wang, S.-H., Zhang, Y.-D.: Covid-19 diagnosis by WE-SAJ. Syst. Sci. Control Eng. **10**(1), 325–335 (2022). https://doi.org/10.1080/21642583.2022.2045645
2. Huang, C., Wang, W., Zhang, X., Wang, S.-H., Zhang, Y.-D.: Tuberculosis diagnosis using deep transferred EfficientNet. IEEE/ACM Trans. Comput. Biol. Bioinf. (2022). https://doi.org/10.1109/TCBB.2022.3199572
3. Nikseresht, M., Mollamotalebi, M.: Providing a CoAP-based technique to get wireless sensor data via IoT gateway. Comput. Commun. **172**(2), 155–168 (2021)
4. Peng, C., Chen, J., Vijayakumar, P., et al.: Efficient distributed decryption scheme for IoT gateway-based applications. ACM Trans. Internet Technol. **21**(1), 1–23 (2021)
5. Cui, E., Yang, D., Wang, H., et al.: Learning-based deep neural network inference task offloading in multi-device and multi-server collaborative edge computing. Trans. Emerging Telecommun. Technol. **33**(7), 4485–4505 (2022)
6. Huang, L., Ran, J., Wang, W., et al.: A multi-channel anomaly detection method with feature selection and multi-scale analysis. Comput. Netw. **185**(8), 107645 (2020)
7. Song, L., Zheng, T., Wang, J., et al.: An improvement growing neural gas method for online anomaly detection of aerospace payloads. Soft. Comput. **24**(6), 1–13 (2020)
8. Jiang, Y., Yu, Y., Peng, X.: Online anomaly detection in DC/DC converters by statistical feature estimation using GPR and GA. IEEE Trans. Power Electron. **35**(10), 10945–10957 (2020)
9. Bhuvaneswari, A., Selvakumar, S.: Anomaly detection framework for Internet of Things traffic using vector convolutional deep learning approach in fog environment. Futur. Gener. Comput. Syst. **113**(1), 255–265 (2020)
10. Podgorelec, B., Turkanovi, M., Karakati, S.: A Machine learning-based method for automated blockchain transaction signing including personalized anomaly detection. Sens. (Basel, Switzerland) **20**(1), 147 (2020)
11. Tanuska, P., Spendla, L., Kebisek, M., et al.: Smart anomaly detection and prediction for assembly process maintenance in compliance with industry 4.0. Sensors **21**(7), 2376 (2021)
12. Shen, H.M., Zhou, G.J.: Repair of erasure codes of distributed storage data based on decision tree model. Comput. Simul. **39**(6), 473–477 (2022)
13. You, X., Hu, X., Feng, Z., et al.: Recognizing protein-metal ion ligands binding residues by random forest algorithm with adding orthogonal properties. Comput. Biol. Chem. **98**(1), 1–5 (2022)
14. Cui, X., Wang, S., Jiang, N., et al.: Establishment of prediction models for COVID-19 patients in different age groups based on Random Forest algorithm. QJM Mon. J. Assoc. Phys. **114**(11), 795–801 (2021)
15. Hosseinzadeh, M., Rahmani, A.M., Vo, B., et al.: Improving security using SVM-based anomaly detection: issues and challenges. Soft. Comput. **25**(4), 3195–3223 (2021)

Research on Fast Encryption of Electronic Health Record Data Based on Privacy Protection

Tianlin Fu[1], Juanfen Shi[2], and Haipeng Ke[3(✉)]

[1] College of Mathematics and Data Science, Minjiang University, Fuzhou 350000, China
[2] School of Electronic Engineering, Henan Information Engineering School, Henan 450008, China
[3] Fujian Zhangzhou No.1 Vocational Secondary School, Zhangzhou 363000, China
kehaipeng@163.com

Abstract. Electronic health records data has the characteristics of massive, multi-modal, heterogeneous, but electronic health records data is easy to be invaded, leading to the disclosure of patient personal information. Health record management systems often ignore the security problems when patients interact with other roles, and the traditional encryption methods have been difficult to effectively meet the security needs of modern privacy data. Therefore, a fast encryption method of electronic health record data based on privacy protection is proposed. Mainly through the combination of privacy protection and homomorphic encryption technology to achieve distributed user privacy data protection, the mining effect of privacy protection is effectively improved, and the data security is guaranteed. The effectiveness and practicability of this method in data privacy security protection are verified by experiments.

Keywords: Privacy Protection · Electronic Health Records · Health Records · Archival Data · Fast Encryption · Encryption Research

1 Introduction

Electronic health records began to be used as early as the end of the 1960s. It records the occurrence, development and treatment outcome of individual diseases, and has high medical value. Electronic health record data has the characteristics of massive, multi-modal and heterogeneous, and its complexity and magnitude of data are far beyond the scope of general data processing tasks. Computer theory, especially the development of emerging technologies such as data storage, machine learning and cloud computing, makes it possible to process massive electronic health archive data and extract useful information such as rules and patterns, which can be used for pathological analysis and disease early warning. However, the information security protection of the medical industry started late, and medical data leakage accidents emerge in endlessly. Hospital managers have absolute control over these electronic health records, which may be maliciously deleted, modified or leaked by internal personnel. If the privacy protection of individuals is not considered, the collection and application of electronic health records data will be greatly hindered [1, 2].

© ICST Institute for Computer Sciences, Social Informatics and Telecommunications Engineering 2023
Published by Springer Nature Switzerland AG 2023. All Rights Reserved
S. Wang (Ed.): IoTCare 2022, LNICST 501, pp. 255–270, 2023.
https://doi.org/10.1007/978-3-031-33545-7_18

The traditional sub health archives data encryption method only uses a single data encryption technology in the data encryption process, resulting in a small coverage of data encryption, a decline in encryption quality, and difficult to meet the security needs of modern privacy data. Therefore, a fast encryption method for electronic health archives data based on privacy protection is proposed. Aiming at the problem of single data encryption method, the distributed user privacy data protection is mainly realized by combining privacy protection with homomorphic encryption technology, which effectively improves the mining effect of privacy protection and ensures data security.

2 Related Work

The extraction and mining of valuable knowledge is realized through big data mining technology in diverse data (with massive and irregular characteristics). The realization methods of mining should be fully considered. The data mining methods based on privacy protection mainly include association rules data mining methods, sequential pattern data mining methods, encryption, and clustering data mining methods. In order to ensure the smooth progress of big data mining, it is necessary to take corresponding restraint measures for different sites to improve their self-restraint management capabilities, and try to avoid the problem of privacy data leakage. In recent years, some academic research results have been achieved, for example, using corresponding data mining methods (based on privacy protection) to improve the execution efficiency and privacy security of data mining based on semi-honest and malicious models; On the basis of in-depth exploration of security protection), a data mining method (based on the hiding of important sequence attributes) is designed, so that the data privacy protection function can be effectively realized; For the distributed environment, a data mining method based on privacy protection is completed. The mining method can effectively solve the problem of privacy leakage in the mining process [3, 4].

3 Methods

3.1 User Privacy Protection

Electronic health record data file management involves user management, authentication, data isolation and other aspects of design. Data isolation can protect individual data, separate the data of different users, and ensure personal privacy, so as to build a user privacy protection structure, as shown in Fig. 1 below:

According to Fig. 1, data sharing can be carried out if permitted. The basic architecture pattern is that a single server is connected to its database and is separated from other architectures. The shared architecture can allow different data information databases, which can be applied to the same a server, users can be distinguished or communicated by ID, with a large degree of freedom and a large capacity, which can effectively ensure the safe communication between users.

The user management of electronic health records is set to the user mode of individual corresponding to their own account. During application, the account and password login is required to ensure the operation safety of the system, and unified management

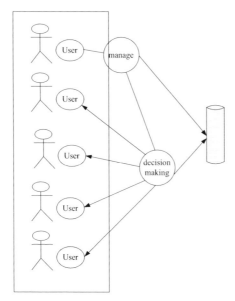

Fig. 1. User privacy protection structure diagram

instructions can be executed. At the same time, the basic information and security of users are guaranteed, and relevant security mechanisms are provided, so as to protect the privacy and precision of users, separate data from the management system, and enhance the information security of users.

3.2 Authority Assignment

The file agent system is mainly used to deal with matters between privacy protection and multi type electronic health record management systems. Different roles have different rights. Through key division, according to the permissions of different files, it can process and retrieve files, write, store and other operations. If necessary, it can be provided to users.

It mainly includes document archives sorting, document storage, information retrieval, access rights design and so on [5].

The program in this paper adjusts the internal management personnel information and system data. The management personnel and the system are divided according to the content and authority scope of their files, and the files are organized to facilitate the user's invocation and rectification [6, 7].

Since the information storage of electronic files involves the access rights of the files, the system design of this paper strengthens the design of the key, makes a reasonable calculation and design for the confidentiality period, and forms a virtual electronic contract to ensure the user's use rights and key confidentiality. Period of security. Build a permission assignment flowchart (Fig. 2):

When users use archives, they need to query and search through the Internet to get the information of relevant archives. Therefore, the retrieval function is an extremely

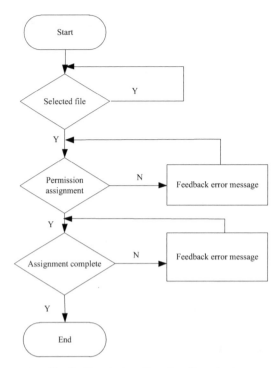

Fig. 2. Permission allocation flow chart

important system design. The application unit puts forward the retrieval request of relevant files to the browser according to the demand, and the request is sent to the processor. Each retrieval unit provides various electronic health files according to the demand, and judges whether to use the key according to the user's role type for security [8].

When the electronic file data is illegally obtained or maliciously tampered, the file agent system can upload the error information, and the administrator can track it through the computer to restore the privacy protected data information file, so that its information security is not infringed. At the same time, a firewall management system is set to protect the integrity of the data. Its working diagram is as follows (Fig. 3):

Set up the encryption model of electronic health records. The application of this model is that electronic health records can complete the information exchange between privacy protection and multi type electronic health record systems, improve the efficiency of information processing and expand the source of information. At the same time, the design of isolation system enhances the security and stability, and ensures the authenticity, reliability and effectiveness of electronic information. The application of cloud computing and smart contract greatly improves the efficiency of data management, realizes the fine management of electronic health records, and has a certain degree of automation ability, reduces the cost of human and material resources and other services, and improves the utilization of resources.

At the same time, the failure of individual data cannot affect the operation of the entire system, which improves the overall security of the system and reduces the possibility

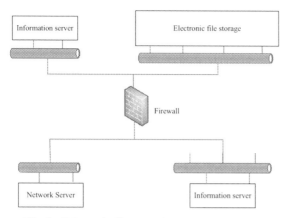

Fig. 3. Schematic diagram of firewall work (Fig. 2)

of illegal access and destruction. Thus, a more complete system software design is constructed.

3.3 Logic Analysis of Electronic Information Resources

Electronic information is stored in the hard disk of the computer. The storage address of each resource in the hard disk has an internal logical relationship. A complete storage area is divided into thousands of storage modules, and each storage module is divided into many levels for encrypted storage of resources. Electronic information includes the basic attribute information, naming, construction time, and logical address of the information. According to the above information, the electronic resources to be stored are logically analyzed. The internal relationship of the same type of electronic resource information has a logical relationship, and different types of resource information has an inverse logical relationship. If different types of resources are stored together, the two resources will consume each other, which is not conducive to the storage of information resources.

Electronic information resources are distributed and stored in different folders of computer hard disk. In order to balance the stability and integrity of information resources in network storage space, this paper optimizes the distribution of electronic information resources through distributed system method. The main working principle of the distributed system method is to convert and identify the format and content of information resources through the signal strength of the information cluster, and finally encrypt the resources according to the identification results. In the process of real-time information storage, the storage location is reasonably distributed to ensure the integrity of resources to the greatest extent. In the process of running, the distributed system converts the format of resources. If the resource is formatted, the format code of information cannot be monitored. When the conversion cannot be carried out, the electronic information resource is directly discarded without content code conversion, which saves the storage space of electronic information resources and improves the storage efficiency of resources. On the other hand, in order to prevent errors in resource conversion, the distributed system will retain the attribute information of information resources in the process of content conversion for electronic information resources with effective format. When resources are extracted and converted incorrectly, it will use artificial intelligence technology and information attributes to restore the original information resources [9, 10].

3.4 Encryption of Electronic Information Resources

Through the above analysis of the logical relationship between electronic resources and the research on the reasonable distribution method of resources, this paper designs an encryption method of electronic information resources based on artificial intelligence technology.

The real-time encryption process of electronic resources studied in this paper is divided into two parts: obtaining the basic information of electronic resources and encrypting electronic resources into the effective encryption area of the computer. The basic information of electronic resources includes attribute information, naming, time information of resource receiving, receiving way and address information of information resources [11]. When reading the basic information of electronic resources, you need to obtain the authority authentication of the resource holder before reading. After reading the resource information, in order to ensure the security of information resources, this paper encrypts the information. Because the resource information is displayed in the form of bytes, and each resource information is represented by a combination of multiple bytes, the core of the encryption of electronic resources is to effectively number the resources. An effective number consists of two 1024 bytes, and the two 1024 byte variables have the same meaning after exchange. Set the two byte read key and the overall key. The specific process is summarized as the following formula:

$$S_i = S_{i-1} + A_{i-1} \tag{1}$$

$$C_i = S_i, X_i + C_{i=1} \tag{2}$$

Among them, A is a byte of 1024; $C_o = 0$; X is the number of the electronic resource.

The above formula is to encrypt the encrypted electronic resource information, but it does not avoid the interference of external signals, which will affect the encryption efficiency of electronic information encryption. Therefore, the level of encryption should be increased to ensure the confidentiality of electronic information encryption [12]. In order to improve the level of information encryption, this paper sets a signal shielding lock in the encryption area of the computer. Once the electronic information is encrypted, the signal shielding lock automatically locks, and cannot receive scheduling information signals other than the computer, and powers the two keys inside the electronic resources. The power processing method without the key is the same, and it is processed by the following formula:

$$r = s - a_b - k \tag{3}$$

where a_b is the key group with two numbers; s is the code of electronic information resources; r is the external interference signal source; k represents the number of power processing of electronic information. Calculate the data of k by substituting the above formula, complete the secondary encryption, improve the real-time encryption method of electronic information resources, and ensure the security of information resources while ensuring the encryption efficiency.

The design of the software part of the hospital file encryption system design based on privacy protection in this paper mainly includes the software program database, the system login program, the web browser and the use of each module inside the system. The specific file encryption process is shown in the following figure (Fig. 4):

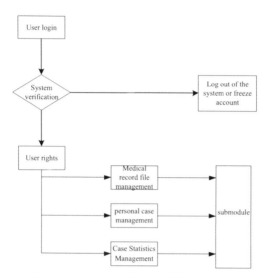

Fig. 4. Encryption process of hospital file encryption system

Database is the core of the file management system. Only with high database security and large memory space, can we ensure the safety of patient information in the hospital. The database is mainly responsible for encrypting the file data and establishing the connection between the file information and various departments. The database E-R diagram is designed. The hospital managers can change and verify the patient information through the identity of the administrator. In the file encryption system, the specific software area program database E-R diagram is as follows (Fig. 5):

The web browser is encrypted by a special code, which can ensure the security of the encrypted data in the hospital file encryption system. The web browser is divided into three browser channels, which are respectively oriented to patients, doctors, and managers, so that the three parties can enter the system at the same time. The login page of the file encryption system software part is registered and logged in through the user's registered mobile phone number, and the system browser is visible to the patient. The hospital doctor also enters the doctor's login browser through the same login page. Through the mutual adjustment between the database of the software system and the various modules in the hardware area, the operation of the browser is maintained, and the stable operation of the file encryption system and the security of file data are guaranteed.

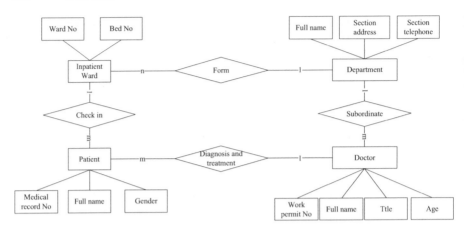

Fig. 5. E-R diagram of the software program database of the hospital file encryption system

The ultimate purpose of designing the hardware area of the hospital file encryption system is to ensure the security of the file encryption system and improve the operation efficiency of the system. Therefore, in order to achieve the design purpose, this paper proposes privacy protection to assist the operation of the encryption function of the system. Privacy protection is an optimized integrated algorithm method of distributed gradient computing. The idea of the algorithm method comes from the gradient lifting iterative decision tree. On the basis of the gradient lifting iterative decision tree algorithm method, the function of computing data encryption by second-order Taylor function is added to improve the encryption speed and accuracy of privacy protection on data files. Specifically, it is completed with the help of the following formula:

$$y_i = \theta(x_i) = \sum_{k=1}^{k} f_k(x_i) \tag{4}$$

Among them, k is the total number of data in the sub-model; y_i is the predicted value of the data sample; x_i is the feature quantity of the input archive data; f_k represents the data encryption regression value of the k cycle of the method.

The above formula introduces the second-order Taylor function to normalize the initial input data to avoid data confusion. In order to calculate the weight value of each file data, this article will refer to the following objective function as follows.

$$0 = 1(y, y_i) + \sum_{k=1}^{k} \beta(f_k) \tag{5}$$

Among them, (y, y_i) integrates the normative model of data; 0 represents the difference between the predicted value of the previous formula and the recorded value of the actual data; β represents the normalization processing coefficient, which is the positive value after calculating the data weight to prevent confusion between data. Use the basic data of deep learning to adjust the state of software encryption method, obtain the state parameters, set the corresponding operation related values, and combine the parameters in deep learning with the operation related values to find the specific encryption address source. Control the transmission direction of private data, guide the basic transmission direction of data by the deep learning function, issue the transmission password to the operation space, and adjust the transmission quantity according to the transmitted code information to maximize the transmission quantity. Set the corresponding transmission adjustment formula as follows:

$$N = c - t \cdot \sqrt{Q^5} \tag{6}$$

In the above formula, N represents the transmission adjustment result data, c represents the data transmission direction data, t represents the transmission password issuing parameter, and Q represents the operation space transmission password parameter.

When the server cannot respond to the transmission operation, it needs to modify its software information, adjust the data status in time, and set the information modification equation as follows:

$$P = v \cdot \frac{w}{K} + \sum A + c^2 \tag{7}$$

In the above formula, P represents the information modification parameter, v represents the transmission operation parameter, K represents the total number of data transmissions, w represents the received data information, A represents the command response parameter, and c represents the data condition adjustment value. In this way, the real performance of the operating system is analyzed, and it is convenient to accurately grasp the system data.

According to the information situation, install the system information device, build the software conversion platform, improve the operability of the software system, and set the corresponding system adjustment equation:

$$T = \sqrt{\frac{u - l}{d}} + \sum P \cdot S^{0.5} \tag{8}$$

In the above formula, T represents the response system adjustment parameter, d represents the installation system information parameter, u represents the operation step readability parameter, l represents the user information parameter, P represents the overall planning value, and S represents the platform construction parameter. According to the obtained parameter information combined with the key operation content, centralized data adjustment operation, improve the privacy data encryption audit method, strengthen the audit strength, and effectively implement data control.

Through the superposition calculation of multiple data, the predicted value of the iterative sample of the data is brought into the loss function, and the calculation result is multiplied by the normalization coefficient, then the final simplified formula of privacy protection is as follows:

$$o^t = \sum_{i=1}^{N} 1 \left(y_i, y^{t-1} + g_i f_i(x_i) + \frac{1}{2} h_i y_i(x_i) \right) + \beta(f_i) \tag{9}$$

Among them, N is the number of integration trees. Encrypt the data files to establish a decision tree. Compare and calculate the input file data with the data in the system database. If the same type of medical record information is retrieved, it will be encrypted in the same encrypted space to facilitate the operation of information call. Integrate and encrypt the redundant data of the decision tree, and finally complete the final management encryption of the data.

4   Experiment

After the realization of the above method design and research, the system improvement operation is carried out according to the designed structure and framework. In order to verify the encryption performance of the encryption method design in this paper, the encryption method design in this paper is compared with the traditional encryption method design, and a comparative experiment is constructed. The experimental comparison indicators are as follows:

(1) Encryption rate
(2) Encryption accuracy

Carry out experimental research according to the above two indicators, build an experimental environment, conduct experimental comparison operations on the basis of software management, pay attention to maintaining system service security when testing the operation status of encryption methods, archive the encrypted electronic health record information, and build a file encryption map (Fig. 6):

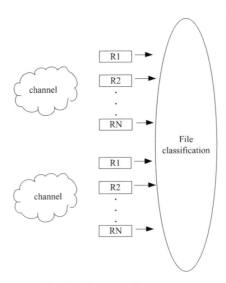

Fig. 6. File encryption diagram

Adjust the final encryption position of the electronic health record data, and set the encryption rate according to the encrypted data results. The comparison table is as follows (Tables 1, 2 and 3):

Table 1. Encryption method design encryption rate table in this paper

Encryption time/d	Encryption rate percentage
10	89%
20	93%
30	96%
40	100%

Table 2. Encryption rate table of traditional encryption method based on SaaS technology

Encryption time/d	Encryption rate percentage
10	77%
20	80%
30	85%
40	89%

Table 3. Traditional encryption method design encryption based on SOA architecture

Encryption time/d	Encryption rate percentage
10	64%
20	72%
30	75%
40	82%

According to the above table, the encryption rate designed by the fast encryption method of electronic health records based on privacy protection technology in this paper is faster than that designed by the other two traditional encryption methods. Because this method uses privacy protection to build a security system in the design process, so as to ensure the security of electronic health records in the transmission process, and adjusts the operation mode of the system according to the obtained security information, it has complete situational operation strength, and can transmit files under different network transmission systems. When the internal part is disturbed by external interference signals in the encryption process, the system will automatically send an alarm signal, and send the alarm signal from the file transmission source point to the file collection end point, so as to prevent abnormal data from invading the encryption method, ensure the complete and safe entry of electronic health file data information, thereby reducing unnecessary system operation waste and improving the overall system encryption rate.

After the above experimental operation is realized, in order to further verify the encryption effect of the system design in this paper, the encryption accuracy of the system is studied. Based on the electronic health record data obtained by the experiment, the error information sent by the system and the correct display information are distinguished, and the information collection is set. Structure diagram (Fig. 7):

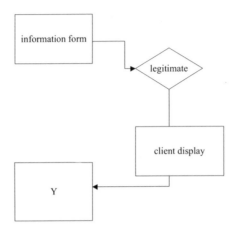

Fig. 7. Information recording structure diagram

According to the experimental information obtained above, the encryption accuracy comparison chart is constructed as follows (Fig. 8):

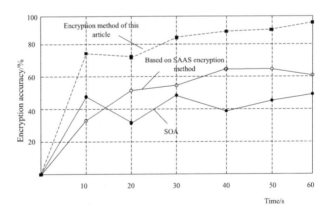

Fig. 8. Encryption accuracy comparison chart

According to the above figure, the encryption accuracy of the fast encryption method of electronic health records based on privacy protection technology in this paper is higher than that of other traditional encryption methods. The reason for this difference is that the software program designed in this paper selects the system encryption mode to manage the electronic health records in transmission, optimizes the encryption structure of the files, simulates the encryption process of the electronic health records, and constructs the encryption model to intuitively reflect the state and operation form of the model, further speed up the overall file encryption operation process, and count the number of electronic health records at any time, Specify the encryption standard of electronic health records according to the passed quantity information. Set up software emergency procedures. When the electronic health records approved by the software cannot be finally encrypted, the emergency procedures can send protection signals, the main system receives signal information, and issues the encryption instructions of electronic health records. Therefore, these electronic health records can complete the final encryption operation. Further realize the mechanism protection operation of electronic health records and improve the accuracy of overall encryption.

To sum up, the design of the fast encryption method for electronic health records based on privacy protection technology in this paper can greatly improve the speed and accuracy of electronic health records encryption, and provide a large amount of data support for the subsequent processing of electronic health records. Has a good operating effect.

After completing the above experimental operations, in order to further test the encryption performance of the encryption system in this paper, set up a secondary system test experiment, first analyze and process the designed system requirements, and provide certain data support for the processed analysis results. When testing the command, place the command information receiver in time to avoid receiving errors caused by poor receiving status. And build the system instruction transmission structure diagram (Fig. 9):

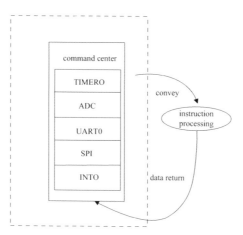

Fig. 9. Encrypted instruction instruction transmission structure diagram

At the same time, allocate the file transmission task at this time, transmit the files in a centralized manner according to different transmission directions, compare the security degree of the files after transmission, and build the encryption security rate comparison table as follows (Tables 4, 5 and 6):

Table 4. Encryption security rate result table of the method designed in this paper

Encryption time/s	Encryption security rate
20	88%
40	94%
60	97%
80	99%

Table 5. Results of system design encryption security rate based on data analysis

Encryption time/s	Encryption security rate
20	67%
40	78%
60	82%
80	86%

Table 6. The result of system design encryption security rate based on file encryption

Encryption time/s	Encryption security rate
20	54%
40	60%
60	66%
80	75%

According to the table of the above experimental comparison results, the file encryption security rate of the hospital file encryption system designed based on privacy protection in this paper is higher than that of the traditional system design, which shows that the system has strong execution and can safely encrypt files. The reason for this difference is that the encryption system in thispaper strengthens the processing of the system hardware structure and assigns different processing information when designing the encryption space. When the external data interference signal is generated, the encryption system will automatically transmit the blocking signal, block and eliminate the interference signal, and ensure the security of the encrypted file. When the hospital archives are in the transmission state, the transmission channel will encrypt and protect the information of this channel, timely collect the security system information related to the encrypted information, and re encrypt the transmitted documents, so as to finally realize the safe transmission of the hospital archives and complete the overall system design and architecture operation. Improve the encryption security rate of the encryption system and enhance the independent protection performance of the system archives.

To sum up, the design of the hospital file encryption system based on privacy protection in this paper has strong file encryption performance, can process complex hospital file information to a certain extent, and query accurate individual files in the complex information flow, which is sustainable. Providing file inspection services can better provide a solid data operation foundation for subsequent research operations.

5 Conclusion

Through the above analysis and the implementation of resource encryption methods, we get the real-time encryption method of electronic health records based on privacy protection. The analysis of information resource logic improves the encryption efficiency of resources, and the research on resource distribution optimization increases the density of real-time encryption of resources to a certain extent. As a new real-time encryption method of resources, it has a very superior application prospect. It is believed that privacy protection technology is an important direction for the development of real-time encryption methods of electronic information resources. In the future, it is necessary to apply the fast encryption of electronic health records data based on privacy protection proposed in this paper to other fields, so as to further expand the application scope of this method, maximize the data security in multiple fields, and promote the further improvement of network security technology.

References

1. Raman, S.R., O'Brien, E.C., Hammill, B.G., et al.: Evaluating fitness-for-use of electronic health records in pragmatic clinical trials: reported practices and recommendations. J. Am. Med. Inf. Assoc. **29**(5), 798–804 (2022)
2. Himmelreich, J., Lucassen, W., Harskamp, R., et al.: Correction:CHARGE-AF in a national routineprimary care electronic health recordsdatabase in the Netherlands: validationfor 5-year risk of atrial fibrillation andimplications for patient selection inatrial fibrillation screening. Open heart **8**(2), 1–10 (2021)
3. Tsai, M.-Y., Cho, H.-H.: A high security symmetric key generation by using genetic algorithm based on a novel similarity model. Mobile Netw. Appl. **26**(3), 1386–1396 (2021). https://doi.org/10.1007/s11036-021-01753-1
4. Xu, W., Zhao, Q., Zhan, Y., Wang, B., Hu, Y.: Privacy-preserving association rule mining based on electronic medical system. Wirel. Netw. **28**(1), 303–317 (2021). https://doi.org/10.1007/s11276-021-02846-1
5. Xu, Z., Luo, M., Kumar, N., et al.: Privacy-protection scheme based on sanitizable signature for smart mobile medical scenarios. Wirel. Commun. Mob. Comput. **20**(1), 1–10 (2020)
6. Chenthara, S.: Healthchain: a novel framework on privacy preservation of electronic health records using blockchain technology. PLoS ONE **15**(12), 105–122 (2020)
7. Yang, Y., Xiao, X., Cai, X., et al.: A secure and privacy-preserving technique based on contrast-enhancement reversible data hiding and plaintext encryption for medical images. IEEE Signal Process. Lett. **27**, 256–260 (2020)
8. Wang, Y., Zhang, L., Zhang, D., et al.: Research on multiple-image encryption scheme based on joint power spectral division multiplexing and ghost imaging. Laser Phys. **31**(5), 055204–055216 (2021)

9. Chen, K., Feng, X., Fu, Y., et al.: Design and implementation of system-on-chip for peripheral component interconnect express encryption card based on multiple algorithms. Circuit World **24**(7), 366–378 (2020)

10. Ay, N., Akpinar Borazan, A., Kuru, D.: Synthesis of boron nitride nanosheets/polyvinyl butyral thin film: an efficient coating for UV protection of extra virgin olive oil in glass bottles. J. Nano Res. **72**(1), 37–51 (2022)

11. Brunekreef, T.E., Otten, H.G., Bosch, S., et al.: Text mining of electronic health records can accurately identify and characterize patients with systemic lupus erythematosus. ACR Open Rheumatol. **15**(3), 1147-158 (2021)

12. Zhang, Y.M.: Mathematical model of network data conformal encryption based on block cipher. Comput. Simul. **39**(3), 466–469 (2022)

Research on Secure Storage of Healthcare Data in the Environment of Internet of Things

Haipeng Ke[1], Juanfen Shi[2(✉)], and Tianlin Fu[3]

[1] Fujian Zhangzhou No. 1 Vocational Secondary School, 363000 Zhangzhou Fujian, China
[2] School of Electronic Engineering, Henan Information Engineering School, Henan 450008, China
hijuanfen@163.com
[3] College of Mathematics and Data Science, Minjiang University, Fuzhou Fujian 350000, China

Abstract. In order to improve the security and storage efficiency of medical care data, a safe storage method of medical care data in the Internet of Things environment is designed. The security analysis of medical care data resources in the Internet of Things environment, and the establishment of trusted identifiers for storage resource provision and use requests, to ensure data security to the greatest extent. Compliance verification of storage resource provision and use requests can solve the problem of data security degradation caused by simple data access methods. For data distance calculation and data division, establish a spatial database, and use distributed storage to realize the safe storage of medical and health care data, in order to solve the problem of low reliability of data storage. The experimental results show that the secure storage method of health care data in the Internet of Things environment studied in this paper not only improves the efficiency of data encryption and retrieval, but also reduces the number of times that data is attacked and stolen, and has a better effect of data secure storage.

Keywords: Internet of Things Environment · Health Care Data · Safe Storage · Constraint Parameters · Trusted Identity · Verification

1 Introduction

With the development of the Internet of Things and the continuous integration of the Internet of Things, the Internet and 3G mobile phones, the degree of intelligence of the Internet of Things will become higher and higher in the future. At the same time, the impact of Internet of Things on security cannot be ignored. The theft of Internet of Things signals will directly affect the information security of the entire Internet of Things. From the perspective of information security and privacy protection, the widespread introduction of Internet of Things terminals not only provides richer information, but also increases the risk of exposing such information [1]. The patient's electronic medical record contains a large amount of privacy information, such as the patient's condition information, consumption records, etc. these information will be centrally stored on the hospital's server, and most hospitals do not attach great importance to information

S. Wang (Ed.): IoTCare 2022, LNICST 501, pp. 271–288, 2023.
https://doi.org/10.1007/978-3-031-33545-7_19

security. There are countless vulnerabilities in the hospital website, so that attackers can easily get the hospital's database and patient information, resulting in the privacy disclosure of users, that is, there is a risk of data disclosure. At the same time, if the attacker deliberately destroys and tampers with the data, it will seriously hinder the availability of the medical system, that is, there is a risk of data tampering.

Some progress has been made in the research on data security storage methods. Reference [2] proposed a data security storage method based on blockchain. In this method, wireless sensor networks and blockchain technologies are used to construct the distribution framework of federated chain sensing nodes and the data storage federated chain model, and data blockchain is formed through the consensus of data acquisition base stations Specific types of hash chains are formed according to data attributes, hash values and other information to facilitate the safe storage of the same type of historical data. Reference [3] proposed a method for medical data security storage based on hybrid encryption. The classical data encryption standard (DES) and asymmetric encryption algorithm (Rivest Shamir Adleman, RSA) are analyzed, and a hybrid encryption method for medical data security storage enhancement is proposed An improved algorithm IBDES is proposed to enhance the security strength through double encryption, and an improved algorithm EPNRSA is proposed to reduce the time complexity of RSA encryption while ensuring the security quality of encryption. An enhanced hybrid encryption method for medical data based on IBDES and EPNRSA is formed to realize the safe storage of data. Reference [4] proposed a design method of hospital financial data security storage system based on homomorphic encryption algorithm. Under the 3-tier hardware structure, two IBMP5570 minicomputers are used to handle the same transaction in a dual cluster mode. Four IBM 3850 servers are used and RADWARE load balancers are configured to automatically distribute workload. Use dual storage disk array cabinets to back up data with each other. Configure SAN switch for data exchange between server and storage. All homomorphic encryption is used to encrypt, decrypt and retrieve the ciphertext files to complete the safe storage of data.

However, the application of the above methods to the safe storage of medical care data has the problems of the security of medical care data and low storage efficiency. In order to solve the problems of traditional methods, a safe storage method of medical care data in the Internet of Things environment is designed to improve the security of hospital data. The main structure of this paper is as follows:

(1) To analyze the security of medical care data resources, on the one hand, the existing asymmetric encryption algorithm is used to verify the identity authenticity of the system participants' nodes, so as to ensure the credibility of transactions on the chain. On the other hand, we design the data structure of the storage resources on the blockchain to provide information and use the request information and carry out trusted identification for them, and design compliance verification methods for the two kinds of information to enhance the credibility of the storage designed in this paper.

(2) Through the analysis of the trusted release of storage resources in the above process, the uniquely identified storage resources are disseminated to other nodes in the P2P network in the form of messages for a certain period of time.

(3) The distance function is established to reasonably divide the spatial data in consideration of the proximity and topological relationship between the spatial element objects, so as to establish a distributed spatial database. The distributed storage method is used to realize the safe storage of medical and health data.
(4) The effectiveness of this method is verified by experiments.
(5) Summarize the full text and draw conclusions.

2 Trusted Identification and Verification of Storage Resource Provision and Use Requests

The research work on the trusted identification and compliance verification of the information provided by the storage resources and the use of the requested information in the network is mainly carried out from two aspects: first, this paper will use the existing asymmetric encryption algorithm to verify the identity authenticity of the system participant nodes, so as to ensure the credibility of the transactions on the chain; The second is to design the data structure of the storage resources on the blockchain to provide information and use the requested information, and carry out trusted identification on it, and design compliance verification methods for the two kinds of information respectively to enhance the credibility of the storage designed in this paper.

2.1 Data resource security analysis.

Before extracting healthcare data, the security of data resources needs to be analyzed, and the main process is as follows:

Represent a hypersphere containing normal sample points as:

$$\min R^2$$
$$s.t.x_i - c^2 \leq R^2, i = 1, \ldots, N \tag{1}$$

In the above formula, R represents the radius of the hypersphere, c represents the spherical center vector, and x_i represents the distance to the spherical center vector.

Since the distance from the data to the spherical center vector is not necessarily less than or equal to the radius, it needs to be corrected. The formula is as follows:

$$\min R^2 + C\sum_{i=1}^{m}\xi_i \tag{2}$$
$$s.t.x_i - c^2 \leq R^2 + \xi_i, \xi_i \geq 0, i = 1, \ldots, N$$

In the above formula, C represents the regularization coefficient, and ξ_i represents the slack variable.

After the correction, set the constraints as follows:

$$f_1(k) = \begin{cases} 1, k = 1, \ldots, N_A \\ 0, k = N_A + 1, \ldots, N_A + M^A \end{cases}$$
$$f_2(k) = \begin{cases} 0, k = 1, \ldots, N_A \\ 1, k = N_A + 1, \ldots, N_A + M^A \end{cases} \tag{3}$$

where, N_A represents the constraint parameter of the A data, and M^A represents the constraint parameter of the A data.

After the above process, the principal components of the information are obtained. During retrieval, it is necessary to establish an inverted index of key features, according to which the location of the information can be quickly detected [5]. In the establishment, all parameter values are searched through the storage address in advance, and then the keyword search is carried out. When a search is completed, the final search results are transmitted to the interactive channel. Retrieval edge weight is an important physical index to measure the retrieval ability of key features of information. The size of edge weight is directly related to the strength of node interaction. The retrieval edge weight value is expressed as:

$$g = 1 - \frac{\left| \dot{k} - \sqrt{(I - U')^x} \right|}{\left| f' \cdot h^2 / l \cdot \bar{\lambda} \right|} \tag{4}$$

In the above formula, l represents the upper limit matching condition parameter of the information in the wireless network, U' is the lower limit matching condition of the information, x represents the statistical coefficient of the power term, h represents the programmed retrieval vector, and l and λ represent the average interaction constant of information nodes respectively. And information priority.

The above process retrieves the key features of the data, and on this basis, processes the data to analyze the security of the data resources. The specific process is as follows:

Step1: Using unsupervised clustering algorithm, allocate nodes, assume that the collected sample set is $M = (m_1, m_2, m_3, \ldots, m_n)$, define set as $A(I)$ to accumulate the sum of sample vectors belonging to various types, and define one of the counters $B(I)$ to register the number of corresponding normal sample categories;

Step2: Divide the cost function in the unsupervised clustering algorithm and calculate the density index of the collected data sample points. The calculation formula is as follows:

$$D_u = \sum_{i=q} d \exp\left(\frac{\|x_i - x_j\|}{d/2}\right) \tag{5}$$

In formula (5), $\sum_{i=q} d$ is the density index of node i, $\|x_i - x_j\|$ is the calculation factor of the density index size of the sample point, and exp is the neighborhood radius of the collected data.

Step3: Calculate each remaining sample point above and determine the Euclidean distance of the unsupervised clustering center. If $r \leq d_2$, this sample point will be classified into the corresponding class of the unsupervised clustering center. If $r \geq d_2$, it will not be classified temporarily, where d_2 is the preset threshold. The larger the value, the more the number of clusters, and vice versa;

Step4: Take the unclassified samples in Step3 as a new sample set, re execute the above processes of step1, Step2 and Step3, and repeat this cycle to make a safety judgment on all data [6];

Step5: Calculate the security situation category of each data, and the calculation formula is as follows:

$$c_i = \frac{E(i)}{B(i)}, i = 1, 2, \ldots, n \tag{6}$$

In formula (6), $E(i)$ represents the initial data center in unsupervised clustering, and $B(i)$ is the maximum distance between data nodes in the network.

According to the above process, complete the data clustering [7], according to the clustering results, the data security analysis, the calculation formula is as follows:

$$[D' = RT \frac{a_i}{f * |d|} \tag{7}$$

In formula (7), RT represents data topology, f represents abnormal parameters, $|d|$ represents protection strategy set, and a_i represents collected operation data.

Predict and collect operation data, and then normalize the data to provide the basis for subsequent data storage.

2.2 Trusted Identities for Storage Resource Provision and Use Requests

How to complete the trusted identification of storage resource information and storage resource usage requests in a decentralized cloud storage system needs to be studied and designed from two aspects. On the one hand, it is determined that the node identity verification method of the Ethereum system is adopted in this solution to realize the authenticity verification of the node identity in the decentralized system. Participating nodes in the system can join the blockchain network through an automatically generated key, and obtain an account address that can uniquely identify the node. Based on the above, the trusted identification of storage resource provision and storage resource usage request in the decentralized cloud storage system, as well as the subsequent double verification of authenticity and compliance are realized.

On the other hand, it is also the research focus of this section. Based on the node identity authenticity verification method, the data structure design of the storage resource provision information and storage resource usage request on the blockchain is completed. In this paper, the design of the demand side requesting the use of storage resources is directly completed by the system participants in the form of issuing storage resource use requests for specific storage resources. Therefore, for the trusted identification method of storage resource provision information and storage resource usage request, the focus is on the allocation process of storage resource and the definition of the behavior of issuing storage resource usage request. For the definition of "electronic money" transaction behavior in Bitcoin, the purpose is to bind node behavior and node identity, and nodes cannot deny that they have done their own behavior, and other nodes cannot pretend to be "behavior initiators". Refer to the design of the Uspent Transaction Output (UTXO) model in the Bitcoin system.

The basic definition of an "electronic currency" is a chain of linked digital signatures. When the owner of the "electronic currency" wants to transfer the "electronic currency" to others, its operation process is to connect a new digital signature at the end of the digital signature chain. The specific content of the signature includes obtaining the hash of the last transaction of the "electronic currency" and the public key of the transfer target account. In the process of value transfer, all current accounts can prove their ownership of "e-money" by digitally signing the wallet address of the account in the previous transaction, which can be verified by others to match their public key, as shown in the following figure (Fig. 1):

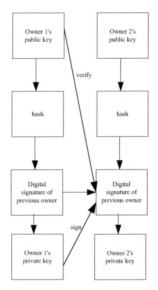

Fig. 1. Data storage structure used in this article

Through the above model analysis, the following will design the data structure of storage resource information and storage resource usage requests. In the solution of decentralized cloud storage resource trust management, storage resource providers hold storage resources and have the qualification of the final storage resource usage authority determination is analogous to the UTXO model. In the data structure design of the storage resource provision information [8], the available attribute information Q of the storage resource and the public key W of the storage resource provider can be used as input, and the output can be provided. The party's open policy for the storage resources held by itself, for example, it can be a set of fixed node public keys, or it can be empty, indicating that the storage resources are only open to a few nodes or completely open. Finally, perform $HASH$ on the above data structure, and then use the provider's private key to digitally sign. Express the formula as:

$$R = T(HASH) * Q * W \tag{8}$$

Through the analysis of the trusted release of storage resources through the above process, the uniquely identified storage resources are spread to other nodes in the P2P network in the form of messages over a certain period of time.

2.3 Compliance Verification of Storage Resource Provision and Usage Requests

Further research and design for its compliance verification method. First of all, the key to verify whether the information provided by the storage resource is legal is to ensure the authenticity of the information provided by the storage resource and the identity of the storage resource provider node. This is also the key link of decentralized trust management in this paper, which is specifically manifested in two points: first, if the provider wants to contribute storage resources in the decentralized system to obtain benefits, the premise is to provide legitimate and trusted storage resources. Before the data is linked, it needs to go through the authenticity verification of node identity and review whether the storage resources it provides are legitimate according to the information provided by the specific storage resources. This is the cornerstone of decentralized cloud storage resource trusted management. Secondly, the data structure that the demand direction sends the use request to meet the required storage resources contains the information provided by the specified storage resources, so it is also necessary to verify the authenticity of the information provided by the storage resources in the compliance verification process of the storage resource use request. The formula is as follows:

$$E = \frac{t}{y} * \sum_{i=1}^{n} h \qquad (9)$$

In the above formula, y represents the resource verification node, and h represents the digital signature information.

After the above processing, for the conversion of plaintext information, the *Hash* function, as the core function in cryptography, can also be called a dispersion function. Through this function, information of varying degrees of complexity can be converted into a fixed language sequence. If the function is represented by H, then the process function of information conversion is $h : h = H(M)$. When it is applied to the actual signature, the information will automatically form a summary of the language. This method can not only reduce the time for handwritten signatures, but also prevent others from counterfeiting signatures and using them to commit crimes [9]. The *Hash* function is used as a password. The basic encryption function of learning ensures the security and reliability of information. Generally, the commonly used *Hash* functions are divided into the following two types: single function and polynomial function. Assuming that the single function $f : X \rightarrow Y$, X and Y are two sets, and any element $x \in X$, you can easily get $Y = f(x) \in Y$, but if the condition is $y \in Y$, you want to require Obtaining $x \in X$ makes $f(x) = Y$ more difficult, then in this case it is a single function, otherwise it is a polynomial function.

Suppose there is a secret S. in order to prevent theft, it is divided into multiple pieces of information, each of which is called a sub secret and owned by a user. It contains the following properties:

(1) Multiple pieces of information can still be reorganized into secrets;
(2) If a fragment is missing, the security barrier of the whole secret has been destroyed and cannot be reconstructed;
(3) Some information fragments cannot predict the main content of the secret;

(4) A user *Alice* takes any point $Ep(a, b)$ on the curve and the other point P as the standard point;

(5) Sets a private password lock $k(0 < k \leq n)$, n is a positive integer greater than 0, and the password Q can be known from $Q=kp$;

(6) Use *Alice* to transport the password Q and the point $Ep(a, b)$ in the curve to another user *Bob* through the standard point;

(7) Acts as the information transmission hub [10], transmits the password and plaintext information to other points M in the curve, and combines with the previous parameters to generate an arbitrary integer set r and $r < n$;

(8) User *Bob* uses the binary algorithm to calculate the point $C1 = M + rQ$, $c2 = rP$;

(9) Uses its own function to return all $C1$ and $C2$ to user *Alice*;

(10) After *Alice* successfully obtains the data information, after obtaining the result of $C1 - kC_2$, all the information of the point M is obtained.

(11) Perform byte transposition operation according to the following formula, and the calculation expression is:

$$b = c' - a'''(C_N + 1) \tag{10}$$

In formula (10), a''' represents plaintext multiple parameters, c' represents fixed transformation parameters, and C_N represents the column element of the N data.

According to the above calculation results, establish the calculation matrix [11]:

$$B = \begin{bmatrix} b_1 \\ b_2 \\ \dots \\ b_n \end{bmatrix} = \begin{bmatrix} 02\ 03\ 01\ 01 \\ 01\ 02\ 03\ 01 \\ 01\ 01\ 03\ 02 \\ 03\ 01\ 01\ 02 \end{bmatrix} \tag{11}$$

After the above process, the plaintext content of the data is converted. After the conversion, the plaintext is obfuscated. The calculation process is as follows:

First, assume that a certain data is x;

Second, operate $x * 01$, and the result is x itself;

Third, the binary operation of $x * 02$ and x moves to the left, and the right side is filled with 0. If the highest binary bit of x is 1, the next step is calculated;

Fourth, the obfuscation calculation is completed in this way, and the result of $x * x$ is obtained.

After the above calculation, the accurate plaintext information is obtained.

3   Implementation of Secure Storage of Healthcare Data

3.1   Data Distance Calculation

Through the above process of data clustering and key distribution, on this basis, the next prediction is made through the probability left by each data, and the distance function is determined based on the gradual reduction of its probability to find the dynamic changes of the data. The premise of establishing the function is to ensure the heredity between the data. The distance function can be defined as:

$$f = \sum_{k}^{i=1} \sum_{n}^{j=1} wd_{ij}^2 \tag{12}$$

Among them, w represents the distance factor, d_{ij}^2 represents the squared distance between adjacent data, and $d_{ij} = x_j - y_i$, y_i represent the average distance between matrix parameters, C_i represents the parameter type, then there is a formula:

$$w_{ij} = \begin{cases} 1, \text{ The n object belongs to the } C_i \text{ class} \\ 0, \text{ The n object does not belong to the } C_i \text{ class} \end{cases} \tag{13}$$

Combined with the irreversibility of clustering data, the formula can be transformed into:

$$f = \sum_{j=1}^{k} \sum_{x \in ci} d_{ij}^2 \tag{14}$$

Because the above formula is carried out on the basis of constant distance, it can also be called distance difference criterion function. Due to the diversity of data mining, the most common type is the mixed type [12], including numbers and images, so the constraint formula restricting the mixed type is:

When $x_i = x_j$, there is $d_{ij} \geq 0$; when $i, j, k \geq 0$, there is $d_{ij} \leq d_{ik} + d_{kj}$, then the distance function formula for clustering is:

$$d_{ij} = \left(\sum_{k=1}^{m} |x_{ik} - x_{jk}|^m \right)^{\frac{1}{p}}, p > 0 \tag{15}$$

In the formula, p represents displacement. When the value of p continues to increase, causing the distance between cluster centers to be farther, the formula becomes:

$$d_{ij} = \left(\sum_{k=1}^{n} |x_{ik} - x_{jk}|^4 \right)^{\frac{1}{2}} \tag{16}$$

When specifying the criteria for the same clustering center, it is necessary to ensure that the same species are clustered with each other to further improve the quality of data mining. If there is an error, iterative calculation can be performed continuously. Then the functional equation that limits the occurrence of the error is:

$$Z_C = \sum_{j=1}^{c} \sum_{k=1}^{n_j} x_k^{(j)} - md_j^2 \tag{17}$$

where Z represents the error and d_j represents the displacement out of range. The dynamic data has the same characteristics as the samples. When the function is determined, the more complex the feature vector is, the greater the error will be, and the result will be greatly different from the prediction. The density of data is related to the number of samples collected. Only by ensuring that the dynamic data is within a certain range can the error be minimized. Therefore, the final clustering function is:

$$W = \sum_{i=1}^{k} \sum_{x_j < c} x_j - c_i^2 \tag{18}$$

Based on the above process, a dynamic distance function is established to analyze the dynamic changes of data and provide a basis for subsequent data storage.

3.2 Spatial Data Division

The data distributed storage mode in the Internet of Things environment should be analyzed according to the specific form of data, and then the spatial data should be divided. The quality of spatial data division directly affects the load of each storage node and the overall performance of spatial data management system. If the stored data to be divided is simple data, divide the data into several parts, and each node in the computer can store certain data. If the object to be divided is complex, the data to be allocated is divided according to the critical matrix. Considering the diversity of spatial data, a jdio curve division method is proposed to ensure the storage balance between each storage node, estimate the number of nodes required according to the amount of data and the calculated workload, and migrate dynamic data between nodes to ensure load balance. Using the distributed storage method of data layer segmentation, the whole spatial area is divided into initial grids. Each grid must contain multiple spatial element objects. Each coordinate in the spatial object is searched through the layer segmentation algorithm. If the amount of spatial object data is large, the data is encoded, and the code of the grid through which the jdio curve passes is taken as the corresponding element object code in the grid, form one or one to many relationships with spatial objects [13]. On this basis, the spatial element objects are sorted according to the initial curve, the data volume of the spatial element objects in the corresponding grid is accumulated from the sub-grid of the initial coding, and each element is divided according to the storage node information of the computer., if the accumulated amount at this time exceeds the corresponding storage node, the grid will be decomposed multiple times until the corresponding data is divided into the specified nodes, and each data in the space is allocated to the space element according to the above process. Subset of objects. The data of spatial division is allocated to storage nodes. At this time, the initial grid is decomposed hierarchically, and the number of objects of spatial elements is greater than the number of storage nodes, so as to improve the division efficiency of spatial element objects. For hierarchical decomposition, the termination order is set. When the division reaches this order, the division is stopped, which can improve the efficiency without affecting the balance of the divided spatial data. The division algorithm is as follows:

$$Q_x = \frac{\omega(W_i)}{F \cdot v(j_0 + 1)} \tag{19}$$

In formula (1), Q_x represents the size of spatial elements, j_0 represents the total number of spatial element objects to be divided, W_i represents the set termination order, and ω represents the curve division order corresponding to the current sub grid. No directional analysis will be done in this calculation.

Through the above formula, the division of spatial data is completed, and the efficiency of distributed storage can be improved through the division of spatial data, which provides a basis for establishing a spatial database in the next step.

3.3 Establish a Spatial Database

Based on the above spatial data division, a distributed spatial database is established. Considering the proximity and topological relationship between spatial element objects, the spatial data is divided reasonably [14]. The database structure is shown in the following figure (Fig. 2):

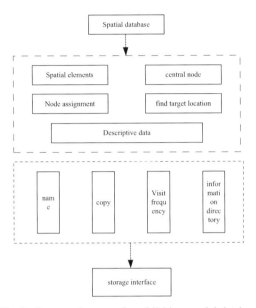

Fig. 2. Process diagram of establishing spatial database

The above figure is the process diagram of spatial database, which is designed according to the above key points when designing the database, so as to meet the characteristics of independence between storage nodes, reduce data transmission between nodes, and improve efficiency. In the distributed database, a node is designed as the central node to maintain the metadata information of the whole network. When a node in the database makes a request, the data node should be processed by the central node. After the task is assigned to other nodes, after the processing is completed, it returns to the target location, takes the database as local data, constructs a global schema, and describes the data from local data, query and process the distributed data, and provide users with a unified data storage interface for the distributed database, so as to realize the transparency of distributed data storage. In addition, the name node server is designed to store and manage the namespace of the file system and the access requests between users, and regularly store the sent data. In order to ensure the reliability of the data, the data should be copied before storage. In order to ensure that the database is damaged or lost when it is stored. On this basis, each node and user storage information directory are managed, and the user access frequency is optimized to optimize the optimal storage of data, so as to complete the design of distributed storage management database. In order to improve the capacity of distributed storage, the database is optimized in the next step.

3.4 Realize Distributed Storage of Cyberspace Data

On the basis of the completion of the database design, in order to increase the database capacity, the database capacity is designed, and the random mechanism is used to distribute the distributed massive data source data packets in cloud computing to all nodes in the distributed system according to a certain reception probability. The storage data packets are formed in the nodes, and the data packets are classified according to the repeatability and access rules of the distributed data, which are divided into hot, cold and repeated storage data packet areas, and partition storage according to the characteristics of different types of data activity factors. The distributed network in cloud computing consists of n nodes, and v nodes are data nodes. Different nodes generate data packets with their own characteristics, and the remaining data nodes are used to store and distribute data. The distributed network is regarded as a random image, the data nodes are described by the fixed points of the graph, and the process of transmitting each data packet to another node according to the transmission mechanism is described by the random walk on the random graph. In order to ensure the random graph They are connected with the maximum probability, and the communication radius of the data node satisfies the following conditions:

$$r \geq \left(sdgt / \lambda o \right)^{1/2} \tag{20}$$

In formula (20), g represents the interference factor during data node communication, and o represents the random image, so the coverage of the random walk to the random image is:

$$DO_y = \sum_r t\sqrt{1 - e^i} \tag{21}$$

In formula (21), e^i represents the efficiency of different vertex numbers of random walks, and O_y represents the coverage time of random walks. No orientation analysis is performed in this calculation.

The coverage rate of the random graph is calculated through the above formula. From the coverage rate, we can know the coverage rate of the data nodes in the distributed network. When the distributed processing platform processes the data, according to the above calculation method, different data can be stored, and the data of different nodes can be called through the corresponding functions, so as to increase the storage capacity of spatial data.

Finally, according to the relationship between the information, the files in the system are clustered. The specific process is as follows.

Suppose, $F = \{f_1, f_2, \ldots, f_n\}$ represents a total of n merged high-density information sets, and the set F is divided by the agent hierarchy to obtain l information clusters $N = \{n_1, n_2, \ldots, n_3\}$. Measure the semantic approximation between high-density information data in ships, measure information by the approximation between entities, and finally take the reciprocal of high-density information to obtain the approximation between information and information, namely:

$$Sim(q_i, q_j) = 1 + \left\{ 1 + dist(q_i, q_j) \right\} \tag{22}$$

In formula (22), q_i and q_j respectively represent the high-density information in the hospital, $dist$ represents the probability measure of being visited in the system, and Sim represents the approximation of the visit form.

Cluster high-density information according to the above process. On this basis, for high-density information storage, store clustered file nodes according to storage space and energy allocation, and set node threshold to prevent a node in the system from bearing too much file storage data. Use the following formula to calculate the grid number, namely:

$$\begin{cases} X = (x_1 - x_2)/L \\ Y = (y_1 - y_2)/L \end{cases} \tag{23}$$

In formula (23), x_1, x_2, y_1, and y_2 respectively represent the geographic coordinates describing the cluster file, X and Y respectively represent the origin of the coordinate system, and L represent the side length of the grid.

On this basis, a multi-threshold prediction mechanism is adopted to ensure the load balance of the high-density information security storage system. The calculation formula is as follows:

$$fit = \frac{sn}{SU(P_i) * bck} \tag{24}$$

In formula (24), fit represents the number of storage information nodes in the system, $SU(P_i)$ represents grid expansion information, bck represents the measurement index of system information, and sn represents storage information.

When the new high-density information is stored, the file is sent to the original saturated grid for storage, so as to realize the safe storage of data.

4   Experimental Analysis

In order to verify the effectiveness of the proposed data storage method, experiments are carried out to verify the proposed method through various aspects. This experiment mainly includes two aspects, one is to analyze the efficiency of the proposed method, that is, the efficiency of data encryption, etc., and the second is to analyze the effect of data security storage, that is, the number of attacks.

The experiment is carried out in the ubuntu10.10 environment of the Vmware Workstation virtual machine, and the cloudsim platform is used to conduct the simulation experiment, and use it to create a data center to provide the basis for the experiment. The traditional data security storage method based on blockchain is used as an experimental comparison method.

4.1   Initialization Time Overhead

When encrypting information, multiple attributes need to be authorized, which will increase the time of data initialization, thus affecting the performance of the entire encryption technology. Therefore, the time cost of information initialization processing

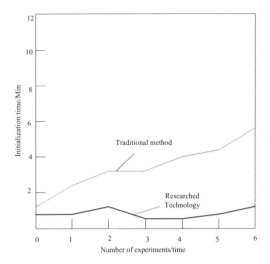

Fig. 3. Initialization time overhead

is taken as the comparison object. The initialization time cost of the proposed method and the traditional method in information encryption is shown in the following figure (Fig. 3):

It can be seen from the above figure that the studied secure storage method takes less time because the studied technology processes the data in advance, reducing the number of attribute authorization institutions, thereby reducing the time cost of initialization processing.

4.2 Key Distribution Time Overhead

The key distribution times for the three methods are as follows (Fig. 4):

Compared with the above figure, it can be found that the proposed data secure storage method spends less time on key distribution. The reason for the less time spent on key distribution of the studied method is that the encryption operation is performed before the file is uploaded and does not involve the generation of attribute keys, so the time for key distribution is less.

4.3 Encryption Time Overhead

The comparison results of the encryption time overhead between the proposed method and the traditional method are shown in the following figure (Fig. 5):

It can be seen from the above figure that the encryption time of the proposed method is less because the proposed method measures the distance between the data, reduces the occurrence of data encryption duplication, and thus reduces the encryption time of the data.

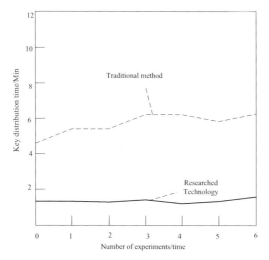

Fig. 4. Key distribution time overhead

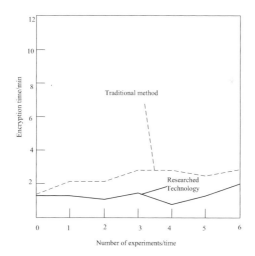

Fig. 5. Encryption time overhead

4.4 Retrieval Time Overhead

The comparison results of the time cost of the proposed method and the traditional method in data retrieval are shown in the figure below (Fig. 6):

Analyzing the above figure, it can be found that the information retrieval time of the two methods is quite different, because the encryption technology studied is not complicated, which reduces the information retrieval time.

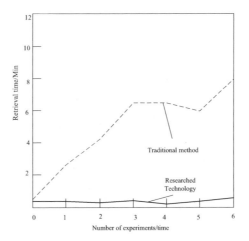

Fig. 6. Retrieval time overhead

4.5 Comparison of Encrypted Information Theft

Comparing the security of the information after the two methods of encryption, the information is stolen as shown in the following figure (Table 1):

Table 1. Stolen situation of encrypted information

Number of experiments/time	The number of times that the researched technical information has been stolen	The number of times the traditional method has been stolen/time
1	0	2
2	1	3
3	0	3
4	0	3
5	0	2
6	0	2
7	0	3
8	1	1
9	0	2
10	0	3

By analyzing the above table, we can find that traditional storage methods have information stolen, and the amount of stolen information is large. After the storage method studied, the information is stolen less, only twice, which can prove that the storage technology studied can improve the security of information storage.

4.6 Comparison of Information Changed

By analyzing the table below, we can find that the information is changed in both methods. The security storage method studied is changed once, and the traditional method is changed many times. The encryption effect is poor, and no research has been done. The storage method is safe (Table 2).

Table 2. Comparison of changes in information

Number of experiments/time	Number of times the technical information studied has been changed / time	The traditional method has been changed times / time
1	0	2
2	1	5
3	0	6
4	0	6
5	0	6
6	0	6
7	0	5
8	0	8
9	0	6
10	0	5

In conclusion, the researched data security storage method can not only reduce the information encryption time, but also improve the information security.

5 Conclusion

The medical data platform designed in this paper can not only realize the distributed storage of medical data, but also ensure the rights control of medical data by patients, and also realize the sharing application of medical data by third-party users. The data allocation strategy is a centralized strategy, which puts forward higher requirements on the computing power, storage capacity and security of the network center node, and further analysis is needed in the follow-up research.

References

1. Huang, J.C., Shu, M.H., Hsu, B.M., et al.: Service architecture of IoT terminal connection based on blockchain identity authentication system. Comput. Commun. **160**(8), 411–422 (2020)
2. Zhang, L.H., Jiang, T.F., Jiang, P.P., et al.: Secure storage scheme for high speed railway monitoring data based on blockchain. Computer Eng. Design **41**(4), 933–938 (2020)

3. Kang, H.Y., Deng, J.: Hybrid encryption method for secure storage of medical data. Trans. Beijing Instit. Technol. **41**(10), 1058–1068 (2021)
4. Deng, Y.X.: Hospital financial data secure storage system based on full homomorphic encryption algorithm. Tech. Autom. Appli. **41**(7), 44–47 (2022)
5. Reppucci, M.L., Acker, S.N., Emily, C., et al.: Improved identification of severely injured pediatric trauma patients using reverse shock index multiplied by Glasgow Coma Scale. J. Trauma Acute Care Surgery **92**(1), 69–73 (2022)
6. Dupuy, B., Romdhane, A., Eliasson, P., Yan, H.: Combined geophysical and rock physics workflow for quantitative co2 monitoring. Int. J. Greenhouse Gas Control **106**(3), 103217–103229 (2021)
7. Li, J., Yan, H., Zhang, Y.: Certificateless public integrity checking of group shared data on cloud storage. IEEE Trans. Serv. Comput. **14**(1), 71–81 (2021)
8. Gokulraj, J., Senthilkumar, J., Suresh, Y., et al.: Data consistency matrix based data processing model for efficient data storage in wireless sensor networks. Comput. Commun. **151**(1), 172–182 (2020)
9. Vuppala, A., Roshan, R.S., Nawaz, S., Ravindra, J.: An efficient optimization and secured triple data encryption standard using enhanced key scheduling algorithm. Procedia Comput. Sci. **1712**, 1054–1063 (2020)
10. Jeong, B.G., Youn, T.Y., Jho, N.S., Sang, U.S.: Blockchain-based data sharing and trading model for the connected car. Sensors **20**(11), 3141–3153 (2020)
11. Hua, D.A., Zheng, Q.A., Qw, B., Zg, B., Yz, C.: Flexible attribute-based proxy re-encryption for efficient data sharing. Inf. Sci. **511**(3), 94–113 (2020)
12. Manikandan, V.M., Bini, A.A.: An improved reversible data hiding through encryption scheme with block prechecking. Proc. Comput. Sci. **171**(1), 951–958 (2020)
13. Geetha, R., Padmavathy, T., Thilagam, T., Lallithasree, A.: Tamilian cryptography: an efficient hybrid symmetric key encryption algorithm. Wireless Pers. Commun. **112**(1), 21–36 (2020)
14. Bao, K.J., Zhang, X.J.: Simulation of remote sharing of database information based on particle swarm optimization. Comput. Simul. **39**(2), 487–49,495 (2022)

Architecture of Wide Area Health Monitoring System

Xiaohan Liu[1,2]([⊠]), Talatu Suri[3], Xiaoyun Zhao[4], Shilong Zhang[1,2], Ou Li[1,2], Yi Yang[1,2], Xiaochao Shi[5], Ping Liang[2], and Kuangyang Shu[1]

[1] CASET Quzhou Research Institute Co. Ltd., Quzhou, China
xhliu@giet.ac.cn

[2] Guangzhou Electronic Technology Co. Ltd., Chinese Academy of Sciences, Guangzhou, China

[3] Minzu University of China, Beijing, China

[4] Tianjin Chest Hospital, Tianjin, China

[5] PLA Strategic Support Force Characteristic Medical Center, Beijing, China

Abstract. Wearable health monitoring system has significant progress with the development of Internet of Things (IOT) technologies. In this manuscript, we discuss the collaborative architecture for distributed wide area health monitoring system. Heterogeneous communication, system modularization, and edge computing are three important aspects for the architecture. A real-world system has been developed, which includes three components: wearable sensor, wireless sensor network, and edge computing terminal, and we performed a series of experiments. We also discuss the collaborative mechanism for heterogeneous and homogeneous health monitoring systems in complex emergency environment.

Keywords: Health Monitoring · Distributed System · Internet of Things · Edge Computing · Collaborative System

1 Introduction

Wearable health monitoring technology has significant progress with the development of information, computing, and communication technologies in the past 20 years. Internet of Things (IOT), 5G/B5G communication, edge computing, satellite constellation internet, Artificial Intelligence (AI) provide more intelligent and rapid support for wearable health monitoring in wide area field environment [1–5].

Especially, health monitoring in extreme or natural disaster environment is important for both victims and rescue workers [6–11]. In wide area environment, we often apply heterogenous and independent information and communication systems at the meantime, the interoperability and scalability problems often make the health monitoring process inefficient and costly.

S. Wang (Ed.): IoTCare 2022, LNICST 501, pp. 289–298, 2023.
https://doi.org/10.1007/978-3-031-33545-7_20

In this manuscript, we discuss the architecture for wide area health monitoring system, as is shown in Fig. 1. We concern three aspects:

(1) Heterogeneous communication: cellular communication, such as LTE, NB-IOT, and 5G are widely applied in urban environment; while Wireless Sensor Networks (WSN), Low Power Wide Area Network (LPWAN), and satellite communication could be applied in rural areas;
(2) System modularization: in complex environment, modular system using open standards could provide better compatibility. Relative open standards such as OGC Sensor Web, Linux EdgeX Foundry, IEEE 1888, oneM2M are well discussed these years;
(3) Edge computing: we perform health data analysis and statistics, and system configuration in the system edge.

This paper is organized as follows: in Sect. 2, we discuss wide area health monitoring system architecture; Sect. 3 introduces a real-world system setup and experiments, and we discuss the collaborative mechanism for heterogeneous and homogeneous systems; in Sect. 4, we introduce the outcomes and discuss important topics on on-going research.

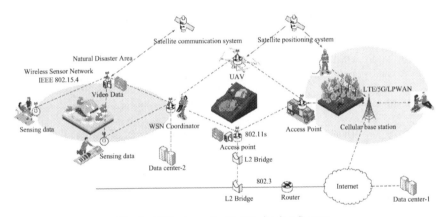

Fig. 1. Wide Area Health Monitoring System

2   System Architecture

For centralized health monitoring system, monitoring terminal such as smart watch, smart wrist band, or a WSN coordinator, transmits data to mobile phone or cloud server. For distributed system, gateway node collects and transmits data to certified cloud server using open protocols. Figure 1 shows a hybrid health monitoring system, which has a centralized system data center (Data center-1), and a distributed system data center (Data center-2).

Figure 2 shows the collaborate architecture for wide area health monitoring system. The gateway collects data from multi nodes through various of capillary communications, such as LPWAN, IEEE 802.15.4 WSN, IEEE 802.11s mesh network, or satellite network, and then communicates with the edge/cloud server through cellular or capillary communication. The system collaboration platform includes registration component, centralized configuration component, cooperation component, computing component, visualization component, etc. Various of applications, such as health, rescue, training, and management, connect with the platform and acquire data from proper cloud server and data center.

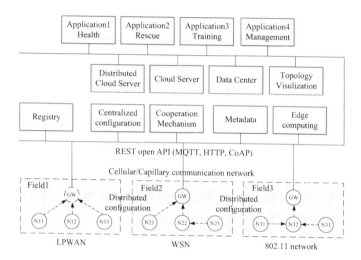

Fig. 2. System architecture

Figure 3 shows the system's working process:

Registration: the sensing node, gateway, edge/cloud server, and application unit first register ID, content information, and metadata to the collaboration platform;

Centralized configuration: the cooperation component implements resource allocation and collaborative computing on the base of registered application, then the centralized configuration component transmits configuration information to the registered unit, and each unit configures its parameters such as data model or edge/cloud server addresses;

Computing and application: the sensing node, gateway, and edge/cloud server calculate and transmit the effective data using configured model/algorithm, and then the applications acquire data from the edge/cloud servers.

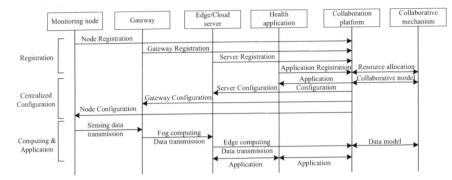

Fig. 3. Health monitoring system's working process

3 System Implementation

A. System Composition and Working Process

A health monitoring system composition is shown in Fig. 4. The system hardware composition is shown in Fig. 5.

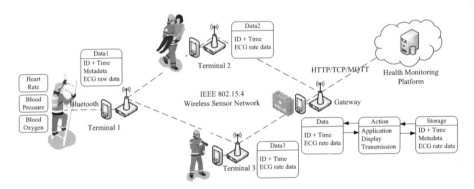

Fig. 4. System composition

The health monitoring process includes 4 steps:

Step 1: we apply wearable sensors to acquire ECG, blood pressure, and blood oxygen raw data. User ID, time, metadata, and monitoring raw data are then sent to fog system using Bluetooth communication;

Step 2: a fog terminal implements data processing, display, transmission, and storage functions. The effective data such as heart rate are calculated from the ECG raw data, and data set *D(ID, time, metadata, ECG rate)* is then stored in the fog terminal memory;

Step 3: the fog terminal connects with a WSN router node, and multi nodes' health data (Data1, Data2, and Data3) are sent to a WSN coordinator (gateway) using IEEE 802.15.4 or IEEE 802.11s mesh communication;

Step 4: the WSN coordinator/gateway node connects with an edge terminal, which implement edge computing, storage and application functions. The edge terminal interacts with collaboration cloud platform using HTTP, TCP, or MQTT internet protocols.

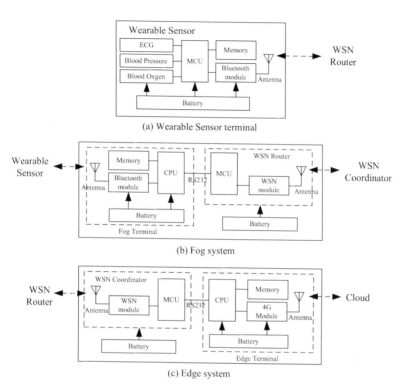

(a) Wearable Sensor terminal

(b) Fog system

(c) Edge system

Fig. 5. System hardware composition

Table 1. Specification of a Health Monitoring System

Item	Specification
Wearable Sensor	Oranger Mi-Rhythm ECG sensor ECG range: 30 bpm–300 bpm; Channe l:1; Size: 45 * 25 * 7 mm; Weight: 10 g ± 1 g
Fog Terminal	CPU: Hisilicon Kirin 710F; OS: Harmony; Maximum frequency: 2.2 GHz; RAM: 4 GB; ROM: 64 GB
WSN module	Digi XBee wireless module Frequency: 900 MHz; Data Rate: 200 kbps
Edge Terminal	CPU: Hisilicon Kirin 659; OS: Harmony; Maximum frequency: 1.7 GHz; RAM: 4 GB; ROM: 64 GB

B. System Implementation

We set up a real-world system, and the system specification is shown in Table 1. We use Oranger Mi-Rhythm ECG sensor to monitor 30–300 bps ECG data; we develop series of software using Harmony OS in fog and edge terminal; we use Digi Xbee wireless module to implement the IEEE 802.15.4 WSN router and coordinator.

Figure 6 (right) shows the fog terminal and software user interface; Fig. 6 (left) shows the acquired ECG raw data and calculated heart rate data.

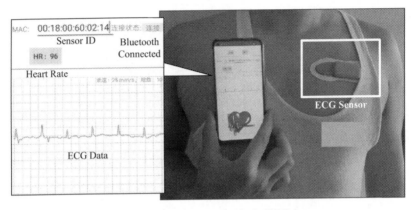

Fig. 6. Fog Terminal and sample ECG data

The prototype edge system is shown in Fig. 7, includes an edge terminal and a WSN coordinator. The edge terminal software user interface includes the comparison of data from multi terminals (fog terminal 1 and fog terminal 2), and data analysis for each terminal.

Figure 8 (a) shows the working process of the WSN router nodes. The router node refresh the network topology on the base of received configuration and link information packet, and transmit both link data and sensing data to the coordinator;

Figure 8 (b) shows the working process of the WSN coordinator. The coordinator refreshes the WSN network topology, and sends configuration and link information packets to all WSN router nodes, then transmits received sensing data to the edge terminal.

C. Heterogeneous Systems' Collaboration

On the base of the proposed architecture and developed single system, we design the collaboration mechanism for multi domain systems, including homogeneous system, heterogeneous system, and general collaborative system.

(1) Homogeneous systems' collaboration: the monitoring terminal and gateway nodes adopt unified open standards for data sensing and transmission, and the nodes could interact data with each other directly. The user could design various of collaboration algorithms according to the application requirements.

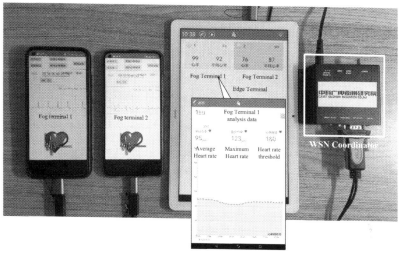

Fig. 7. Edge terminal and sample heart rate data

(2) Heterogeneous systems' collaboration: the gateway nodes adopt different standards for data sensing and transmission, so we need to develop software or hardware middleware in the north direction of the gateway node. And the gateway node could interact with other system using the middleware.

(3) General collaborative system: in a general system, homogeneous and heterogeneous systems from multi domain collaborate with each other for complex task. The hierarchical structure is shown in Fig. 9, and we concern the three types system collaboration.

There are three kinds of computing servers: the edge collaboration server implements the control and configuration function; the data server implements the data interaction function; the general emergency server implements the application function. The edge collaborative server transmits configuration information to registered gateway or middleware nodes, which compose systems' control chain; each gateway or middleware node interact with the cloud/edge data server, and compose systems' data chain.

The homogeneous system A and C's gateway nodes, heterogeneous system B's middleware node perform data interaction on the base of the configuration information. The unregistered heterogeneous system D's middleware node, and homogeneous system E's gateway node, interact with system C's gateway node, and join the inter systems' data chain. The sub-layer terminal nodes are managed by the gateway node.

We concern three parameters for the collaborative data chain: location of the disaster area and people, location of the gateway node of homogeneous system or the middleware node of heterogeneous system, and network connectivity condition. The network connectivity status is confirmed by the network topology update module. During one clock cycle, the gateway or middleware node broadcasts "Hello message", which includes ID and node's location. The receiver sends back an "ACK message", which includes receiver's ID and location, and after handshake we confirm the sender and receiver have neighborhood relationship, then the network topology is updated. For a new registered

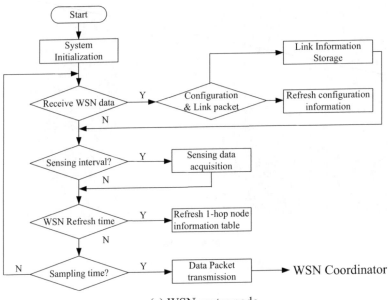

(a) WSN router node

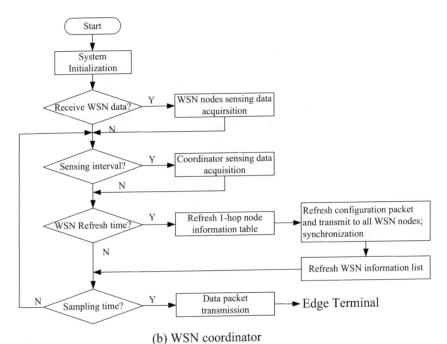

(b) WSN coordinator

Fig. 8. WSN working process

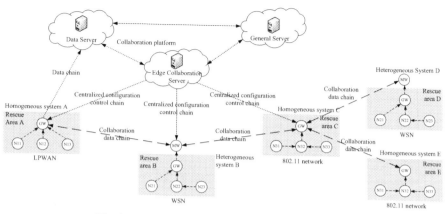

Fig. 9. Hierarchical structure of collaboration systems

gateway or middleware node, the destination is affected by disaster area and people's location, and neighbor node's location. The location parameters "pull" the node periodically. When all the nodes come into a "stable status" according to the application requirement, we consider that the system has completed the emergency task.

4 Discussion

In the proposed system architecture, each system's configuration could be centralized informed from the collaboration platform according to the application requirements, and each system proceeds the configuration in a distributed manner. Therefore the architecture has advantages in at least two following aspects:

(1) Scalability: the sensing and computing algorithm could be modularized, and heterogenous and homogeneous systems could work together using the architecture and open standards. Sensing units could update algorithms/models for different applications with the support of middleware.

(2) Resilient system: in wide area environment, when a sub-system is destroyed or moved, the applications could delete or mark the sub-system records in the registration list easily. Since the communication status is unpredictable, Delay Tolerant Network (DTN) mode command, and routing algorithms could be configured from the collaboration platform to the sub-system.

Currently, only ECG sensor is applied in the system, more sensors will be applied in future development. In Sect. 3 (a)–(b), we introduce the development of an "end-to-edge" health monitoring system. Based on the mechanism introduced in Sect. 3 (c), we are developing the "edge-to-Cloud" collaboration system using docker technology, and the micro services include: data receiving interface service, registration service, collaboration model service, health data output API interface service, system topology service, etc. A sample output data set could be described as *Data (ID, Type, No. of terminals, Communication radius, area width, area length, No. of monitored people, people's location)*.

5   Conclusions

In this manuscript, we propose a collaborative architecture for distributed wide area health monitoring system, and we concern 3 aspects: heterogeneous communication, system modularization and open standards, and edge computing. A real-world ECG monitoring system has been implemented, which includes ECG sensor, Wireless Sensor Networks, and fog/edge terminals. An "End-to-edge" collaboration mechanism and a series of experiments have been performed. Also we discuss the "edge-to-cloud" collaboration mechanism and implementation for heterogeneous and homogeneous systems in complex wide area environment.

The proposed architecture and real-world system implementation provide guidelines for wide area data sensing and communication system construction in IOT and 5G/B5G era. We are focusing on general integrated emergency sensing system on on-going research.

Acknowledgment. This research is supported by Science and Technology Project grant of Quzhou city (No. 2020K13).

References

1. Qadri, Y.A., Nauman, A., Zikria, Y.B., Vasilakos, A.V., Kim, S.W.: The future of healthcare internet of things: a survey of emerging technologies. IEEE Commun. Surv. Tutorials **22**(2), 1121–1167 (2020)
2. Tataria, H., Shafi, M., Molisch, A.F., Dohler, M., Sjoland, H., Tufvesson, F.: 6G wireless systems: vision, requirements, challenges, insights, and opportunities. Proc. IEEE **109**(7), 1166–1199 (2021)
3. Chang, Z., Liu, S., Xiong, X., Cai, Z., Tu, G.: A survey of recent advances in edge-computing-powered artificial intelligence of things. IEEE Internet Things J. **8**(18), 13849–13875 (2021)
4. Kodheli, O., et al.: Satellite communications in the new space era: a survey and future challenges. IEEE Commun. Surv. Tutorials **23**(1), 70–109 (2021)
5. Liu, G.: Data collection in MI-assisted wireless powered underground sensor networks: directions, recent advances, and challenges. IEEE Commun. Mag. **59**(4), 132–138 (2021)
6. Pathak, N., Misra, S., Mukherjee, A., Kumar, N.: HeDI: healthcare device interoperability for IoT-based e-Health platforms. IEEE Internet Things J. **8**(23), 16845–16852 (2021)
7. Ding, X., et al.: Wearable sensing and telehealth technology with potential applications in the coronavirus pandemic. IEEE Rev. Biomed. Eng. **14**, 48–70 (2020)
8. Vedaei, S.S.: COVID-SAFE: an IoT-based system for automated health monitoring and surveillance in post-pandemic life. IEEE Access **8**, 188538–188551 (2020)
9. Wu, Q., Chen, X., Zhou, Z., Zhang, J.: FedHome: cloud-edge based personalized federated learning for in-home health monitoring. IEEE Trans. Mob. Comput. **21**(8), 2818–2832 (2022)
10. Wei, K., Zhang, L., Guo, Y., Jiang, X.: Health Monitoring based on internet of medical things: architecture, enabling technologies, and applications. IEEE Access **8**, 27468–27478 (2020)
11. Liu, J., Miao, F., Yin, L., Pang, Z., Li, Y.: A noncontact ballistocardiography-based IoMT system for cardiopulmonary health monitoring of discharged COVID-19 patients. IEEE Internet Things J. **8**(21), 15807–15817 (2021)

Internet of Things Technologies in Healthcare for People with Hearing Impairments

Bader Alsharif[✉] and Mohammad Ilyas

Florida Atlantic University, Boca Raton, FL 33431, USA
{Balsharif2020,ilyas}@fau.edu

Abstract. The Internet of Things (IoT) is a technology that connects physical objects, software, and hardware for interacting with each other and exchanging valuable data. In the healthcare sector, those data can be used by physicians, vendors, health organizations, and researchers to improve healthcare quality and reduce annual healthcare spending. Consequently, the emergence of the IoT in the healthcare field has led to transformative growth in activity and creativity. The rapid proliferation of IoT devices and applications can assist people of all ages with hearing difficulties in their daily activities to improve their and their caregivers' quality of life. People with disabilities, particularly those with hearing impairments, have fewer opportunities for social interactions, education, and access to modern technologies. These aspects are crucial factors in developing their learning capacity and cognitive skills. IoT technology can be oriented to assist people with hearing disabilities to enhance their quality of life without relying on assistance from others and that is a noble goal of our research.

Keywords: Internet of Things (IoT) · IoT in healthcare · Hearing Impairments · Wearable devices · security · privacy

1 Introduction

The Internet of Things (IoT) is a rapidly growing technology that connects hardware, software, physical objects/things, and computing devices for interacting, collecting, sending, and receiving data without human intervention [1]. These connected objects and devices join this sophisticated network with uniquely identifiable IP addresses. Most people think that the use of IoT applications and devices are only associated with smart homes and cities for users' comfort, privacy, and security. In fact, however, the development and growth of the IoT has opened up a new era in the healthcare, education, energy, transportation, and agricultural sectors as well as many other sectors [3]. By 2025, more than 75 billion IoT devices will join the Internet to provide significant computational resources and services for many different fields [2]. The emergence of the IoT in the healthcare field has led to transformative growth in activity and creativity. The rapid proliferation of IoT devices and applications can assist people of all ages with hearing difficulties in their daily activities to improve their and their caregivers' quality of life [4].

S. Wang (Ed.): IoTCare 2022, LNICST 501, pp. 299–308, 2023.
https://doi.org/10.1007/978-3-031-33545-7_21

According to the World Health Organization, hearing loss affects more than 1.5 billion people worldwide, and by 2050 it is estimated that approximately 700 million people will be added to the number of those with disabling hearing loss. As a result, the rate of hearing impairments among the population has risen and is increasing the annual costs of the healthcare sectors of many countries [5]. This vast number of people with hearing deficiency or loss need assistance with using today's technology. IoT technology should be oriented to assist people with hearing disabilities to enhance their quality of life without relying on assistance from others.

People with hearing sensory impairments cannot socialize effectively with ordinary people because they do not have one of the most important and frequently used senses [7]. Hearing sense strongly relates to speaking, and people who are affected with hearing impairments can be deterred from speaking or verbally communicating. To compare this condition to a computing device, if there are no inputs there will be no outputs, and so these individuals cannot gain any cognition or development from hearing. This can lead to mental disorders due to social isolation, frustration, and loneliness. Furthermore, students with hearing impairments have lower educational levels than ordinary students [6, 7]. The most effective way for people with hearing loss to communicate with one another is by using sign language. Sign language is the act of expressing oneself through hand gestures, eyes, face, lips, and body [12]. Similarly, normal people need to learn sign language to communicate with deaf people or use interpreters. In all cases, communication between deaf people must be live and visible to each other to convey messages and meaning. Many conditions can cause people to develop hearing disabilities. The most common cause of hearing loss is congenital and is present at birth due to genetic circumstances. The second most common factor that causes hearing loss is aging. Chronic middle ear infections and damage to the inner ear caused by ototoxic drugs or accidents are other causes of hearing loss [5]. The last condition of developing hearing disabilities is exposure to loud noise or loud music for a long time, which can damage the inner ear's nerve [5].

Cochlear implants and hearing aids are important solutions for people who are suffering from hearing deficiency, as they allow them to improve their oral communication for language acquisition and enhance their sound awareness. There are four levels of

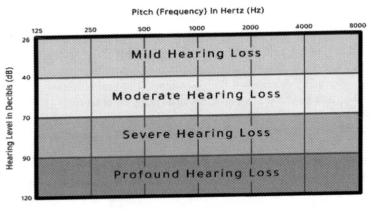

Fig. 1. Degrees of Hearing Loss

hearing loss as seen in Fig. 1: mild (26–40 dB), moderate (41–70 dB), severe (71–90 dB), and profound (above 91 dB) [13]. Indeed, many deaf people are not able to use either cochlear implants or hearing aids due to their level of hearing deficiency not being supported [10]. Additionally, many people who have had cochlear implants or use hearing aids are not satisfied with these solutions due to many reasons related to background noise, fit and comfort, the inferior quality of hearing and the risk of surgery failing [11].

2 The Internet of Things (IoT): An Overview

As previously mentioned, the IoT comprises different gadgets and devices that make up a network of constantly communicating items. Some examples of items that can be included within IoT-based technology are sensors, wearable devices, controllers, actuators, and laser scanners [1, 14]. When these items interact and communicate in a constant fashion, they form a spectrum that can best be described as a network. According to [15], "the Internet of Things is the concept of connecting any device (so long as it has an on/off switch) to the Internet and to other connected devices. The IoT is a giant network of connected things – all of which collect and share data about the way they are used and about the environment around them". The items in the IoT can interact together even outside of human participation, though some components of the IoT may require human actions to perform certain specific functions [16].

Today, several applications of the IoT have contributed to improving the human experience. For instance, smart homes, offices, cities, smart farms, smart cars, smart industries, pollution and waste control, automated gates and garage doors, traffic monitoring, and management, energy-saving thermostats and humidity controllers, and last but not least smoke and fire alarms all have been enabled by the interaction of different technologies within IoT networks [15]. Other phenomena that have improved the human experience by using the IoT include wearable devices that can track and monitor users' health and fitness [14, 17]. The majority of modern devices interact with the IoT in some way enabled by some form of IoT – in fact, due to the sheer range of IoT applications, they cannot all be listed, which only emphasizes the IoT's importance for the contemporary human experience. The most important way the IoT contributes to different technological transformations is by allowing incompatible items to interact meaningfully. Traditional manufacturers of different technologies may deliberately make devices incompatible with others – this is a business model that ensures that only the accessories and parts of the manufacturer's initial product can work with the product, thereby assuring their organization of otherwise peripheral sales [18]. The IoT reverses this conundrum by providing a platform through which different incompatible technologies are not only able to interact and communicate, but also to generate actionable insights as reported by [19]. By bringing different technologies together, the IoT allows the benefits of all the components to be realized at the applicable stage [19]. Alternatively, the IoT also allows the shortcomings and limitations of different technologies to be complemented by other more able components [19] (Fig. 2).

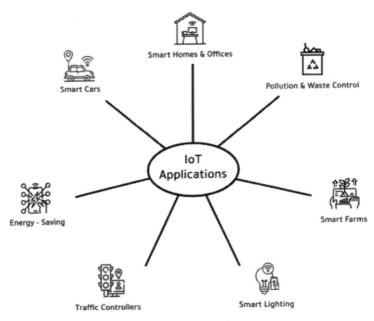

Fig. 2. IoT Applications

2.1 IoT in Healthcare

The IoT also has a vital role to play within the healthcare field. In healthcare, different components in the network can gather and integrate data before performing analyses [14]. Many applications within healthcare make use of the IoT – these range from diagnostic processes requiring the use of interactive devices, the collection of patient information, access to patient medical data, remote tracking of patient developments, and continuous monitoring [14]. According to [20], "The IoT promises many benefits to streamlining and enhancing health care delivery to proactively predict health issues and diagnose, treat, and monitor patients both in and out of the hospital". All these applications contribute to the life-saving capacity of healthcare processes because they ensure the healthcare practitioner makes decisions that are guided by actual actionable knowledge. When analysis of data from different components on the network is achieved, the most valuable information can be gleaned and then used to promote evidence-based practice. [16] states that, "the Internet of Things (IoT) has been widely applied to interconnect available medical resources and provide reliable, effective, smart healthcare services". It is possible to discern patterns, draw inferences, identify potential issues, and make appropriate recommendations when healthcare practitioners are equipped with credible information obtained from accredited healthcare technologies [14, 16]. For example, it is possible for a healthcare practitioner to determine whether patients are at an increased risk of developing certain conditions through monitoring their cholesterol levels – in this instance, the statistics regarding the patient's cholesterol levels provide valuable and actionable information. Therefore, the IoT generates information and records that healthcare practitioners are able to use to ensure they reach desirable outcomes.

Within healthcare, the IoT enables the uninterrupted and constant collection of patient data. Most research opines that patient data become more credible and useful if gathered in a continuous stream instead of taking sporadic measurements [21]. This perspective is also held by [22], who postulates that uninterrupted information collection is crucial for the healthcare practitioner to reach meaningful conclusions. The IoT, by virtue of not requiring human intervention to function effectively, is able to ensure constant engagement by all its components as previously stated; once all the components are switched on, they continue to function for as long as they are able to acquire battery or some form of electric power [20]. Therefore, the IoT facilitates the uninterrupted collection of patient records, data, and information in a way that makes all resultant insights more credible than those collected outside of the IoT (Fig. 3).

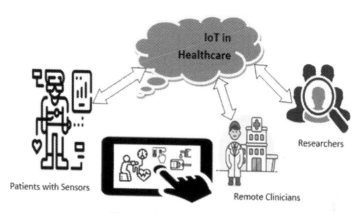

Fig. 3. The IoT in Healthcare

The focus of this survey paper is to outline and examine some IoT devices, applications, and systems utilized for people with hearing impairments as well as some obstacles and challenges that must be addressed. In fact, without reliable technology, people with hearing problems cannot communicate effectively with ordinary people unless they have certain communication abilities or technologies [9]. Therefore, we must ensure they have widespread access to modern technologies to satisfy their needs and concerns.

3 Related Work

Various research studies are available in the literature concentrating on how IoT technology interventions and development can provide the opportunity for people with disabilities, especially hearing impairments, to overcome traditional impediments. IoT technology solutions are used to facilitate their everyday activities and increase their social integration in daily life. IoT technology in healthcare has developed different applications and wearable devices that are used to manage hearing impairment complications as well as hearing loss in addition to increasing dependency on technologies as assistive tools. These devices and applications enable personalized healthcare, which can assist in remote monitoring, screening, diagnosis, and the early detection of hearing loss [1].

Wearable devices in particular have significant potential for use with speech recognition applications to assist people with hearing difficulties due to their lightweight and low cost [7]. Wearable devices with tangible interfaces are an alternative solution when it comes to mobility as auxiliary communication. [28] stated that using voice recognition to convert voice to text is an important implementation when communicating between ordinary people and deaf people without using sign language. The text data are transferred to Arduino over Bluetooth, where they are interpreted using ASCII characters and displayed on the wearable device as text.

People with hearing impairments cannot hear any sounds from the surrounding environment to improve their awareness. In this case, we cannot communicate or get their attention to raise the alert about dangerous situations unless we are visible to each other. In [8], the authors developed a wearable device that can sense and detect sounds in real-time such as a phone or bell ringing, alarm sounds, brake sounds, dogs barking, other sounds related to the audio fingerprint method and human sounds. When the wearable device detects and identifies one of these sounds, it directly transmits these data to the user through vibrations. Each of the above-listed sounds has distinct levels of vibration and intensity, which allows deaf people to easily distinguish between the various vibrations related to each sound. This system, [8] uses speech recognition methodology, but instead of translating spoken language into text, they translate sounds into vibrations in a wearable device. In addition, they use a microphone to process ambient sounds. Finally, for coding, they rely on Python programming language. Their system achieves an accuracy rate of 99% for identifying an alarm sound and a phone ringing, 98% for a doorbell ringing, 97% success in identifying a human voice, 96% success in identifying dog sounds and other sounds using the audio fingerprint method, and 93% success in identifying brake sounds. Those numbers are significant achievements for sound recognition and classification in real-time performance. In the end, [8] tried to enable and promote the use of IoT technology in healthcare with little equipment cost to protect people with hearing problems in an outdoor or indoor environment. In [12], the authors mentioned a smart bear for children that can sense and measure body temperature, blood pressure, oxygen levels, and heart rate. These vital data can be sent directly to the parents' smartphones via wireless communication technologies. The organization that invented the "Teddy the Guardian" smart bear can easily use their idea to address the hearing difficulties of deaf people and their caregivers. Many IoT applications and technologies are being developed to serve normal people. However, if manufacturers put more effort into orienting IoT technology to people with hearing impairments they could get many potential benefits and high profits.

Many researchers nowadays are focusing on how to facilitate communication between normal people and deaf people using today's technology. The work presented in [29–31] is a glove equipped with wireless communication technology and sensors that allows hearing-impaired people to interact with others who are not familiar with or do not understand American Sign Language. The job of the wireless glove is to sense and record the fingers flexion of the ASL and send the data to a smartphone programmed application using Bluetooth technology to convert the sign language received data into text and voice (Table 1).

Table 1. Summary of IoT Services for People with Hearing Impairments.

IoT services	IoT devices	Gateway	Communication type
29	Speech-to-text	Arduino	Bluetooth
8	Real-Time Detection	Raspberry Pi	USB
12	Smart bear	Mobile phone	Bluetooth
30,31,32	Glove	Mobile phone	Bluetooth

4   Challenges and Future Work

The first major issue associated with the application of the IoT in deafness and hearing loss management stems from security. As an unconventional network, it is possible for the IoT to be breached, leading to unauthorized access to information – cyber-attacks are becoming an increasing problem in the contemporary world, and healthcare has not been spared [23]. Different components of the IoT present various levels of risk for security vulnerabilities – for instance, wearable devices (which are relatively simple technologies without electronic encryptions) can be easily hijacked by unauthorized parties [23]. Alternatively, servers containing sensitive information may be hacked to provide unauthorized access to unscrupulous parties [24]. Therefore, this presents a challenge for the IoT-reliant healthcare profession, and the management of deafness and hearing loss is no different.

Legal issues also need to be considered in the use of the IoT in the management of deafness and healthcare. The US has laws such as HITECH and HIPAA that govern the access and use of patient health records see Fig. 4 for privacy rule and security requirements – when unauthorized access to this information occurs, the healthcare organization can be held legally liable and face litigation [25]. The protection of all manner of healthcare IoT is therefore a requirement for all healthcare organizations, especially considering that they generate both soft and hard copies of patient medical records [24]. Security challenges that result in unauthorized access to private (and sensitive) patient information and records can lead to violations of the aforementioned data privacy laws, fines and a loss of licensure. Alternatively, the patient can file a lawsuit against the healthcare organization, leading to compensatory payments [24]. Therefore, healthcare organizations that rely on the IoT to manage deafness and hearing loss have to contend with the legal framework surrounding its usage.

The last major issue relating to the use of the IoT in the management of deafness and hearing loss is poor connectivity. As indicated in the definition of the IoT, the devices involved in the network function in a wireless capacity – this can create issues when the different healthcare technologies are not compatible, to begin with [26]. As previously mentioned, a method commonly used by manufacturers is to ensure that the accessories and different spare parts they construct for their products are exclusive, thus assuring them of peripheral sales as posited by Kessler [26].

The view that connectivity issues can affect the IoT during the management of different medical conditions is also shared by [14]. This view is also shared by Yin et al., who cite completely incompatible healthcare technologies as compromising the effectiveness of IoT networks [16]. Therefore, different components may be completely incompatible as per the manufacturers' intentions, hence limiting the effectiveness of the IoT.

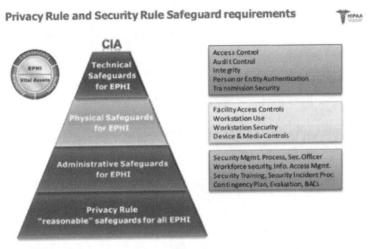

Fig. 4. Privacy Rule and Security Requirements [25]

Every connected device and application has potential security issues. When it comes to the security challenges facing IoT networks in the management of deafness and hearing loss, approaches involving high-end encryptions can be applied. The most recent development that can be employed by healthcare organizations is the use of blockchain technology – IBM states that "In most blockchains or distributed ledger technologies (DLT), the data is structured into blocks and each block contains a transaction or bundle of transactions. Each new block connects to all the blocks before it in a cryptographic chain in such a way that it is impossible to tamper with" [27]. Granted, blockchain technology is not completely foolproof, as it has some security shortcomings. However, its basis on decentralization and cryptography provides a robust foundation that cannot be easily breached, making it perhaps the most secure approach for the IoT [27]. Healthcare organizations should therefore invest in blockchain technology to protect the structural integrity of the IoT.

For future work, we are working on building an automated sign language recognition system using deep learning algorithms to recognize hand gestures. The system will assist in communication between ordinary individuals and hard-of-hearing people.

5   Conclusion

The development of IoT technology continues to meaningfully contribute to the healthcare sector, opening new possibilities for improving people's quality of life. People with disabilities, particularly those with hearing impairments, have fewer opportunities for social interactions, education, and access to modern technologies. These aspects are crucial factors in developing their learning capacity and cognitive skills. Deafness and hearing loss are among the most understated public health concerns across the world. There are millions of people across the world who suffer from some form of hearing loss. Despite the obviously debilitating nature of these conditions, as demonstrated by many research papers using Google Scholar, a number of researchers have worked on improving and expanding the use of IoT technology in healthcare to serve deaf people. Not only do deafness and hearing loss lower the individual's quality of life, t but also compromise their potential for academic and professional achievement. It is for this reason that this group requires assistive technologies that can deliver sound signals in a format they can comprehend and interpret. We are working on building a recognition system that can help in translating sign language to normal people and the reverse.

References

1. Kashani, M.H., Madanipour, M., Nikravan, M., Asghari, P., Mahdipour, E.: A systematic review of IoT in healthcare: applications, techniques, and trends. J. Netw. Comput. Appl. **192**, 103164 (2021)
2. Zhang, P., Zhang, J., Elsabbagh, A.: Lower limb motion intention recognition based on sEMG fusion features. IEEE Sens. J. **22**(7), 7005–7014 (2022)
3. Islam, S.R., Kwak, D., Kabir, M.H., Hossain, M., Kwak, K.-S.: The internet of things for health care: a comprehensive survey. IEEE Access **3**, 678–708 (2015)
4. Antonić, M.: IoT technologies offer new potentials for people with disabilities. In: 2021 International Conference on Software, Telecommunications and Computer Networks (SoftCOM), pp. 1–6. IEEE (2021)
5. World Health Organization (2021)
6. Haile, L.M., et al.: Hearing loss prevalence and years lived with disability, 1990–2019: findings from the Global Burden of Disease Study 2019. Lancet **397**(10278), 996–1009 (2021)
7. Yağanoğlu, M.: Real time wearable speech recognition system for deaf persons. Comput. Electr. Eng. **91**, 107026 (2021)
8. Yağanoğlu, M., Köse, C.: Real-time detection of important sounds with a wearable vibration based device for hearing-impaired people. Electronics **7**(4), 50 (2018)
9. Pothong, K., Turner, S.: Living with hearing loss in a connected home: white paper (2020)
10. Sicong, L., Zhou Zimu, D., Junzhao, S.L., Han, J., Wang, X.: UbiEar: bringing location-independent sound awareness to the hard-of-hearing people with smartphones. Proc. ACM Interact. Mobile Wearable Ubiquit. Technol. **1**(2), 1–21 (2017)
11. McCormack, A., Fortnum, H.: Why do people fitted with hearing aids not wear them? Int. J. Audiol. **52**(5), 360–368 (2013)
12. Cano, S., Peñeñory, V., Collazos, C.A., Albiol-Pérez, S.: Designing internet of tangible things for children with hearing impairment. Information **11**(2), 70 (2020)
13. Law, E.L.-C., Roto, V., Hassenzahl, M., Vermeeren, A.P., Kort, J.: Understanding, scoping and defining user experience: a survey approach. In: Proceedings of the SIGCHI Conference on Human Factors in Computing Systems, pp. 719–728 (2009)
14. Yang, X., et al.: Exploring emerging IoT technologies in smart health research: a knowledge graph analysis. BMC Med. Inform. Decis. Mak. **20**, 1–12 (2020)
15. Clark, J.: What is the internet of things, and how does it work. IBM Business Operations Blog, Nov. 17 (2016)
16. Yuehong, Y.I.N., Zeng, Y., Chen, X., Fan, Y.: The internet of things in healthcare: an overview. J. Ind. Inf. Integr. **1**, 3–13 (2016)

17. Nižetić, S., Šolić, P., González-De, D.-I., Patrono, L.: Internet of things (IoT): opportunities, issues and challenges towards a smart and sustainable future. J. Clean. Prod. **274**, 122877 (2020)
18. Kumar, S., Tiwari, P., Zymbler, M.: Internet of things is a revolutionary approach for future technology enhancement: a review. J. Big Data **6**(1), 1–21 (2019). https://doi.org/10.1186/s40537-019-0268-2
19. Khalid, L.F., Ameen, S.Y.: Secure Iot integration in daily lives: a review. J. Inf. Technol. Inform. **1**(1), 6–12 (2021)
20. Kelly, J.T., Campbell, K.L., Gong, E., Scuffham, P.: The internet of things: impact and implications for health care delivery. J. Med. Internet Res. **22**(11), e20135 (2020)
21. El Zouka, H.A., Hosni, M.M.: Secure IoT communications for smart healthcare monitoring system. Internet of Things **13**, 100036 (2021)
22. Xu, G.: IoT-assisted ECG monitoring framework with secure data transmission for health care applications. IEEE Access **8**, 74586–74594 (2020)
23. Somasundaram, R., Thirugnanam, M.: Review of security challenges in healthcare internet of things. Wirel. Netw. **27**(8), 5503–5509 (2020). https://doi.org/10.1007/s11276-020-02340-0
24. Williams, P.A., McCauley, V.: Always connected: the security challenges of the healthcare internet of things. In: 2016 IEEE 3rd World Forum on Internet of Things (WF-IoT), pp. 30–35. IEEE (2016)
25. CDC: Health Insurance Portability and Accountability Act of 1996 (HIPAA)|CDC (2020). https://www.cdc.gov/phlp/publications/topic/hipaa.html. Accessed 26 Mar 2022
26. Kessler, M.: Incompatible tech confuses consumers Lack of uniform standards leave many frustrated. https://www.forbes.com/feeds/general/2005/01/07
27. Muzammal, S.M., Murugesan, R.K.: A study on leveraging blockchain technology for IoT security enhancement. In: 2018 Fourth International Conference on Advances in Computing, Communication & Automation (ICACCA), pp. 1–6. IEEE (2018)
28. Bansal, M., Garg, S.: Internet of Things (IoT) based assistive devices. In: 2021 6th International Conference on Inventive Computation Technologies (ICICT), pp. 1006–1009. IEEE (2021)
29. Peng, S., Zhou, Y., Cao, L., Shui, Y., Niu, J., Jia, W.: Influence analysis in social networks: a survey. J. Netw. Comput. Appl. **106**, 17–32 (2018)
30. Sarji, D.K.: HandTalk: assistive technology for the deaf. Computer **41**(7), 84–86 (2008)
31. Singh, B.S.: IOT based smart healthcare applications for people with disabilities. Asian J. Convergence Technol. (AJCT) (2018). ISSN–2350–1146

Artificial Intelligence-Based Early Warning Method for Abnormal Operation and Maintenance Data of Medical and Health Equipment

Xuan Zhang[1](✉), Yihan Ping[2], and Chao Li[3]

[1] Monroe College, New Rochelle, NY 10801, USA
xzhang9979@monroecollege.edu
[2] Georgia Institute of Technology, Atlanta, GA 30332, USA
[3] Department of Information Engineering, Tongling Polytechnic, Tongling 244000, Anhui, China

Abstract. When traditional early-warning methods for abnormal operation and maintenance data of medical care equipment are used to process nonlinear abnormal data in the operation and maintenance process of medical care equipment, the data classification accuracy is poor, resulting in insufficient reconciliation level of early-warning methods. Therefore, an artificial intelligence based early-warning method for abnormal operation and maintenance data of medical care equipment is proposed. First, the article establishes the overall framework of data anomaly early warning, including communication network layer, smart contract layer, equipment layer, and application layer. Based on artificial intelligence technology, it establishes the anomaly data detection model, uses RNN cyclic neural network as the basis, designs the anomaly data detection process, and analyzes whether medical and health care equipment is in an abnormal operating state by comparing the real value of current measurement points with the predicted value of RNN neural network model. The experimental results show that: combined with the experimental results of nonlinear data, it can be determined that the data classification accuracy of the designed early-warning method is high, the early-warning data is more comprehensive and complete, and the detection method is superior to the common detection methods.

Keywords: Artificial Intelligence · Medical and Health Care Equipment · Operation and Maintenance Data · Abnormal Warning

1 Introduction

Medical care equipment is the equipment and tools used in medical care and other work, which can facilitate medical staff to judge patients' symptoms more quickly and accurately. Use medical equipment to treat patients to the greatest extent, so that patients can get rid of the pain as soon as possible. It can be said that medical equipment is the

S. Wang (Ed.): IoTCare 2022, LNICST 501, pp. 309–321, 2023.
https://doi.org/10.1007/978-3-031-33545-7_22

most important means to help hospitals improve medical quality and efficiency [1, 2]. Medical care equipment is the integration of computing, network, detection and medical process. It can realize the safety of the physical world, monitor the patients in use reliably and in real time, and ensure the safety of patients' use. Therefore, it has a wide application prospect in the future medical process. In the process of the development of medical and health care equipment, the continuous development of wireless sensor network, biomedical sensor and cloud computing technology has given birth to the wide application of medical and health care equipment in the medical field. Medical and health care equipment mainly obtains biometric information through sensors, collects and integrates the information, and through a networked intelligent medical system composed of drug delivery medical equipment, all units in the system realize information interaction through communication network, thus realizing the interconnection of medical resources [3].

For the use and management of medical equipment, it is necessary to carry out refined management in the whole life cycle. With the continuous development of medical technology and equipment, it is necessary to carry out periodic operation and maintenance for medical and health care equipment. In the process of operation and maintenance, if the relevant data is abnormal, it means that there is a certain risk of failure inside the equipment, and it is prone to danger when people use it [4]. Therefore, early warning of the abnormal operation and maintenance data of medical and health care equipment is an important prerequisite to ensure the normal work of medical and health care equipment and improve the safety and efficiency in the medical process [5]. When the traditional early warning method of medical and health care equipment operation and maintenance data abnormality deals with the nonlinear data in the process of medical and health care equipment operation and maintenance, the accuracy of data classification is poor, which leads to the insufficient reconciliation level of the early warning method. Therefore, this paper proposes an early warning method of medical and health care equipment operation and maintenance data abnormality based on artificial intelligence.

2 Research on Abnormal Early Warning of Medical and Health Care Equipment Operation and Maintenance Data

2.1 Establish the Overall Framework of Data Anomaly Warning

Based on artificial intelligence, the abnormal data early warning of medical and health care equipment operation and maintenance is mainly aimed at the security problems of medical and health care equipment tools in recent years, and the information data security diagnosis, traceability and abnormal information early warning during equipment application are studied [6, 7]. From the overall structure of the early warning method, it can be divided into data layer, network layer, intelligent contract layer, equipment platform layer and application layer, as shown in Fig. 1.

In the whole early warning method, the data layer is the basis of the early warning method, in which the storage of block data, transaction data and hash address is designed. In the communication network layer, the main logic responsible for the abnormal warning of the whole operation and maintenance data has a relatively complete mechanism in

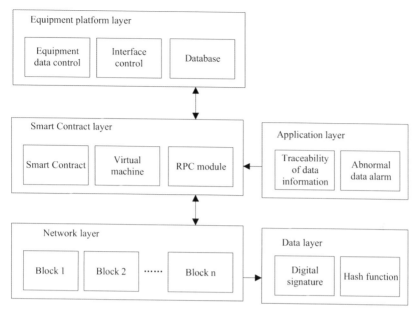

Fig. 1. Framework of early warning method

consensus and verification. In the intelligent contract layer, the interactive RPC module based on JsonStandard RPC is used to realize the request service of the remote medical care equipment program. In the remote state, the block node and consistency processing are regarded as the transaction interaction in the network layer, and the EVM module is used to run the intelligent early warning contract. In the device layer, the RPC module in the contract layer can be called to retrieve the data information of the device and related control instructions [8]. In the application layer, an interface library is designed for information exchange, so as to track the information source of medical and health care equipment and detect abnormal data in advance.

2.2 Establish Abnormal Data Detection Model Based on Artificial Intelligence Technology

Under the joint action of external factors and internal factors, the data have an impact and then form fluctuation indicators. Therefore, SPSS statistical software is used to draw the box diagram of equipment operation and maintenance data changes, from which the basically unchanged index data are found and eliminated. One of the indicators is the upper quartile, expressed as Q_u, that is, the indicator sequence is divided into four parts on average, and the calculation formula is:

$$Q_u = \frac{n+1}{4} \tag{1}$$

The value of n is determined according to the actual situation, and Q_u is further calculated. Another index is the quartile distance of IQR, and the calculation formula is:

$$IQR = 3 \times \frac{n+1}{4} - Q_u \tag{2}$$

In the box chart, the upper and lower limits are the minimum and maximum values within the non-abnormal data range, and the relevant calculation formula is:

$$\begin{cases} T_{\min} = Q_u - 1.5IQR \\ T_{\max} = Q_u + 1.5IQR \end{cases} \tag{3}$$

The biggest advantage of box chart is that it is not affected by outliers, and it can describe the discrete distribution of data in a relatively stable way [9]. By observing the box chart, we can preliminarily eliminate the non-fluctuating indicators with outliers close to 0. Normalize the remaining indexes with fluctuating data, and continue to analyze the abnormal degree of their data. The expected risky abnormal data must have the characteristics of persistence and relevance at the same time. Based on the characteristics of risky abnormal data, the continuity of indicators is first studied. Four kinds of scatter distributions can be obtained by drawing the corresponding scatter plots of each group of data in EXCEL for regression analysis.

In the model established in this paper, recurrent neural network is mainly used as the basis of artificial intelligence calculation. In the neural network, the neural network layers, including the input layer, the hidden layer and the output layer, are all connected, but the neurons in the same layer are not related to each other. The time series data is dependent on the information before and after the change of time, and the prediction of time series data using neural network model will not cause information omission [10]. The reason why RN is called a recurrent neural network is that the hidden layer information of the current moment is retained to participate in the calculation of the next network, and the historical information is continuously transmitted through the interconnected hidden layers in each network. The following Fig. 2 shows the structure diagram of RNN in chronological order:

As can be seen from the figure, corresponding to the time relationship of data, the hidden layer in the middle of RNN is also sequential from left to right. The workflow of RN can be roughly divided into the following steps:

(1) x_t indicates the input at time t, which indicates a multi-dimensional vector.
(2) s_t indicates the hidden layer state at time t, which has the function of information memory, storage and transmission. The layer value is determined by the accumulated information of the hidden layer in the previous time and the input information of this layer. The value of the first hidden layer state s_0 is generally 0 after initialization. Expressed by the formula:

$$s_t = f(Ux_t + Ws_{t-1}) \tag{4}$$

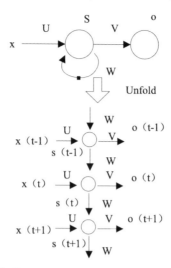

Fig. 2. RNN neural network structure diagram

In the above formula, f represents the nonlinear activation function.

(3) o_t indicates the device output at time t.

Through the above test of volatility data continuity, the index that abnormal data meet the continuity condition is obtained. These indicators are extracted, Pearson correlation coefficient is obtained by SPSS, and correlation analysis is carried out to test the linkage [11, 12]. Six groups of abnormal risk data were obtained. By using Python for programming, calculation and analysis, we can get the specific risk abnormal points of each group of data, and then we can get the abnormal degree score.

2.3 Medical and Health Care Equipment Operation and Maintenance Data Abnormal Warning

The analysis of current measuring points in medical and health care equipment is not only of great significance for the detection of the running state of the equipment, but also an essential component for the comprehensive evaluation of the medical and health care equipment and even the overall physical function of the patient. In the process of operation and maintenance of medical equipment, it will be affected by real-time environmental factors, and the operation process is quite different in different situations. The data early warning mainly includes two aspects: one is the identification of abnormal data caused by the abnormal work of sensors inside the equipment; On the other hand, in the process of communication, the identification of data tampering caused by device IoT blockchain attack. Therefore, the traditional rated threshold can't be used in the early warning process, and the threshold needs to be updated and managed with reference to the running state of the current day. The current data model of medical care equipment is established based on the data in the normal and stable operation process. The estimated value of the current measuring point at the next moment can be obtained by acquiring the data change and development law from the historical data of equipment operation and learning. When the medical care equipment is in normal operation, the actual value of the current measuring point is very close to the predicted value, and the deviation can be guaranteed within a certain range. Therefore, by comparing the real value of current measuring point with the predicted value of RNN neural network model, it is analyzed whether the medical and health care equipment is in abnormal operation. The deviation index of equipment current measuring point is defined as the ratio of the actual value of the equipment, the difference between the predicted value and the predicted value, and the formula is as follows:

$$D_e = \left| \frac{Y_t - Y_m}{Y_m} \right| \tag{5}$$

In the above formula, Y_t represents the real value obtained by the measuring tool, and Y_m represents the predicted value output by the measuring point prediction model. When the predicted equipment is in normal operation, the deviation index is very low, and the curve is drawn as shown in the following Fig. 3:

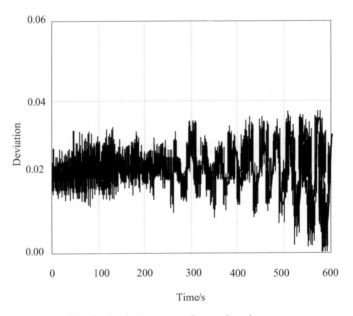

Fig. 3. Deviation curve of normal equipment

When it is within the threshold, no alarm is needed; When the predicted equipment is in abnormal operation, the real value differs greatly from the predicted value, and the deviation index will increase significantly, so it is necessary to send out an alarm. Observing the deviation curve of normal equipment, it is found that the deviation is always below 2% during operation. When external conditions or internal faults fluctuate, the burr in the deviation curve exceeds 2%, but it will soon return to below 2%. Therefore, a value of D_e of 10% is set as the first alarm threshold, and a value of D_e of 20% is set as the second alarm threshold. For the predicted equipment, calculate the deviation of the actual value of the current measuring point. If it is lower than the threshold, it is normal; if it is higher than the threshold, it is abnormal.

In order to prevent the data of each link in the process of operation and maintenance from being tampered with, while recording the data in each link, the intelligent contract is called to realize homomorphic encryption. Smart contracts can't directly operate data with the blockchain built into healthcare devices, so they need to be connected by triggers. When the operation and maintenance work is completed and data encryption is needed, the trigger will send the address of the smart contract interface with full homomorphic encryption and the data to be encrypted. When the data encryption is completed, the trigger sends the contract address and ciphertext to the blockchain network. For the abnormal data generated when the sensor is in abnormal working state, this paper uses confidence interval to identify the possible abnormal data points in the data. In the normal working state of the sensor, the sampled value fluctuates in a small range. However, when the abnormal state occurs, the sampling value will appear obvious deviation. Using this principle, firstly, K normal data are stored for each link of sensors, and according to these data and the preset confidence A, the approximate interval estimation of the total sample can be obtained $\{LCL, UCL\}$. When the data $R(t)$ at a certain time satisfies the following two expressions, it indicates that the value is abnormal data:

$$\begin{cases} LCL \leq R(t) \leq UCL \\ R(t) = R(t-1) \end{cases} \tag{6}$$

In the above formula, LCL represents the lower limit of the confidence interval, and UCL represents the upper limit of the confidence interval. Because the blockchain attack of medical and health care equipment in the Internet of Things is concealed, in order to prevent the blockchain data anomaly caused by the attack, the attack process is divided

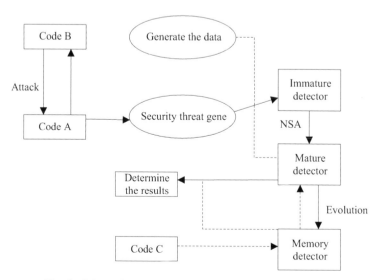

Fig. 4. Schematic diagram of abnormal data detection process

and prevented one by one. Attacks can be divided into three stages: pre-restart, restart and after restart. When the victim node B restarts, it is detected that its incoming and outgoing connections are intercepted by the attacking node A.. This indicates that the attacking node A successfully launched the attack before the node B restarted. Therefore, it is necessary to collect the data sent by node A to node B before node B restarts, so as to constitute a security threat gene. The attack detection module is divided into two parts: the first part is an immature detector, and the second part is a mature detector. The security threat gene and the data randomly generated according to its format are used as the training samples of immature detectors, and NSA algorithm is used for training until it evolves into a mature detector. After a certain number of tests, the maturity detector will evolve into a memory detector. The data detection process of a node in the device is shown in the following Fig. 4:

The node data detection process in the figure above: firstly, it is matched with the memory detector. If the matching is successful, it indicates that the node has abnormal data, and it is put into the security threat gene pool to participate in the training of the immature detector; If not, it is sent to the maturity detector for detection. When the mature detector matches successfully, it indicates that the node has abnormal data, and the security threat gene is also put in; If it doesn't match, it means that the node has no abnormal data.

3 Performance Test of Data Anomaly Early Warning Method

3.1 Preparation of Experimental Data

After the design of the abnormal early warning method of medical and health care equipment operation and maintenance data based on artificial intelligence is completed, a performance test method is designed according to the application characteristics of the early warning method. In the performance test, real medical and health care equipment operation and maintenance data are used for simulation and editing, mainly including user information, medical records, patient functions and other related information. The selected data set characteristics are shown in Table 1.

Based on the above data, aiming at the problems existing in common data anomaly early warning methods, a nonlinear data classification experiment is designed to verify the actual performance of the early warning methods. In the experiment, another data anomaly warning method is selected as a comparison, namely, the anomaly warning method based on deep learning and the anomaly warning method based on transfer learning. The proposed warning method is placed under the same experimental conditions for nonlinear data experimental analysis and early warning evaluation analysis, and the application level of each warning method is analyzed according to the experimental results.

3.2 Experimental Results of Nonlinear Data

In order to further verify the data processing ability of the anomaly early warning method, a nonlinear data experiment is designed, and two kinds of nonlinear data are constructed

Table 1. Data set characteristics

Data set	Attribute number	sample number	Category number	Data type	Whether the default
Voltage constant value	16	20000	26	numeric type	N
Current constant value	19	2561	7	numeric type	Y
running mode	8	743	2	numeric type	Y
performance period	9	632	2	mixed type	Y
User heart rate	4	492	3	numeric type	Y
The user blood pressure	166	352	2	numeric type	N
Fault indicator data	34	269	2	mixed type	Y

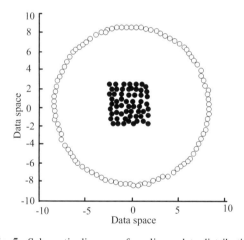

Fig. 5. Schematic diagram of nonlinear data distribution

in the same space, one is distributed in a ring with the origin as the center, and the other is distributed in a square shape. The specific distribution is shown in Fig. 5.

The Gaussian kernel parameter is set to 0.4, and the initialization center point is (0, 0). Three different abnormal data warning methods are used to process nonlinear data, and the third-party software is used to output the experimental results. The details are shown in Fig. 6.

According to the experimental results shown in the figure, when the data anomaly detection method deals with nonlinear data, the data classification results of the experimental results of the early warning method based on deep learning are not ideal. The data distributed in the ring are fused in the square, and there is no clear dividing line

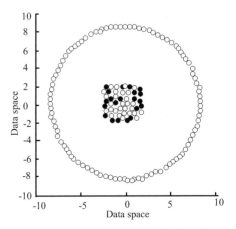

(a) Experimental results of early warning method based on deep learning

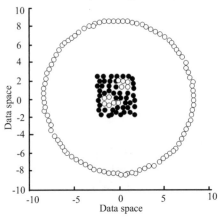

(b)Experimental results of early warning method based on transfer learning

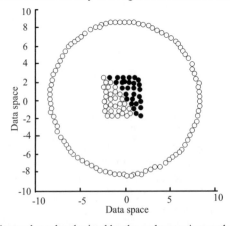

(c)The experimental results obtained by the early warning method in this paper

Fig. 6. Experimental results of different data anomaly detection methods

between the two data. The early warning method based on transfer learning has the same problem. In the experimental results, the data distributed in the ring is distributed in the square, which is aggregated and not completely separated. In contrast, the experimental results of the proposed early warning method show that the nonlinear data classification is more obvious and disjoint, and the nonlinear data classification effect is better. To sum up, the proposed data anomaly early warning method has higher data classification accuracy, and can efficiently process various types of data.

3.3   Experimental Results and Analysis of Anomaly Detection and Evaluation

In the abnormal early warning and evaluation, it is mainly based on the experimental results of the above nonlinear data and the early warning performance of the early warning method itself. In the experiment, the recall rate and precision rate are used as index variables, and the F value is calculated according to these two sets of values, which indicates the harmonic average level of anomaly detection methods. The relevant calculation formula is as follows:

$$Pre = \frac{w^+}{w^+ + c^+} \tag{7}$$

$$Rec = \frac{w^+}{w^+ + c^-} \tag{8}$$

$$F = \frac{2Pre \cdot Rec}{Pre + Rec} \tag{9}$$

In the formula, Pre indicates the precision rate, w^+ indicates the correct warning example, Rec indicates the recall rate, c^+ indicates the positive warning error example, and c^- indicates the negative warning error example. Three different data anomaly warning methods are used to process the experimental data, and after the warning is completed, the experimental results of each method are output. As shown in Fig. 7.

In Fig. 7, Method 1 and Method 2 are two common early warning methods, and Method 3 represents the data anomaly early warning method proposed in this paper. In the three groups of experimental results, the proposed detection method is calculated to determine that the F value is 0.536, the F value of method 1 is 0.253, the F value of method 2 is 0.328, and the F value of method 3 is 0.421. Combined with the changes of recall and precision in the above figure, it can be seen that the recall and precision are higher than those of common detection methods, and the F value is also higher, which indicates that the medical care equipment operation and maintenance data anomaly warning based on artificial intelligence proposed in this paper. Combined with the experimental results of nonlinear data, it can be determined that the data classification accuracy of this early warning method is high, and the early warning data is more comprehensive and complete. This detection method is superior to common detection methods.

To sum up, the artificial intelligence based early warning method for abnormal operation and maintenance data of medical and health care equipment studied has higher data classification accuracy, more comprehensive and complete data that can be alerted, and can efficiently process various types of data.

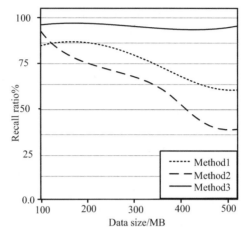

(a) Experimental results of data early warning recall rate

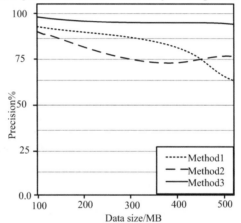

(b) Experimental results of data early warning precision rate

Fig. 7. Experimental results of different data anomaly detection methods

4 Concluding Remarks

In this paper, artificial intelligence technology is applied to the abnormal warning of medical equipment operation and maintenance data. Through the combination of RNN neural network and early warning, the data transmission and detection between equipment nodes are realized. At the same time, the detection model of abnormal data is constructed by using the principle of artificial intelligence learning, so as to realize the early warning of abnormal data. After testing, the scheme proposed in this paper can better realize the detection and early warning of nonlinear data.

References

1. Siamak, H., Ali, S., Ghanbari, A.T.: An artificial intelligence-based prediction way to describe flowing a Newtonian liquid/gas on a permeable flat surface. J. Therm. Anal. Calorim. **147**(6), 4403–4409 (2022)
2. Wang, J., Pei, L.: Anomaly detection and multi-stage risk pre-warning technology of power grid control system based on deep learning. J. Shenyang Univ. Technol. **43**(06), 601–607 (2021)
3. Zhang, S., Zheng, J., Shen, X., et al.: Anomaly detection of ADS-B air position data and statistical analysis. Electron. Opt. Control **29**(04), 101–105 (2022)
4. Khosravi, A., Laukkanen, T., Saari, K., et al.: An artificial intelligence based-model for heat transfer modeling of 5G smart poles. Case Stud. Therm. Eng. **28**(12), 101–113 (2021)
5. Chen, Y.-q., Sun, T., Zhang, Q.-y.: Intelligent engine room multi-source data detecting method based on DBSCAN cluster algorithm. Ship Sci. Technol. **43**(17), 156–160 (2021)
6. Meng, H., Li, Y.: Anomaly detection and relation extraction for time series data based on transformer reconstruction. Comput. Eng. **47**(02), 69–76 (2021)
7. Turner, D., Pera, A., et al.: Wearable internet of medical things sensor devices, big healthcare data, and artificial intelligence-based diagnostic algorithms in real-time COVID-19 detection and monitoring systems. Am. J. Med. Res. **8**(2), 132–145 (2021)
8. Zhang, S., Li, D., Sun, Y., et al.: Unified anomaly detection for syntactically diverse logs in cloud datacenter. J. Comput. Res. Dev. **57**(04), 778–790 (2020)
9. Qiu, K., Jiang, Y.: A service running data anomaly detection method based on weighted LOF and context judgment in cloud environment. Comput. Eng. Sci. **42**(06), 951–958 (2020)
10. Rafiei, H., Akbarzadeh-T, M.-R., Pariz, N., Akbarzadeh, A.: Expert systems and the prospects of artificial intelligence for the automatic supervisory control of salinity gradient solar ponds. Solar Energy **246**(1), 281–293 (2022)
11. Yu, M., Yang, F.: Field failure operation and maintenance simulation of automation equipment based on information link technology. Comput. Simul. **38**(12), 475–479 (2021)
12. Daly, T.T.W.: Artificial intelligence, deep aging clocks, and the advent of 'biological age': a Christian critique of AI-powered longevity medicine with particular reference to fasting. Religions **13**(4), 334–342 (2022)

Abnormal Signal Recognition Method of Wearable Sensor Based on Machine Learning

Chao Li[1][(✉)] and Xuan Zhang[2]

[1] Department of Information Engineering, Tongling Polytechnic, Tongling 244000, Anhui, China
llcc222@yeah.net
[2] Monroe College, New Rochelle, NY 10801, USA

Abstract. The recognition of abnormal signal of wearable sensor is of great significance to the application value of the device. In order to improve the accuracy of abnormal signal recognition of wearable sensors and indirectly ensure the safety of wearable sensor devices, a method of abnormal signal recognition of wearable sensors based on machine learning was proposed. According to the different abnormal types and principles of wearable sensors, the signal abnormal judgment criteria are set. The wearable sensor signal is collected, and the initial signal is preprocessed by Kalman filtering, normalization and weighted fusion. The machine learning algorithm is used to extract the features of sensor signals, and the recognition results of the abnormal type, abnormal semaphore and abnormal location of sensor signals are obtained through feature matching. Through the identification performance test experiment, it is obtained that the average abnormal type error detection rate of the optimization design identification method is 0.86%, and the average statistical error of abnormal semaphore is 0.22 db, lower than the preset value.

Keywords: Machine Learning · Wearable Sensor · Abnormal Signal · Signal Identification

1 Introduction

Sensor is a kind of detection device, which can feel the measured information, and can transform the sensed information into electrical signals or other required forms of information output according to a certain law, so as to meet the requirements of information transmission, processing, storage, display, recording and control. The characteristics of the sensor include miniaturization, digitalization, intellectualization, multifunction, systematization and networking. It is the primary link to realize automatic detection and automatic control [1]. The existence and development of sensors make objects have senses such as touch, taste and smell, and make objects slowly become alive. According to their basic sensing functions, they are usually divided into ten categories: thermal sensors, photosensitive sensors, gas sensors, force sensors, magnetic sensors, humidity

© ICST Institute for Computer Sciences, Social Informatics and Telecommunications Engineering 2023
Published by Springer Nature Switzerland AG 2023. All Rights Reserved
S. Wang (Ed.): IoTCare 2022, LNICST 501, pp. 322–338, 2023.
https://doi.org/10.1007/978-3-031-33545-7_23

sensors, sound sensors, radiation sensors, color sensors and taste sensors. In the environment of rapid expansion of information, more and more people have an increasing demand for the speed and frequency of information exchange. People are using mobile personal computers or mobile phones to receive, process and send all kinds of messages at any time. This dependence on electronic devices makes the relationship between people and machines become closer and closer, making portable wearable devices inevitable for the development of the times. The main application fields of wearable sensors include: medical fields represented by blood glucose, blood pressure and heart rate monitoring, health care fields represented by sports monitoring, consumption fields represented by information entertainment, and industrial and military fields represented by data acquisition and display. Relevant data points out that wearable devices in the health care and medical fields account for 60% of the market share this year, and the share may be further increased in the future.

Due to the aging of the internal components of the wearable sensor, the wrong installation of the sensor and other reasons, the abnormal state of the wearable sensor will not only affect the user's experience, but also may bring potential safety hazards such as electric leakage and magnetic leakage. Therefore, it is necessary to identify and detect the abnormal real-time signals of wearable sensors, so as to provide valuable reference data for the timely maintenance of sensors. Anomaly recognition is one of the important topics in the research of data analysis technology. Its main task is to find the anomaly in time, so that we can quickly take measures to early warn the anomaly and assist scientific decision-making. At present, the more mature sensor abnormal signal recognition methods include: abnormal recognition method based on the principle of electrical impedance, abnormal recognition method based on static fault tree and abnormal recognition method based on steady-state fault quantity. However, the above abnormal signal recognition methods can not recognize the type and location of abnormal signals at the same time, and the abnormal signal recognition results have large errors, which is lack of reference value for the maintenance of wearable sensors. Therefore, machine learning algorithm have been introduced.

Machine learning is an interdisciplinary subject involving probability theory, statistics, approximation theory, convex analysis, algorithm complexity theory and other disciplines. It specializes in studying how computers simulate or realize human learning behavior, so as to acquire new knowledge or skills, reorganize the existing knowledge structure and constantly improve its own performance. It is the core of artificial intelligence and the fundamental way to make computers intelligent. Machine learning methods based on statistical features can be divided into supervised learning and unsupervised learning according to learning methods. Supervised learning is to train the marked data, generate models, and then test and classify. This method has a high prediction accuracy, but it can not classify unknown categories. Common methods include Bayesian, decision tree, etc. The other is semi supervised learning, which can use labeled and unlabeled samples for training at the same time. Compared with it, it has more room for development, but it is still in the state of research. Select the appropriate machine learning algorithm and apply it to the optimization of the abnormal signal recognition method of wearable sensors, in order to improve the accuracy of abnormal signal recognition of wearable sensors and indirectly ensure the safety of wearable sensor devices.

2 Design of Abnormal Signal Recognition Method of Wearable Sensor

2.1 Set the Judgment Standard of Wearable Sensor Abnormality

Wearable sensor anomalies mainly include: complete failure anomaly, fixed deviation anomaly, drift deviation anomaly and accuracy degradation. Among them, failure anomaly refers to the sudden failure of sensor measurement, and the measured value has always been a certain constant; Deviation anomaly mainly refers to a kind of anomaly that the measured value of the sensor differs from the real value by a certain constant; Drift anomaly is a kind of anomaly that the difference between the measured value and the real value of the sensor changes with time; The decrease of accuracy refers to the deterioration of the measuring ability and accuracy of the sensor. When the accuracy level is reduced, the average value of the measurement does not change, but the variance of the measurement changes [2]. Both fixed deviation anomaly and drift anomaly are not easy to find, which will cause a series of unpredictable problems in the process of anomaly occurrence, so that the control system can not function normally for a long time. The types of abnormal signals of some wearable sensors and their causes are shown in Table 1.

Table 1. Description of abnormal signal types of wearable sensors

Serial number	Sensor abnormal signal type	Cause of abnormal signal
1	Stuck exception an exception caused by a stuck sensor running program	Stuck exception an exception caused by a stuck sensor running program
2	Abnormal gain: the working frequency or signal of the sensor changes with a constant gain due to the aging of the sensor element	Abnormal gain: the working frequency or signal of the sensor changes with a constant gain due to the aging of the sensor element
3	Abnormal deviation due to the abnormal connection of the sensor, the working signal has a fixed deviation	Abnormal deviation due to the abnormal connection of the sensor, the working signal has a fixed deviation
4	Abnormal short circuit the output signal is close to zero due to the short circuit of the sensor circuit and other reasons	Abnormal short circuit the output signal is close to zero due to the short circuit of the sensor circuit and other reasons
5	Abnormal open circuit. The output signal is close to the maximum value due to the open circuit of the sensor output circuit and other reasons	Abnormal open circuit. The output signal is close to the maximum value due to the open circuit of the sensor output circuit and other reasons

(continued)

Table 1. (*continued*)

Serial number	Sensor abnormal signal type	Cause of abnormal signal
6	The offset abnormal sensor is disturbed by a stable signal	The offset abnormal sensor is disturbed by a stable signal
7	The original output signal of the periodic abnormal sensor is interfered by the periodic signal of a certain frequency	The original output signal of the periodic abnormal sensor is interfered by the periodic signal of a certain frequency
8	Random abnormal sensor is disturbed by a random signal	Random abnormal sensor is disturbed by a random signal
9	The output signal offset signal caused by abnormal zero drift, temperature drift, sensitivity drift, etc	The output signal offset signal caused by abnormal zero drift, temperature drift, sensitivity drift, etc
10	Abnormal impact abnormal impact is caused by the interference of a pulse signal on the sensor	Abnormal impact abnormal impact is caused by the interference of a pulse signal on the sensor

The wearable sensor is stuck abnormally, the gain abnormally and the deviation abnormally meet the following characteristics:

$$x_\psi(t) = \begin{cases} c, \psi \in U_{\text{Stuck}} \\ \beta_i x(t), \psi \in U_{\text{gain}} \\ x(t) + \Delta\varepsilon, \psi \in U_{\text{deviation}} \end{cases} \qquad (1)$$

where c is constant, β_i and $\Delta\varepsilon$ are constant gain and constant deviation respectively, and U_{Stuck}, U_{gain} and $U_{\text{deviation}}$ correspond to the set of stuck abnormal, gain abnormal and deviation abnormal signals. According to the above method, the standard characteristics of all abnormal signals of wearable sensors can be obtained, which can be used as the comparison standard to determine the signal type of wearable sensors.

2.2 Collect Wearable Sensor Signal

Wearable sensors are mainly divided into three parts from the physical structure: detection coil, analog circuit board and digital circuit board. In terms of circuit structure, it is mainly divided into: resonant input excitation resonant circuit, detection circuit, primary amplification and filtering, secondary amplification and filtering, AD sampling and digital signal processing, as shown in Fig. 1.

OP1, AD1, op2, OP3, ad2 and OP4 in Fig. 1 are the output signals that can be collected by the sensor. In practical engineering, only AD1 and ad2 signals are used. Since the four detection coils of the sensor are placed in space according to certain rules, the output of the four channel resonant circuit has a certain correlation. As described in Sect. 2, the output four channel OP signals differ by one quarter of the periodic phase in sequence, and the two channel ad signals differ by one half of the periodic phase [3].

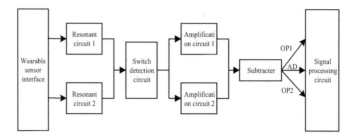

Fig. 1. Circuit structure diagram of wearable sensor

The output signal of a normal sensor is a sinusoidal like periodic signal. When the gap between the sensor and the track is certain, the amplitude of the sensor output signal remains unchanged. If the amplitude of the sensor output signal changes, or there is no output signal, it indicates that the sensor has failed. Take the wearable sensor shown in Fig. 1 as the target to collect the real-time data generated by the sensor, and the acquisition process of angular velocity and acceleration signals is shown in Fig. 2.

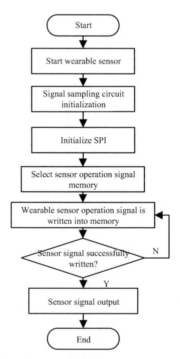

Fig. 2. Flow chart of wearable sensor signal acquisition

Similarly, the acquisition result of wearable sensor position signal can be obtained, which can be quantitatively expressed as:

$$\begin{cases} X = (R + H) \cos \delta \cos \sigma \\ Y = (R + H) \cos \delta \sin \sigma \\ Z = \left(\frac{\kappa_1^2}{\kappa_0^2} R + H \right) \sin \delta \end{cases} \tag{2}$$

In the above formula, the variables R and H respectively represent the height of the radius of curvature charge relative to the surface of the ellipsoid, δ and σ correspond to latitude and longitude, κ_0 and κ_1 are the long and short semi axis parameters describing the earth as a reference ellipsoid. According to the above methods, the real-time acquisition results of wearable sensor operation signals can be obtained.

2.3 Fusion Processing of Wearable Sensor Signals

Wearable sensor signal acquisition process will be polluted by different degrees of noise, so that the obtained sensor data is also mixed with noise information, so that useful signals can not be directly detected [4]. Kalman filter can be used to estimate the necessary useful signals, so as to detect the abnormal occurrence of sensor data. Kalman filter adopts linear minimum variance estimation, which encapsulates the state quantity in the corresponding state space in the filtering process, and then obtains the state estimator in real time through continuous iteration. This method is very suitable for dealing with the estimation of multi-dimensional random variables. And only through the state equation of the observation system and the statistical characteristics of noise can be used to express the statistical characteristics of the actual state quantity and noise, which does not need to grasp the error changes between the observation and the real state quantity in real time. The Kalman filter processing process of wearable sensor signals can be expressed as:

$$\begin{cases} X_k = BX_{k-1} + An_{k-1} \\ Y_k = GX_k + N_k \end{cases} \tag{3}$$

In the above formula, X_k and Y_k are the state variables and observation variables of the wearable sensor signal respectively, B, A, G and N correspond to the state transfer matrix, interference transfer matrix, observation noise matrix and observation matrix, and n_{k-1} represents the input noise value in the signal [5]. By substituting all the signal acquisition data into formula 3, the noise signal suppression processing in the initial acquisition signal can be realized. Normalize the noise signal, and the processing process can be expressed as:

$$x = \frac{x_{max} - x}{x_{max} - x_{min}} \tag{4}$$

x_{max} and x_{min} correspond to the maximum and minimum values of wearable sensor signals. On this basis, the data processing results are fused, and the processing results are as follows:

$$x_{fuse} = \frac{\kappa_{fuse}(x_i + x_j) + (\kappa_{fuse} - 1)^2 x_i x_j}{1 + \kappa_{fuse}^2 - (\kappa_{fuse} - 1)^2 (x_i - x_j)^2} \tag{5}$$

where x_i and x_j are the i and j signal processing results of the wearable sensor respectively, and κ_{fuse} is the fusion coefficient between the data. Complete the fusion and processing of wearable sensor signals according to the above process.

2.4 Extracting Sensor Signal Characteristics Using Machine Learning Algorithm

BP neural network in machine learning is selected as the technical support for feature extraction of sensor signals. The network topology of BP neural network is composed of three parts, which are input layer, hidden layer and output layer respectively. The connection relationship is shown in Fig. 3.

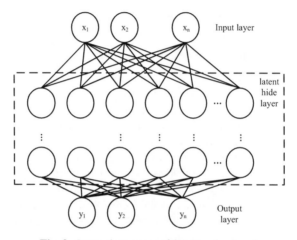

Fig. 3. Internal structure of BP neural network

The calculation process of each neural unit in Fig. 3 can be expressed as:

$$
\begin{cases}
u_1^{(2)} = g\left(\varpi_{11}^{(1)} x_1 + \varpi_{12}^{(1)} x_2 + \lambda_1^{(1)} \right) \\
u_2^{(2)} = g\left(\varpi_{21}^{(1)} x_1 + \varpi_{22}^{(1)} x_2 + \lambda_2^{(1)} \right) \\
u_3^{(3)} = g\left(\varpi_{31}^{(1)} x_1 + \varpi_{32}^{(1)} x_2 + \lambda_3^{(1)} \right) \\
u_1^{(3)} = g\left(u^{(2)} + u_2^{(2)} + u_3^{(2)} + \lambda_1^{(2)} \right)
\end{cases}
\tag{6}
$$

The output result $u_i^{(j)}$ of formula 6 represents the i neural unit of the j layer in BP neural network, ϖ and λ represent the weight value of the neural unit respectively, and $g()$ is the activation function. Its numerical expression is as follows:

$$
g(x) = \frac{1}{1 + \exp^{-e}}
\tag{7}
$$

The calculation result of formula 7 is substituted into formula 6. After integration, the relationship between the input and output of BP neural network is as follows:

$$
u^{(l+1)} = g\left(\varpi^{(l)} x^{(l)} + \lambda^{(l)} \right)
\tag{8}
$$

In the network training phase, wearable sensors train the network weights according to the given training mode in four processes: "forward propagation of mode" → "reverse propagation of error" → "memory training" → "learning convergence". In the working stage of the network, according to the trained network weight value and the given input vector, the solution of the output vector corresponding to the input vector is obtained in the way of "mode forward propagation". The input signal is transmitted from the input layer node to each hidden layer node in turn, and then to the output layer node. If the expected output cannot be obtained at the output layer, it will turn to reverse propagation, return the error signal along the original path, and modify the weights of neurons at each layer through learning to minimize the error signal. In the process of BP network learning, first adjust the connection weight between the output layer and the hidden layer, then adjust the connection weight between the intermediate hidden layer, and finally adjust the connection weight between the hidden layer and the input layer. In the actual training and learning iteration process, the fusion processing results of wearable sensor signals are substituted into the input layer of BP neural network, and these information is continued to be transmitted to the hidden layer nodes of the middle layer connected later. The middle layer loads the internal information processing of neural network, which is the core part of the network. It mainly transforms the input information according to the requirements of information change, The number of intermediate layers can also be changed according to the requirements of transformation, using a single hidden layer or multiple hidden layers structure; The last hidden layer transmits the processed information to the nodes of the output layer. After further conversion and processing, the output layer finally outputs the information processing results of this neural network forward learning to the outside world [6]. When the output value of the neural network does not match the expected output value, the neural network will carry out error back propagation to change the learning process of the network connection weight. The error starts from the output layer, and the weight of each layer in the network is modified according to the gradient descent method of the error, and gradually passes back to the hidden layer and input layer of the network. After repeated cycles and multiple above learning processes, the connection weights of each layer of the network are continuously adjusted according to the difference between the network output and the actual output of the sample, so that the output of the network is closer to the actual value of the system. This process is the training and learning process of the neural network. In neural networks, the steepest descent method is widely used as its learning rule, and the network parameters are continuously adjusted through the back propagation of the difference between the network output and the actual output of the sample. This process takes the sum of squared errors of the network output as the evaluation standard, and this process will not be terminated until the difference between the network output and the actual output of the sample meets the accuracy requirements or the number of network learning and training reaches the preset value [7]. In the process of multiple learning iterations, the weights and offsets of neurons will change dynamically, so it is necessary to use formula 9 to update all neural units in BP neural network.

$$\begin{cases} \varpi_{new} = \varpi - \frac{\partial \varphi}{\partial \varpi} \\ \lambda_{new} = \lambda - \frac{\partial \varphi}{\partial \lambda} \end{cases} \tag{9}$$

In the above formula, φ is the update cost function. Finally, according to the process shown in Fig. 4, the forward and back propagation are repeated to complete the learning iteration process of BP neural network.

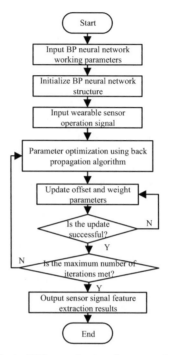

Fig. 4. Flow chart of BP neural network propagation and learning

For the sensing signal with the overall downward depression of signal amplitude, take the ordinate value of the peak point with higher value as the baseline, and take the area covered between the data curve between the two peaks and the baseline. The calculation formula of this characteristic parameter is as follows:

$$\chi = \sum_{t=1}^{N_{\text{collection}}} \{x(t) - \min[x(t)]\} \tag{10}$$

where $N_{\text{collection}}$ represents the collected signal quantity of the wearable sensor, and min() is the minimum value calculation function [8]. Similarly, the feature extraction results of signal peak value, valley value, average value, valley spacing, peak spacing, signal area, signal surface energy, signal length, signal width and so on can be obtained and output in the form of feature vector.

2.5   Realize Abnormal Signal Recognition of Wearable Sensor

Combined with the sensor signal characteristics extracted by machine learning algorithm, the abnormal signal type, signal quantity and abnormal location of the current wearable sensor are determined through feature matching, signal statistics and other technologies.

Identify the Abnormal Type of Signal

The identification of abnormal type of wearable sensor signal is to match the real-time collected and extracted operation signal with the set abnormal standard, and calculate the similarity between them using formula 11.

$$\phi = \sqrt{(\chi_{set} - \chi_{draw})^2} \tag{11}$$

where χ_{set} and χ_{draw} correspond to the set abnormal signal characteristics and the extracted wearable sensor signal characteristics [9]. Set the determination threshold of the abnormal signal type as ϕ_0. if the calculation result obtained from formula 11 is higher than ϕ_0, it is determined that the current wearable sensor signal characteristics are consistent with the abnormal signal characteristics, so that the abnormal recognition result of the current wearable sensor signal is the abnormal type corresponding to the χ_{draw} feature. Otherwise, it needs to be re determined until the determination conditions are met.

Statistical Abnormal Semaphore

The statistical process of abnormal semaphores of wearable sensors can be expressed as:

$$M_{abnormal} = \sum_{i=1}^{num_{satisfy}} m_i \tag{12}$$

In the above formula, m_i is the number of the i signal that meets the abnormal condition. The wearable sensor signals identified as abnormal state are counted according to formula 12, and the quantitative statistical results of abnormal signal quantity are obtained.

Determine the Abnormal Position of the Signal

Figure 5 shows the identification principle of abnormal signal position of wearable sensor.

In order to monitor the condition of each sensor, the following three decision functions can be formed by using formula 13:

$$\begin{cases} F_1 = d_1 d_3 \\ F_2 = d_1 d_2 \\ F_3 = d_2 d_3 \end{cases} \tag{13}$$

When the wearable sensor operates in the normal state, the error of the state variable estimated by the filter is very small, so the value of d_i fluctuates around zero, and the

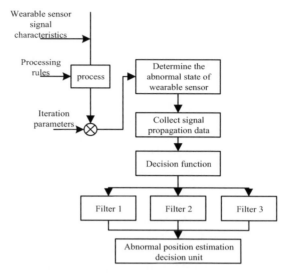

Fig. 5. Schematic diagram of abnormal signal positioning of wearable sensor

value of F_i also fluctuates around zero. When a sensor is abnormal at a certain time, the error of the state variable estimated by the state variable estimated by the first filter will be large, so the values of d_1 and d_3 will increase correspondingly, and the value of F_1 will also increase a lot compared with F_2 and F_3. Similarly, when sensor 2 is abnormal, the value of F_2 will also increase a lot compared with F_1 and F_3, so that the abnormal position of the sensor can be determined by the change of the decision function, realize the positioning of abnormal wearable sensors.

3   Experimental Analysis of Recognition Performance Test

In order to test the recognition performance of the optimized wearable sensor abnormal signal recognition method based on machine learning, different types of wearable sensors are selected as the research object for testing. Through the control of sensor working parameters and working environment, the setting samples of sensor abnormal signals are obtained. Through the comparison between the output results of the design recognition method and the setting data, the test results reflecting the performance of the abnormal signal recognition method of the optimized wearable sensor are obtained.

3.1   Prepare Wearable Sensor Research Samples

Wearable heart rate sensor, temperature sensor, gyroscope and pressure sensor are selected as the research objects in this experiment. The model of heart rate sensor is KEYENCE and the model of temperature sensor is PT100. In addition, the models of gyroscope and pressure sensor research samples are pa-arc-0050 and pt124g-111 respectively. The total number of research samples prepared for this experiment is 80, and the number of samples of each wearable sensor is 20. Before starting the experiment, they debug the prepared wearable sensor research samples to ensure that the initially prepared research samples are in a normal state.

3.2 Configure the Experimental Environment

The test bench is equipped with a secondary coil, which is connected in series with the Programmable Potentiometer on the hardware circuit of the control box. The control box controls the resistance of the Programmable Potentiometer to change regularly through the hardware program, and the programmable potentiometer is used as the load to affect the equivalent load of the coil of the relative position sensor. At the same time, the control box collects data in real time from the sensor communication interface, and sends it to the upper computer in real time through serial port to USB interface after simple digital signal processing. The upper computer displays and stores the received sensor data in real time and diagnoses the sensor fault. The test bench is mainly used to load the relative position sensor and the secondary coil. The size design of the test bench refers to the overall size of the potting coil at the bottom of the relative position sensor, with a width of 114mm. Wearable sensors are always a pair of redundant structures, which can be used to switch sensors when the train is too long stator track joints, so as to ensure the reliability of positioning and speed measurement signals. The interval between each pair of sensors is just the width of one sensor. Therefore, in order to better simulate the actual working conditions of the sensors, this test platform has designed the same installation position size as the sensors on the train, and is conducive to the development of off-line test experiments of wearable sensor signal switching. The excitation frequency of the coil of the relative position sensor is 3.2 MHz and 2.5 MHz high-frequency signals. The test bench works in a high-frequency electromagnetic field environment, so the material of the test bench cannot be metal materials with strong conductivity and magnetic conductivity. At the same time, in order to consider the convenience of processing, the test environment selected polyoxymethylene resin as the material. Polyoxymethylene resin has good insulation performance and high hardness, which is suitable for machining and meets the needs of testing environment.

3.3 Generate Wearable Sensor Signal

By controlling the working parameters and environment of the wearable sensor, the abnormal signal of the wearable sensor is generated. The initial signal generation results of the heart rate sensor numbered A01 and the temperature sensor numbered B01 are shown in Fig. 6.

Before data analysis, it is necessary to normalize the sample data. Neural network trains and predicts the network based on the statistical distribution probability of samples in events. Normalization is the statistical coordinate distribution unified between intervals $[-1,1]$. In addition, normalization is also to speed up the training speed of neural network and the convergence of network.

3.4 Input Machine Learning Algorithm Working Parameters

Because the optimized wearable sensor abnormal signal recognition method uses the BP neural network algorithm of machine learning algorithm, it is necessary to set the

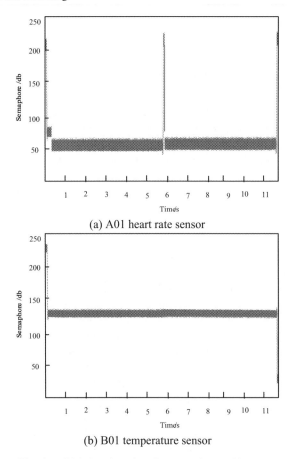

(a) A01 heart rate sensor

(b) B01 temperature sensor

Fig. 6. Initial signal setting diagram of wearable sensor

relevant working parameters. Set the learning rate and attenuation index of BP neural network to 0.0001 and 0.4 respectively, the regularization parameter to 10, the number of neurons in input layer and output layer to 50, the number of neurons in hidden layer to 100, and the number of neural network layers to 5. The maximum number of iterations of BP neural network is 20, and the weight initialization is 0.2. Finally, the above working parameters are input into the operation program of the wearable sensor abnormal signal recognition method.

3.5 Describe the Performance Test Process

Use the synchronous data acquisition instrument to collect data, use the designed circuit board to analyze the collected data through programming, and display the analysis results on the 256*128 LCD screen. Figure 7 shows the abnormal signal output results of the heart rate sensor numbered A01 and the temperature sensor numbered B01.

Similarly, the abnormal signal recognition results of all wearable sensor research objects can be obtained.

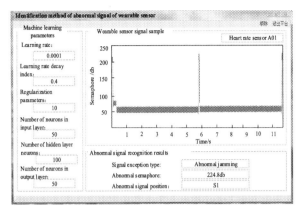

(a) A01 heart rate sensor

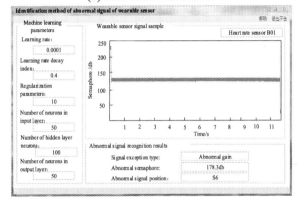

(b) B01 temperature sensor

Fig. 7. Recognition results of abnormal signals of wearable sensors

3.6 Set Identification Performance Quantitative Test Indicators

In the experiment, two indicators, the false detection rate of abnormal types of sensors and the statistical error of abnormal signals of sensors, are set as quantitative test indicators to test the recognition performance. The numerical results of the false detection rate of abnormal types are as follows:

$$\eta_w = \frac{n_e}{n_{all}} \times 100\% \tag{14}$$

In the formula, the variables n_e and n_{all} are the semaphore of the sensor abnormal type identification error and the total amount of sensor signal samples prepared. The specific value of n_e is determined by comparing the identification output results with the setting data. In addition, the test result of the statistical error of the abnormal signal of the sensor can be expressed as:

$$\varepsilon_{signal} = M_{set} - M_{distinguish} \tag{15}$$

In the above formula, M_{set} and $M_{distinguish}$ are the set abnormal semaphore and the actually recognized abnormal semaphore respectively. In order to ensure the optimization effect of the wearable sensor abnormal signal recognition method based on machine learning, it is required that the error detection rate of the abnormal type of the design method should not be higher than 1%, and the statistical error of the abnormal signal should not be higher than 0.5 dB.

3.7 Analysis of Experimental Results

Through the statistics of relevant data, the test results of the false detection rate of sensor abnormal types are obtained, as shown in Table 2.

Table 2. Test data of sensor abnormal type and false detection rate

Wearable sensor number	Total sensor signal /db	Abnormal type identification correct semaphore /db	Abnormal type identification error semaphore /db
A01	240	237.3	2.7
A02	180	178.6	1.4
A03	220	217.9	2.1
B01	250	248.3	1.7
B02	270	267.5	2.5
B03	190	188.5	1.5
C01	150	148.7	1.3
C02	260	257.8	2.2
D01	170	168.6	1.4
D02	200	198.4	1.6

Numbers a, B, C and D in Table 1 represent heart rate sensor, temperature sensor, gyroscope and pressure sensor respectively. By substituting the data in Table 1 into formula 14, it is calculated that the average false detection rate of sensor abnormal type is 0.86%, which is lower than the preset value. The error detection rate of the design method shall not be higher than 1%. This is because the method in this paper sets the signal anomaly judgment standard according to different types and principles of wearable sensors. The wearable sensor signals are collected, and the initial signals are preprocessed through Kalman filtering, normalization and weighted fusion. In addition, the test results of the statistical error of the abnormal signal of the sensor are shown in Table 3.

By substituting the data in Table 2 into formula 15, the average value of the statistical error of the abnormal signal of the sensor in the optimal design method is 0.22 db. The statistical error of the abnormal signal of the design method is not higher than 0.5 dB. This is because the method in this paper uses machine learning algorithm to extract the

Table 3. Test results of statistical error of sensor abnormal signal

Wearable sensor number	Set sensor abnormal semaphore /db	Identify sensor abnormal semaphore /db
A01	225.0	224.8
A02	178.5	178.3
A03	204.2	204.0
B01	238.7	238.5
B02	266.4	266.1
B03	179.5	179.2
C01	144.9	144.6
C02	252.6	252.4
D01	158.4	158.2
D02	188.2	188.1

features of sensor signals, and obtains the recognition results of the abnormal types, abnormal signals and abnormal positions of sensor signals through feature matching.

4 Conclusion

Wearable sensors have important application value in medical monitoring, human motion recognition, medical rehabilitation and other fields. Abnormal signal is an important embodiment of the real-time running state of wearable sensors. The key of abnormal data recognition is how to form a characteristic contour of the normal activity of the sensor. The self-learning habit and adaptability of neural network have attracted more and more scholars to study how to apply it to anomaly detection. It mainly trains a large number of samples, constantly learns and adjusts the subject's feature pattern, so as to build an adaptive feature contour. On this basis, the wearable sensor real-time running signal features are matched with the normal active feature contour to obtain accurate anomaly recognition results. From the experimental results, it can be seen that the recognition method of optimized design meets the preset requirements in two aspects: the false detection rate of abnormal signal types and the statistical error of abnormal semaphores, so it can be applied to the daily maintenance and monitoring of wearable sensors.

Fund Project. 2021 Anhui Provincial Natural Science Research Key Project (KJ2021A1384).

References

1. Loginov, V.A., Elnikov, A.V.: Method of signal identification based on wavelet analysis. In: IOP Conference Series: Materials Science and Engineering, vol. 921, no. 1, p. 012014 (2020). (6pp)

2. Lam, H.F., Adeagbo, M.O.: An enhanced sequential sensor optimization scheme and its application in the system identification of a rail-sleeper-ballast system. Mech. Syst. Signal Process. **163**(3), 108188 (2022)
3. Qin, D., Zhang, J.: A new identification method of underground excavation based on velocity estimation using double point synchronous measurements. IEEE Access **8**, 3910–39112 (2020)
4. Liu, Y., Zhang, S., Li, Z., et al.: Abnormal behavior recognition based on key points of human skeleton. IFAC-PapersOnLine **53**(5), 441–445 (2020)
5. Qian, H., Zhou, X., Zheng, M.: Abnormal behavior detection and recognition method based on improved ResNet model. Comput. Mater. Continua **65**(3), 2153–2167 (2020)
6. Kai, Z., Tw, D., Cw, D., et al.: Skeleton based abnormal behavior recognition using spatio-temporal convolution and attention-based LSTM. Procedia Comput. Sci. **174**, 424–432 (2020)
7. Li, Z., Mu, J., Mo, X.: Research on outlier identification of FPGA data processing based on sequential CNN. Comput. Simul. **39**(05), 409–412, 422 (2022)
8. Maity, A., Mandal, D., Misra, I.S.: A simple proposition for heart sound signal de-noising for effective components identification in normal and abnormal cases. Biomed. Signal Process. Control **71**, 103264 (2022)
9. Huang, D., Liu, Y., Liu, Y.H., et al.: Identification of sources with abnormal radon exhalation rates based on radon concentrations in underground environments. Sci. Total Environ. **807**, 150800 (2022)

Author Index

A
Alsharif, Bader   299

B
Boubacar, Habiboulaye Amadou   3

C
Chen, Lizhi   191, 206
Chen, Zhongwei   73, 88

D
Degila, Jules   3
Deng, Xuchu   191, 206

F
Fu, Tianlin   255, 271

G
Guo, Te   20

H
Hu, Yi   221, 239
Huang, Zhichang   73

I
Ilyas, Mohammad   299
Ismaïl, Lawani   3

K
Ke, Haipeng   255, 271

L
Lai, Zongying   191
Laoualy Chaharou, Ibrahim Mouazamou   3
Li, Chao   309, 322
Li, Helin   102, 117
Li, Ou   289
Li, Xiang   49, 61
Li, Xiaofeng   73, 88
Liang, Ping   289
Liu, Changyan   133, 143

Liu, Wenjian   35
Liu, Xiaohan   289
Liu, Xinyao   221, 239

P
Ping, Yihan   309

S
Shi, Chiyu   35
Shi, Juanfen   255, 271
Shi, Xiaochao   289
Shu, Kuangyang   289
Song, Shiyang   20
Su, Junyu   20, 35
Suri, Talatu   289

T
Tang, Jinhai   20

W
Wan, Qianyi   133
Wan, QianYi   143
Wang, Wennan   20, 35
Wang, Ying   102, 117
Wang, Yu   143

X
Xie, Wenjuan   159, 178

Y
Yang, Yi   289

Z
Zhang, Shilong   289
Zhang, Xuan   309, 322
Zhao, Hanxu   35
Zhao, Xiaoyun   289
Zhou, Jin   159, 178
Zhu, Linkai   20
Zhuo, Shufeng   221, 239
Zou, Zixiu   221, 239

© ICST Institute for Computer Sciences, Social Informatics and Telecommunications Engineering 2023
Published by Springer Nature Switzerland AG 2023. All Rights Reserved
S. Wang (Ed.): IoTCare 2022, LNICST 501, p. 339, 2023.
https://doi.org/10.1007/978-3-031-33545-7

Printed in the United States
by Baker & Taylor Publisher Services